Early Child Development: Investing in our Children's Future

Early Child Development: Investing in our Children's Future

Proceedings of a World Bank Conference on Early Child Development: Investing in the Future, Atlanta, Georgia, April 8-9, 1996

Editor:

Mary Eming Young
Human Development Department
The World Bank
Washington, DC, USA

1997

Elsevier

Amsterdam - Lausanne - New York - Oxford - Shannon - Tokyo

International Congress Series No. 1137
ISBN 0-444-82605 x

This book is printed on acid-free paper.

Published by:
Elsevier Science B.V.
P.O. Box 211
1000 AE Amsterdam
The Netherlands

Library of Congress Cataloging in Publication Data:

Printed in the Netherlands

Authors

W. Steven Barnett, Ph.D.
Professor of Economics and Policy
Graduate School of Education
Rutgers—The State University of New Jersey
New Brunswick, New Jersey, U.S.A.

Donald A. P. Bundy, Ph.D.
Deputy Director
Partnership for Child Development
Centre for the Epidemiology of Infectious Disease
Reader in Parasite Epidemiology and
Fellow of Linacre College
University of Oxford
Oxford, England, United Kingdom

Moncrieff Cochran, Ph.D.
Professor
Department of Human Development and Family Studies
College of Human Ecology
Executive Director
Cornell Early Childhood Program
Cornell University
Ithaca, New York, U.S.A.

Judith L. Evans, Ed.D.
Director
The Consultative Group on Early Childhood Care and Development
Haydenville, Massachusetts, U.S.A.

Elena L. Grigorenko, Ph.D.
Associate Research Scientist
Department of Psychology and Child Study Center
Yale University
New Haven, Connecticut, U.S.A.

Cigdem Kagitcibasi, Ph.D.
Professor of Social and Cross-cultural Psychology
Koc University
Istanbul, Turkey

Avima Lombard, Ph.D.
Director of Early Childhood Projects
The NCJW Research Institute for Innovation in Education
Professor Emeritus
School of Education
The Hebrew University of Jerusalem
Jerusalem, Israel

Reynoldo Martorell, Ph.D.
Robert W. Woodruff Professor of International Nutrition
Department of International Health
The Rollins School of Public Health of Emory University
Atlanta, Georgia, U.S.A.

Catherine Nokes, Ph.D.
Coordinator of Cognition Panel
Partnership for Child Development
Centre for the Epidemiology of Infectious Disease
University of Oxford
Oxford, England, United Kingdom

Lawrence J. Schweinhart, Ph.D.
Research Division Chair
High/Scope Educational Research Foundation
Director
High/Scope Quality Head Start Research Center
Ypsilanti, Michigan, U.S.A.

Robert J. Sternberg, Ph.D.
IBM Professor of Psychology and Education
Department of Psychology
Yale University
New Haven, Connecticut, U.S.A.

Jacques van der Gaag, Ph.D.
Advisor
Human Development Department
The World Bank
Washington, D.C., U.S.A.

Mary Eming Young, M.D., Dr.P.H.
Senior Public Health Specialist
Human Development Department
The World Bank
Washington, D.C., U.S.A.

Other Contributors - Panel on Policy Implications*

Armeane M. Choksi, Ph.D., Chair
Vice President
The World Bank
Washington, D.C., U.S.A.

Sir George A. O. Alleyne, M.D., F.R.C.P.
Director
Pan American Health Organization
Washington, D.C., U.S.A.

David de Ferranti, Ph.D.
Director
Human Development Department
The World Bank
Washington, D.C., U.S.A.

William Foege, M.D., M.P.H.
Chairman
Task Force for Child Survival and Development
Atlanta, Georgia, U.S.A.

James Kunder, M.A.
Vice President
Save the Children USA
Westport, Connecticut, U.S.A.

* The panel discussion formed the basis for the chapter on "Policy Issues and Implications of Early Child Development."

Acknowledgments

This proceedings of the World Bank conference, "Early Child Development: Investing in the Future," could not have been developed without the support and contributions of many individuals. Thanks are first extended to the World Bank's senior management, in particular Caio Koch-Weser and Armeane Choksi for their support of children's issues and the early child development program. Sincerest appreciation is given to Elaine Wolfensohn for her personal participation and interest in the Bank's early child development (ECD) initiative.

Special thanks are due to David de Ferranti, director of the Human Development Department, for his support and guidance in planning and organizing the conference. Special thanks also to Jacques van der Gaag, who was one of the first to recognize the global importance of ECD interventions in the developing world and to put this issue on the Bank's agenda.

The conference brought together the world's leading experts, academicians, and practitioners to focus on various aspects of early child development. The conference would not have been possible without the collaboration of the Task Force for Child Survival and Development. William H. Foege, the Task Force's chairperson, and Michael Heissler, the Task Force's program director, are gratefully acknowledged for their recommendation to hold the conference at The Carter Presidential Center in Atlanta, Georgia. Thanks also to Susan Yelton and Debra L. Elovich, of the Task Force, who organized "Child First: A Global Forum," for facilitating linkage of this meeting with the Bank's conference.

Thanks are also extended to the Multilateral Development Department, Royal Ministry of Foreign Affairs, Norway, for funding part of the preparation of the conference background papers. Many thanks are due to the team that helped organize the conference: Ramon Bolanos, Margaret Kajeckas, Euna Osbourne, Elizabeth Sherman, and Jane Thomas. A special note of appreciation goes to Leo Demesmaker for his guidance on conference planning and to Samuel Rachlin for liaison with the media. Thanks also to all 150 participants from 26 countries who made the conference happen and, in particular, to Barbara Bruns, Frans Lenglet, and Margaret Saunders of the Bank's Economic Development Institute for financing the participation of 30 individuals from developing countries. This support helped to expand the global importance of the conference.

Sincerest thanks to Sally McGregor, Heather Weiss, Robert Myers, Maris O'Rourke, and Maria Angelica Kotliarenco for their review of the background papers and cooperation in chairing the conference sessions.

Because the conference focused on descriptions of ECD programs in action and synthesis of the state of knowledge on benefits of early interventions, the participants especially benefited from field practitioners' presentations of country programs. Particular thanks in this regard are extended to Lea Kipkorir and Margaret Kabiru, who described programs in Kenya; Marta Korintus, Hungary; Erlinda Pefianco, Philippines; Adelina Covo de Guerrero, Colombia; and Binoo Sen, India. In addition, special acknowledgments are due to partners from key supporters of early child development: UNICEF, UNESCO, UNDP, WHO, PAHO, USAID, InterAmerican Development Bank, Asian Development Bank, Organization of American States, and nongovernmental organizations, including Bernard van Leer Foundation, Aga Khan Foundation, Save the Children USA, Christian Children's Fund, World Organization for Preschool Education, World Vision, High/Scope Educational Research Foundation, and The Consultative Group on Early Child Care and Development.

Many, many, many thanks to Linda Richardson and Elizabeth Taber for the text editing; without their persistence, meticulous efforts, and superb skills the timely preparation of this proceedings would not have been possible.

Contents

Part III. Investing in early child development: Economic and policy considerations

Early Child Development: Investing in our Children's Future
M.E. Young, editor.

Introduction

Mary Eming Young

Early child development (ECD) programs have been pioneered throughout the world for the past three decades. Evidence shows that these programs are successful. They address effectively some of the most vital issues of human development: malnutrition, stunted cognitive development, and unpreparedness for primary education. They can increase the efficiency of primary and secondary education, contribute to future productivity and income, and reduce the costs of health and other public services. Indirectly, they help reduce gender inequities, increase female participation in the economy, and enhance community development.

What is ECD? It is the provision of services that promote young children's development. The services target children's basic needs: nutrition, protection, health care, *and* interaction, stimulation, affection, and learning. Interventions are based on an understanding that children do not just grow in size; they evolve into unique human beings capable of mastering increasingly complex ideas and activities. Early child development programs thus include nurturing and care as well as physiological, cognitive, and intellectual stimulation to help children develop essential capacities and attain their full educational and productive potential.

Cumulative research indicates that most rapid mental growth occurs during infancy and early childhood and that a child's early years are critical for forming and developing intelligence, personality, and social behavior. Research also indicates that primary school and even kindergarten (for children 4-5 years old) may be too late to counteract negative physical, neurological, psychological, and social factors associated with early deprivation and inadequate stimulation. Children who are exposed to these unhealthy, unstimulating environments and who are not reached at earlier ages often develop poorly and suffer lifetime consequences of slowed or impeded development.

Debates about the advantages and effectiveness of early child development have evolved over the past 30 years as researchers documented the effectiveness of high-quality day-care programs for disadvantaged children. In the United States the first studies, conducted from the late 1960s to the mid-1970s, addressed questions about whether early intervention could have any lasting positive effects. This initial skepticism was overcome as effects were demonstrated. A second set of studies, conducted during the 1980s, investigated whether different program models could have different effects on children's development. Currently, researchers are focusing on identifying the essential elements of effective, small-scale programs and the possibilities for expanding these programs into national efforts.

In April 1996 the World Bank convened a conference, entitled "Early Child Development: Investing in the Future," to assess the state of the art in early child development. This conference, held at The Carter Presidential Center, Atlanta, Georgia, brought together the world's leading experts, researchers, and practitioners in the field. The participants summarized and synthesized knowledge on the benefits of early intervention, the economics of ECD programs, and public policy issues. They focused on the economics of ECD programs and sought to determine whether ECD programs offer a reasonable economic return to investment. Although the success of many ECD programs is well documented, the cost-effectiveness of these programs has not been evaluated systematically. The participants therefore were asked to consider the effectiveness of interventions, range of alternative programs, program costs, and overall cost-effectiveness of early child development.

This volume contains the proceedings of the conference. The chapters consist of papers developed for or subsequent to the conference. They are grouped into three main parts: Nutrition, Health, and Education: Synergistic Effects; Early Child Development: Program Options; and Investing in Early Child Development: Economic and Policy Considerations. Twelve chapters are included. In these chapters, the authors describe current understanding and suggest areas for future study and action. The contributions reflect their appreciation for the historical development of ECD programs, their review of the published literature, and their research and practical experience.

Definitions and Concepts

Before introducing the contents of the chapters, several terms need to be defined for the reader. First, early child development is viewed as encompassing the years 0-8. It includes the periods of early postnatal development, infancy, toddlerhood, preschool, kindergarten, and early primary school. It takes into account the variation in ages when children enter primary school, usually at age 6 but often not until age 8. This conceptualization of early child development also implies a relationship between children's learning at home and at school; these learning environments are mutually supportive, not separate entities. Within the 0-8 year timeframe, the years 0-3 are viewed as critical based on current evidence indicating that children develop certain key capacities, which are difficult to acquire later, during this time.

Second, the term "development" is used in this volume primarily to refer to an individual's growth—physical, mental, and cognitive—rather than the socioeconomic status of an entire country. Third, depending on the context, "environment" refers to the physical environment or the socioemotional and behavioral environment; these environments may be supportive or deleterious for children. Fourth, "human capital" is used to refer to individuals' physical and behavioral endowments which enable them to become productive members of society.

Fifth, the contributing authors agreed to use the terms "developed countries" and "developing countries" when discussing different regions of the world or comparing ECD strategies in different countries. Distinctions among countries always are difficult to convey. For example, all countries can be viewed as developing, with one no more developed than another. Also, use of the terms "industrialized" and "nonindustrialized" implies that industrialization is a preferred goal or ultimate end point. Some of the contributing authors noted preference for the term "Majority World" to refer to countries where most of the world's population resides or where population growth is well above replacement levels (e.g., in Asia, Africa, Latin America). In this volume, "developed" and "developing," which are the terms preferred by the World Bank, are used throughout for consistency.

Nutrition, Health, and Education: Synergistic Effects

The four chapters in part I address the synergistic effects of nutrition, health, and education. In "Health and Early Child Development," Don Bundy explains the relationship between good health and child development. He emphasizes that child survival should not be seen as an end in itself, but as the means by which children can live to benefit from educational opportunities that will enable them to develop their full potential. He notes that the period of 0-8 years of age is a time of rapid development when physical and nutritional inputs have the most profound and lasting consequences. These ages are when many of the most prevalent and infectious diseases occur: acute diarrhea, measles, acute respiratory infections, malaria, and intestinal parasites. He reviews research which shows that stunted physical growth and development are major consequences of ill health and are associated with late or nonenrollment in school, slow progression through school, and enhanced risk of dropping out of school. Stunted growth and development also are associated with reduced physiological capacity and work output. Promotion of early childhood development thus includes recognition of the need for delivering a comprehensive package of interventions that are cost-effective and sustainable.

In "Undernutrition during Pregnancy and Early Childhood: Consequences for Cognitive and Behavioral Development," Reynaldo Martorell reviews the literature on the short- and long-term consequences of undernutrition on behavioral development, educability, work capacity, and reproductive health. He highlights the cost and benefit of certain features characteristic of successful nutrition programs for the early years. Martorell also notes that growth failure occurs almost exclusively during the intrauterine period and in the first 2 years of life and that prevention of stunting, anemia, or vitamin A deficiency therefore requires interventions for very young children. He argues that nutrition programs should be integrated with prenatal and postnatal health care for mothers and children and that psychosocial stimulation, which also affects development, should be incorporated into these programs to enhance the effects of improved nutrition. Martorell reports that an annual investment of US$10-30 per beneficiary is needed to provide an effective, integrated nutrition and health program.

Robert J. Sternberg and colleagues address two related topics. In the first chapter, "Effects of Children's Ill Health on Cognitive Development," written with Elena Grigorenko and Catherine Nokes, the authors note the interplay between genes and environment and review research on the cognitive effects of environmentally provoked conditions of ill health. They discuss the effects of protein-energy malnutrition; short-term food deprivation; micronutrient deficiencies (zinc, iron, iodine, thiamine, vitamin A); viral infections (human immunodeficiency virus, influenza, colds, infectious mononucleosis); bacterial infections (otitis media); helminth infections (hookworm, whipworm, roundworm, schistosome); and environmental toxins (alcohol and drugs, lead, ionization). In their review, the authors highlight the buffering role of children's home environments. Commenting on several problems associated with studying the effects of ill health on cognitive development, the authors note that this research is often not based on a theory of cognitive development or is based on poorly justified theories such as intelligence quotient, which represents only a portion of cognitive abilities. They also note that assessment instruments often reflect the values of developed countries and thus are inappropriate for developing countries and that the etiology and severity of disease are often overlooked when defining "ill health." They propose a cognitive activation model to explain the continuous, interactive relationship between environment and cognitive development.

In a second chapter, "Interventions for Cognitive Development in Children 0-3 Years Old," Sternberg and Grigorenko present evidence to show that cognitive abilities are both heritable and molded by the environment and that environmental interventions can and should be started at an early age. They review the state of knowledge on cognitive abilities, describing alternative models of intelligence as well as types and examples of cognitive interventions. Noting that research has shifted toward examining the effectiveness of such interventions, the authors describe the literature on long-term effectiveness and on negative influences on outcomes. They also consider the methodological drawbacks of this research and evaluation issues. They suggest criteria for designing effective interventions and encourage the use of interventions that both eliminate impediments to cognitive development, such as poor nutrition or ill health, and incorporate positive cognitive-behavioral stimulation. One technique for accomplishing this combined intervention is scaffolding, or the provision of socioemotional, behavioral, and cognitive supports that involve parents and are tailored to a child's needs and capacity.

The conference participants and contributing authors agreed that health and cognitive interventions need to be interactive and designed as integrated programs of nutrition, health, and psychosocial stimulation. They also agreed that the most effective means for establishing and promoting these interventions would be to build onto existing services. In addition, they noted that children develop in recognizable stages, which requires caregivers to provide activities that are appropriate for each stage of development, and that programs that encourage active learning and child-initiated play are most effective.

Early Child Development: Program Options

Five chapters in this part review various options for developing ECD programs. The first three chapters present conceptual frameworks for classifying and considering alternative ECD programs. The first of these chapters presents a framework for tailoring ECD programs to a nation's characteristics and needs, the second summarizes eight strategies for designing ECD programs, and the third identifies elements of quality for ECD programs.

In the first chapter, "Fitting Early Childcare Services to Sociocultural Needs and Characteristics," Moncrieff Cochran emphasizes that nations must organize programs that are responsive to their particular needs and that reflect their values, customs, and traditions. He notes that two major combinations of factors, related to the movement of mothers into the work force and concern about the effects of poverty on children, impel societies to establish childcare policies and programs. Drawing from two previous major studies, Cochran surveys the range and effect of different ECD models. He describes a framework for assessing the needs of a country and for documenting cultural, economic, and social influences on service programs. He then applies this framework to two case examples, Kenya and Colombia. Cochran gives special attention to the tension between the quantity and quality of programs, the need for appropriate infrastructure, and the low priority given to ECD programs. He argues persuasively that ECD programs contribute to the formation of human capital in developing countries, primarily from the multiplier effects produced by training a large number of local citizens in the principles of early child development.

In "Programming in Early Childhood Care and Development," Judith L. Evans delineates the major ECD programming strategies being used to meet both universal and specific developmental needs in different cultures. She affirms that the traditional Western preschool, which focuses on children's mental development, is comparatively expensive, offered late in a child's life, and unsuitable for many countries and settings. Alternative approaches to this Western model initiate ECD intervention before a child is 3 years old, do not adopt a compensatory approach, do not depend on expensive infrastructure or highly trained professional staff, and allow services to be provided to more people for the same cost. Evans describes eight complementary strategies of ECD intervention that are mutually supportive and could be combined for maximal effect. The strategies are: delivering services directly to children, supporting and educating caregivers, promoting community development, strengthening national resources and capabilities, strengthening demand and awareness, developing national childcare and family policies, developing supportive legal and regulatory frameworks, and strengthening international collaboration.

In "Early Childhood Programs: Elements of Quality," Lawrence J. Schweinhart outlines seven essential elements of high-quality ECD programs. These elements, which are derived from research conducted in the United States and other countries, are: a validated child development curriculum, a validated strategy for assessing child development, a low ratio of young children to each teacher, trained staff, systematic inservice training and supervisory support, partnership between parents and teachers, and meeting a child's health and family needs. Schweinhart identifies the level of quality needed for each element and discusses how the level of acceptable quality may vary in situations of competing priorities. In this discussion, he confronts the question, "How can programs stray from ideal quality and still be worth doing?" Arguing that one of the most important effects that an ECD program can have in a developing country is providing a validated curriculum, he rates six curriculum models based on the quality of their documentation, validation, and dissemination. He asserts that all ECD programs should be learner-centered, although he recognizes that this approach may be regarded as countercultural in other, more authoritarian, cultures.

The last two chapters in this part focus on one element of quality that has been shown to maximize the effectiveness of ECD programs: involvement of parents and families. The two chapters describe in detail the success of several ECD programs that incorporate parent education, one in Turkey and two in Israel. These programs, which were designed initially to achieve local goals, have been adapted to other settings and have been expanded to national levels.

In the first chapter, "Parent Education and Child Development," Cigdem Kagitcibasi reviews the literature on the effects of parent education on child development and describes the Turkish Early Enrichment Project (TEEP). Describing programs in the United States and developing countries, she notes similarities and differences in their quality, generalizability, effect, and access. The studies show that programs that target child education as well as parent education and support are more effective, that parental involvement is crucial, and that the quality of implementation affects outcomes. The multifaceted TEEP project showed that educational day care produced the best results on most cognitive measures and in school adjustment and achievement and that the training of mothers through enrichment programs that involved extensive group discussions on childrearing and maternal support was beneficial. Based on the Turkish experience with TEEP and an expanded Mother-Child Education Program (MOCEP), Kagitcibasi suggests seven essential ingredients for successful programs. These include a whole child and contextual approach, multiple goals that are shared, empowerment of parents, optimal timing, and cost-effectiveness. The interaction of these ingredients can generate a positive, dynamic, and self-sustaining cycle that makes investment in ECD worthwhile.

In the next chapter, "Two Home-Based Programs for Early Child Education," Avima Lombard states that the greater part of children's early cognitive learning, including language development and skills, occurs in the home setting. She describes two home-based early education programs developed in Israel: the Home Instruction Program for Preschool Youngsters (HIPPY), which focuses on children ages 3-6, and the Home Activities for Toddlers and their Families (HATAF), which focuses on families with children 10-36 months old. Both programs target parents, and HIPPY incorporates closely planned children's activities. The programs demonstrate three important aspects of home-based programs: they are community-based, they incorporate cultural sensitivity, and they are cost-effective. Lombard emphasizes that home-based programs must address the needs of children and parents, recognize that reaching adults requires different skills than reaching children, and successfully bridge the gap between home and school. Planning for coordinated home-based programs includes assessing the characteristics of the populations to be served, identifying services to be provided, organizing administrative operations, establishing community relationships, and evaluating the programs' cost-effectiveness.

The conference participants and contributing authors agreed that the primary question today is not whether an investment should be made in early child development, but how that investment should be made and at what age. They agreed on the following points: children need to be served in the context of their families; no single model can be imposed on multiple cultures; parents must be involved actively as partners; all programs should adopt an active learning approach; the quality of a program is more important than the type of program; greater attention needs to be paid to inservice training when designing programs in developing countries; the bias toward compensatory programs needs to be overcome; an evaluation component should be incorporated into the design of all programs; a holistic view of early childhood development is required when designing programs to meet health, education, and socialization needs; and establishing clearly understandable goals is crucial.

In discussion, the conference participants emphasized the need for closer coordination among professionals designing health, nutrition, and education programs. They noted that professionals working in different disciplines often have different agendas and, when developing interventions, may omit elements that are known to contribute to children's overall well-being even though, in general, they support the need for holistic approaches. The participants also noted that although definitions of "going to scale" and related programming terms are being refined to allow for greater variety and flexibility, more research is needed to understand fully the issues involved in programming trade-offs. They encouraged greater consideration of the economic dimensions and national histories that influence programming.

Investing in Early Child Development: Economic and Policy Considerations

Three final chapters consider the economic and policy aspects of investing in early child development. Building on the previous chapters, which document the need for and effectiveness of a variety of ECD strategies, the authors present frameworks for weighing the benefits and costs of ECD programs and for stimulating further discussion of key policy issues.

In "Early Child Development: An Economic Perspective," Jacques van der Gaag answers policymakers' questions on "Why invest in ECD programs?" Presented as the keynote address at the conference, this chapter also confronts questions that administrators face in selecting among different strategies and programs. Van der Gaag proposes that benefit-cost analysis is a useful tool for examining ECD programs rationally and rigorously. He presents a hypothetical age-earnings profile for a woman with and without schooling and suggests that similar analysis could be done to demonstrate the productivity potential for an entire cohort of children who do or do not benefit from ECD programs. He emphasizes that the economic returns to investment of these programs could be as, or even more, significant as the returns already shown for education. Van der Gaag reminds us of the grim statistics in the developing world, where infant and child mortality is still very high and where a large proportion of children are not enrolled in primary school or drop out in the early grades. He holds up the promise of ECD interventions to revise these statistics, break the cycle of poverty, and increase the lifetime productivity potential of entire cohorts of children in low-income countries and regions of the world.

In "Costs and Financing of Early Childhood Development Programs," W. Steven Barnett states that local conditions vary so greatly that no single approach for providing or financing ECD programs is desirable universally. The variables of each programming strategy and intervention model (child care and education, nutritional supplementation, health care, parent education) affect potential costs. Service providers is one variable that is common to all models but may have different costs depending on their amount of formal training and credentials and whether or not they are paid. Barnett presents a framework, the Resource Cost Model, for identifying required resources and analyzing their costs. To estimate costs accurately, initial, direct, and indirect costs must be specified per resource unit. Opportunity costs also must be measured; for example, the current market values for staff may not be applicable in economies where these persons would otherwise be under- or unemployed. Barnett also describes major determinants of cost, relative costs of formal and informal programs, two approaches for evaluating program benefits, and measurable benefit indicators for ECD programs. The most important benefit indicators are likely to be a child's physical health and development, school success and progress, parental employment and earnings, and family size and structure. To achieve these benefits and meet the costs of early child development, public and private resources are needed, as well as international support.

In the concluding chapter, "Policy Issues and Implications of Early Child Development," Mary Eming Young summarizes key themes reiterated throughout the volume and identifies policy issues and implications for further discussion. Drawing on a final panel session at the conference, she notes that governments will be moved to create policies that support young children only when local communities encourage these policies and when policymakers are convinced that their actions will influence the development of human capital and the well-being of children. Promotion of early child development requires, first and foremost, the formulation of clearly stated and shared goals, that is, a unified message that can be communicated at local, national, and international levels. It also involves the commitment of multiple stakeholders (public and private sectors, nongovernmental organizations, bilateral and multilateral agencies); emphasis on a child's entire well-being, with simultaneous attention to survival and nonsurvival needs; and priority for the most needy children and families. With this direction, national interest and resources can be generated to enable already-proven programs to "go to scale" and to continue to design effective programs based on increased knowledge and understanding of the needs of children. The ultimate goal, of course, is to help all children develop to their fullest potential, thus enabling them, their families and communities, and their societies to thrive.

I. Nutrition, Health, and Education: Synergistic Effects

Health and Early Child Development

D. A. P. Bundy

Current estimates by the United Nations Children's Fund (UNICEF) indicate that more than 90 percent of the world's children now survive beyond infancy (UNICEF 1995). This success of child survival programs has led to greater focus on the needs of survivors and to increasing emphasis on the prevention of morbidity as well as mortality (Rhode 1988). The 1993 World Development Report, *Investing in Health*, has brought this issue into sharper focus by emphasizing the enormous global burden of ill health that persists despite the continuing fall in child mortality rates (World Bank 1993).

Recognition of the scale of morbidity has also led to a reassessment of the implications of ill health for human development. Reducing this burden of morbidity is now seen not as an end in itself, but as a means to allow individuals to achieve their full potential, and as a method to promote the development of human capital. The aim is not only to achieve and sustain good health, but by doing so to promote the overall development of individuals and societies.

From this perspective, ill health is viewed as a constraint on development, implying the need to develop health strategies that maximize developmental outcomes rather than target the most severe illness. Although in many cases these aims are coincident, and particularly so in early childhood, this perspective has given much greater prominence to highly prevalent but non-life-threatening conditions and to targeting the life stages which are most crucial to development. This expanded focus does not imply the abandonment of clinical services, but rather their supplementation by programs that seek a broader developmental goal.

Human development is a continuous process and justification can be made for its support at every stage. Even before conception the promotion of parental health can contribute to the physiological inheritance of a future child even, arguably, over multiple generations. Maternal health programs can contribute to intrauterine growth and development, as well as to subsequent development (Rondo and Tomkins 1993), while antenatal, perinatal, neonatal, infant, early childhood, school-age, adolescent, and adult health programs may all help ensure that the developmental gains are sustained. Given the finite capacity of health systems, however, which of these approaches, or combination of approaches, provides the greatest developmental return on investment needs to be explored.

For many of these approaches well-documented programmatic experience and institutional support exist, but programs to promote early child development, and development at school age, have received less attention. This chapter aims to help redress this balance by assessing the impact on subsequent development of ill health during early childhood and by reviewing the options for intervention. The following sections review the importance of early life, the effects of ill health on development, the consequences of early insults for later outcomes of relevance to human capital development, and appropriate health interventions that might contribute to an early child development (ECD) strategy.

Subsequent chapters in this volume address the effect of nutrition and nutritional interventions on cognitive and behavioral development (Martorell, this volume) and the effect of ill health on cognitive development (Sternberg, Grigorenko, and Nokes, this volume). The present chapter necessarily overlaps with these and others, particularly in relation to nutrition, since growth is used here as a proxy for development and since dietary supplementation, particularly with micronutrients, is an increasingly important component of health interventions.

The Importance of Early Life

Neonatologists, pediatricians, and educators are all likely to offer different definitions of early childhood. In this volume, early childhood is defined as the period extending from birth to 8 years of age (Young 1995). There can be little controversy about the start point, or about the inclusion of the first 3 years of life, when the rate of physical development is most rapid. The end point, however, is more arbitrary and is defined by programmatic concerns rather than by physiological stage. The natural end point is the age at which a child enters school, since ECD programs are intended to serve as the precursor for school health programs, or at least as a means of promoting child development in preparation for basic education. For a majority of countries enrollment becomes legally possible at age 5 or 6, but in practice most children enroll several years later. Figure 1 shows this discrepancy for enrolled and nonenrolled children in rural Tanzania.

Defining development from a health perspective is also difficult and tends to rely primarily on measures of physical growth as a proxy for overall physiological development (Martorell, this volume, 1995b). Measures of height and weight and their combined indices are considered to provide an integral of past experience of health insults, although for older children they may be a lagged indicator, reflecting conditions some years previously (Beaton and others 1990). Other anthropometric measures, particularly those related to fat stores, are considered more reflective of current experiences (Martorell 1995b). The apparent precision of growth measures is, however, somewhat confounded in practical applications by the complex interaction between body weight and height (Nabarro and others 1988).

The age dependency of growth rates provides a particularly strong argument for ensuring good health in early childhood, when the growth rate is most rapid. Insults during the first years of life cause growth faltering in which children may fall 2 standard deviations below the age-specific growth standards in as short a period as 6 months. This effect suggests that there are particular benefits in preventing early ill health. And remediation during this early period results in more rapid rehabilitation of a child, which suggests that palliative or curative interventions also are likely to be most beneficial when provided in early life.

These observations have encouraged the perception that early growth faltering "programs" a child to a lower growth trajectory from which there is no recovery, and which results in similar growth deficits in the adult to those seen in the child. Although there is substantial evidence for early growth failure, the evidence for lack of plasticity in

Figure 1. Age Distribution of Enrolled and Nonenrolled Children in Rural Tanzania

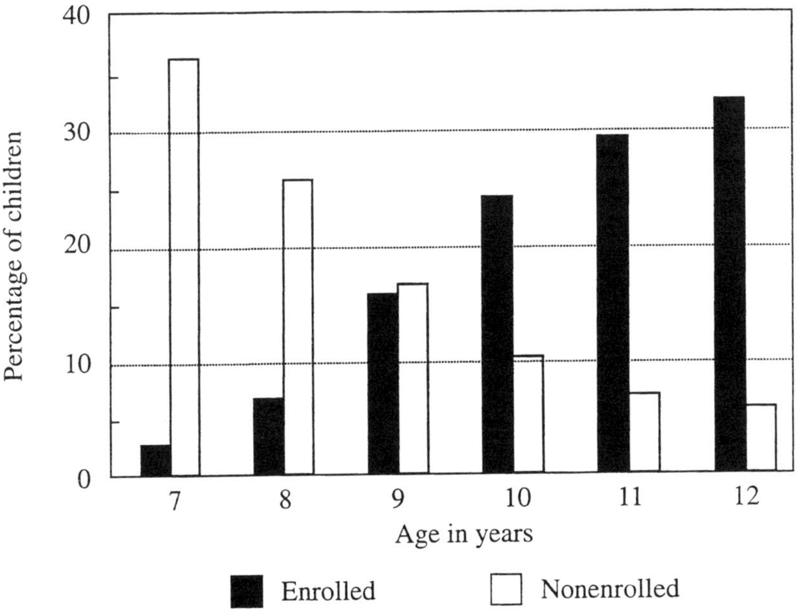

Source: Beasley 1995.

growth in later childhood is based on relatively few studies (Martorell and others 1995; Satyanarayana and others 1979). Furthermore, evidence shows that catch-up growth can occur in late childhood provided that improvements in circumstances are sustained (Golden 1994), but it is uncertain whether this catch-up is sufficient to fully restore attained adult height (Martorell, Khan, and Schroeder 1994). Evidence also shows that sustained low growth velocity across the boundary from early to late childhood can result in further growth deficit, although this deficit occurs at a rate which is inevitably much slower than that seen with insults in early childhood. Since knowledge about growth during later childhood and adolescence is limited (Martorell and others 1995), the apparent absence of catch-up growth may reflect what has been observed in the limited studies available rather than what might be possible with appropriate intervention (Golden 1994).

As an example, figure 2 reports growth deficits for school-age children in Tanzania. The first graph (*A*) shows the mean height-for-age Z scores (± 1 standard deviation) of the U. S. National Center for Health Statistics (NCHS) standards for 227 girls aged 7-12 years from villages in the Tanga region. The heights were converted to Z scores based on the nearest year-age estimate. The sample sizes of each year-age class are given in parentheses. The data indicate a significant change in Z score with age (general linear model, F=7.83, df=5, p=0.0001).

The second graph (*B*) shows the mean height velocity (± 1 standard deviation) in centimeters per 6 months for a subsample of 127 girls aged 7-12 years. Paired standing measurements taken 120±5 days apart were converted to 6-month velocities for each age

Figure 2. Growth Deficits in School-age Children in Tanzania

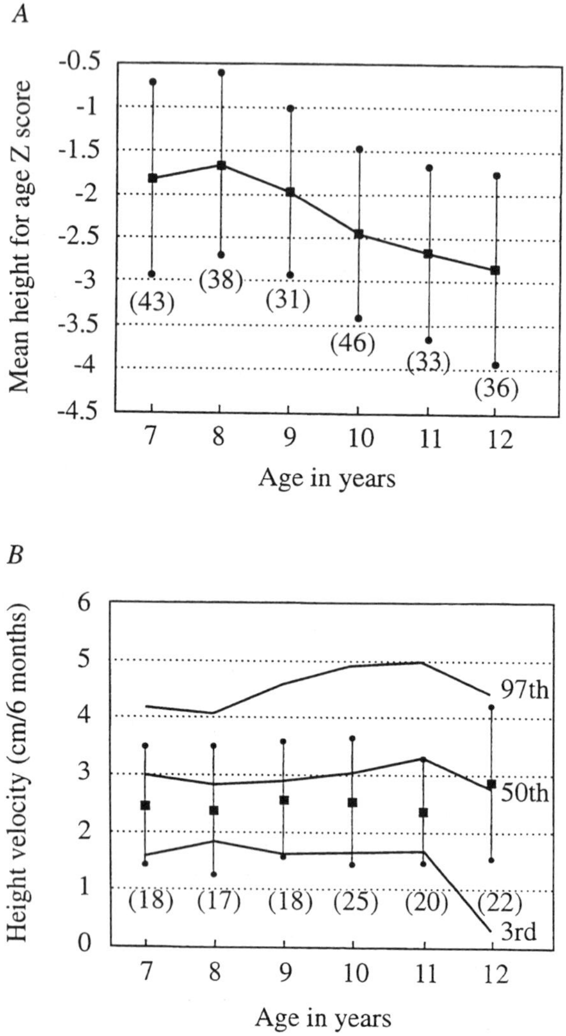

Source: Beasley 1995.

class. The sample sizes of each year class are given in parentheses. Continuous lines denote the 3rd, 50th, and 97th percentiles of 6-month height velocity reference standards (Roche and Himes 1980). The majority of height velocities are significantly lower than the reference medium (sign test, $Z^+ = 3.286$, $p<0.002$).

Overall, the use of growth as a measure of development suggests two conclusions. First, that insults during the earliest years have the most profound consequences for development. And, second, that the opportunities for remediation during the later period of early childhood have yet to be fully understood or exploited.

Physical growth is a useful proxy for development and one that is used extensively in this review. It should be recognized, however, that physical growth can only capture a narrow segment of the complex of factors that change during the development of a child. Health constraints in early childhood also have consequences for cognitive and mental development (Simeon and Grantham-McGregor 1990), as further explored by Sternberg and colleagues (this volume). The effects of ill health on this aspect of child development have been long recognized, but have only recently become again a focus of investigation (Pollitt, 1990). The association between cognitive deficit and some of the most prevalent consequences of, and contributors to, ill health in early childhood, such as micronutrient deficiency, suggests that the silent burden of cognitive and mental underdevelopment may be as large and important as the more widely acknowledged physical burden.

Health and Physical Development

Many health conditions affect child development during the early years of life. These range from acute episodes, for example of diarrheic disease, that often have strikingly rapid consequences for growth, to chronic infections, for example with parasitic helminths, that have more insidious effects. These multiple insults often occur concurrently so that it is difficult, or impossible, to attribute risk with any precision (Guerrant and others 1983). Furthermore, they typically occur against a background of other, predisposing factors such as malnutrition. For example, an African child at the end of the rainy season and before the harvest may be subjected simultaneously to the worst nutritional consequences of the "hungry" period and to the highest rates of transmission of malaria, gastrointestinal pathogens, and acute respiratory tract infections. Development is thus constrained by a complex of factors which may operate simultaneously. A program that seeks to improve development under these circumstances must recognize the need for an approach that is sufficiently comprehensive to, at the least, address the multiple primary causes of ill health.

The period of early childhood encompasses the age range when many of the most prevalent conditions attain their highest incidence. Furthermore, the peak incidence of different conditions typically occurs at different ages, such that a child is subjected to multiple, sequential insults throughout the early years of life. Figure 3 illustrates the exposure of children to a sequence of potential insults in early life. Infection-specific morbidity is scaled on the figure as a proportion of the peak value observed for that infection. Morbidity for diarrhea is estimated from the percentage of time with diarrhea, for malaria and measles from case incidence, and for *Trichuris* (whipworm) from infection intensity. With the exception of the two malaria syndromes, the data are from separate studies in different countries (Martorell 1989; Hill and others 1991; Chen and others 1994; Bundy and others 1987). The data indicate not only that early childhood is a period of particular health risk, but also that preventive or curative measures must be appropriately age-targeted.

The following sections consider some of the more prevalent conditions and infections of early childhood. These include diarrhea, measles, acute respiratory tract infections (ARI), malaria, intestinal parasitic worm infections, and other conditions such as asthma,

Figure 3. Age Distribution of Infection-specific Morbidity During Early Childhood

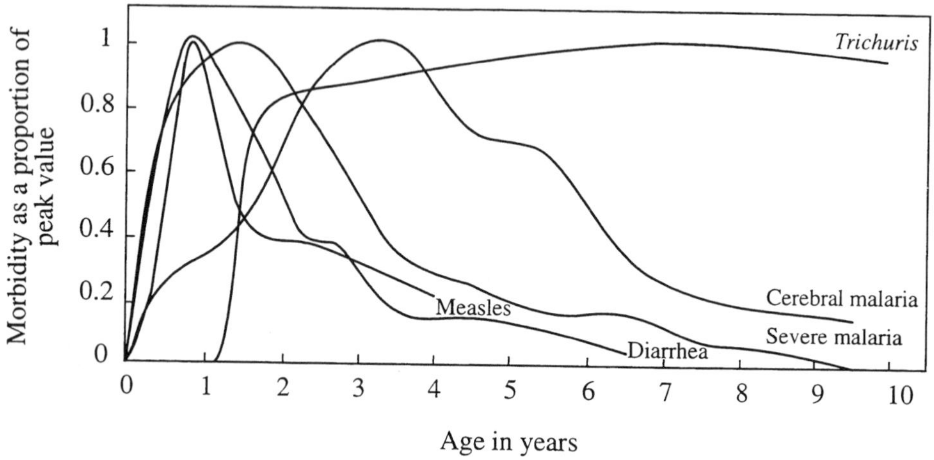

Source: Martorell 1989; Hill and others 1991; Chen and others 1994; Bundy and others 1987.

disability, and blindness. These infections and conditions are considered here as single insults, but in practice often occur simultaneously.

Diarrhea

Acute diarrhea is the most common of all illnesses in children in developing societies. Its prevalence is highest toward the end of the first year and in the second year of life (figure 3). Most episodes have a duration of 3-7 days, and it is not unusual for 10 to 20 percent of children to be affected on any one day (Martorell and others 1975). Persistent diarrhea, with a duration longer than 14 days, is less common than acute diarrhea but is associated with greater mortality and nutritional consequences (Tomkins, Behrens, and Roy 1993; Black 1993). Diarrhea results from infection by any one of a wide range of viral, bacterial, and protozoal enteric pathogens transmitted by the fecal-oral route. It is a major source of mortality and morbidity.

Growth faltering appears to follow multiple, sequential episodes of diarrhea, often involving different pathogens. Figure 4 shows such faltering in one young boy who experienced multiple infectious episodes from 1-3 years of age. On the figure, the length of each horizontal line indicates the duration of each infectious episode. Evidence from Bangladesh shows that one episode predisposes to another (Chowdhury and others 1990).

Whether nutritional status per se predisposes to diarrhea appears to vary geographically. Evidence shows an association with diarrhea incidence in Central America and Africa (Sepulveda, Willett, and Munoz 1988; Tomkins 1981) and an association with increased duration, but not incidence, in the Indian subcontinent (Black, Brown, and Becker 1984). Recent intervention studies in Africa indicate that vitamin A supplementation reduces the severity of episodes, hospital admissions, and diarrheal deaths (Filteau and others 1995).

Figure 4. Weight and Episodes of Infectious Disease in a Rural Guatemalan Boy

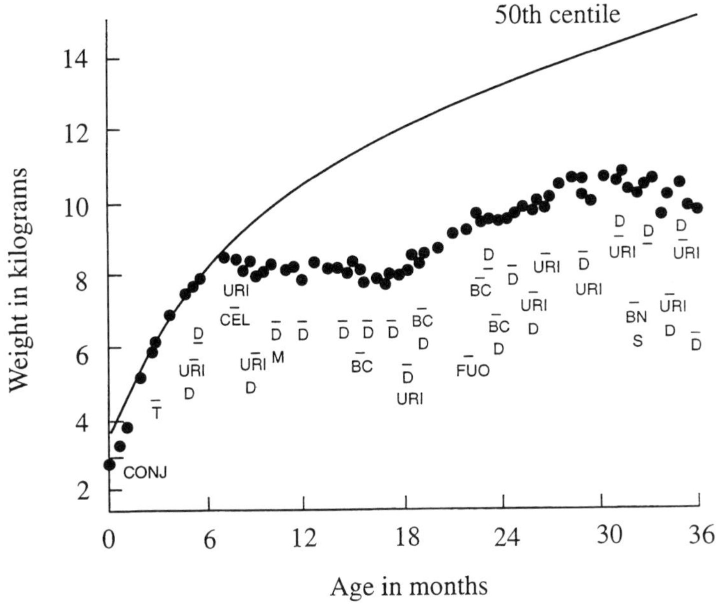

Note: *D*, diarrhea; *URI*, upper respiratory infections; *BC*, bronchitis; *M*, measles; *T*, oral thrush; *BN*, bronchopneumonia; *CONJ*, conjunctivitus; *CEL*, cellulitis; *S*, stomatitis; *FUO*, fever of unknown origin.

Source: Mata and others 1977.

In some settings, such as Latin America (figure 4), quantitative studies indicate that infectious diarrhea is more important than food availability as a cause of growth faltering in early childhood (Martorell and others 1980; Schorling and Guerrant 1990). In other areas, such as Bangladesh, inadequate food availability may be more important, although diarrhea still plays a role (Briend 1990). A review of studies of this issue (Tomkins 1992) suggests that the relative importance of diet and infection varies locally, depending on the balance between infection epidemiology and food availability as well as on the degree of effort made by caretakers to compensate for the anorexia resulting from infection.

Measles

In common with diarrhea, measles is a major source of early mortality and morbidity. It has its highest incidence in the first year of life (figure 3) in most developing societies and often precipitates severe protein-energy malnutrition (PEM). The age distribution of infection varies with population density and vaccination coverage, and infection in middle and late childhood occurs in some areas (Foster, McFarland, and Meredith John 1993). The infection is acute but is characteristically followed by several weeks of profound anorexia, often leading to secondary dysenteric complications. The postmeasles dysentery phase is associated with growth faltering (figure 4), although the temporal and symptomatic similarities may prevent its differentiation from the affects of diarrhea in general. Unlike an episode of diarrhea, the growth faltering precipitated by an acute attack of measles has an extended period during which no catch-up growth occurs. In a study in Africa, deficits in weight and length persisted for 6 months after an acute attack, particularly in children less than 1 year old (Van Lerberghe 1990).

The postmeasles phase is also associated with vitamin A deficiency because of the general metabolic response to infection, and the combination of these two is the most common cause of blindness in children in many parts of Africa (Tomkins 1992). Vitamin A deficiency has profound consequences for mucosa, and particularly for the conjunctiva, and there is evidence for increased risk of xerophthalmia following diarrhea (Sommer and others 1983).

ARI

ARI is the most frequent illness globally and a leading cause of death in developing societies (Stansfield and Shepard 1993). ARI cause an estimated 4 million deaths annually in children under 5 years old. More than 75 percent of mortality is ascribed to pneumonia, and the observation that the death rate from this disease is 10-50 times higher in developing societies indicates opportunities for improvement (WHO 1984). Control of ARI aims primarily at mortality reduction rather than promotion of child development, but is considered here because of its considerable importance to health in early childhood and because of its focus on the same age group as ECD strategies. ARI also forms part of the complex of early insults that may contribute to growth faltering (figure 4).

ARI includes a complex of clinical conditions of varying etiology and severity, including relatively minor upper respiratory tract infections, such as colds and sore throats, and more serious acute lower respiratory tract infections, such as pneumonia and bronchiolitis. The predominant causes of ARI mortality are bacterial and viral pneumonia, measles (see above), and pertussis. Diphtheria, bacterial pharyngitis, and "opportunistic" viral bacterial infections are also considered important, but their relative contribution to mortality has yet to be quantified.

Incidence peaks at four to nine infections in each of the first 2 years of life, falling to three to four infections per year by school age. The case-fatality ratio is highest in the youngest children, with pneumonia occurring 1.5-1.8 times as frequently in infants as in children 2-4 years of age (Berman and McIntosh 1985). ARI is also a major contributor to morbidity; children under 5 years spend on average 22 to 40 percent of observed weeks with ARI in general and 1 to 14 percent of weeks with the more serious lower respiratory tract infection. The case rate is several orders of magnitude higher in malnourished children and the very young.

In developing societies, evaluation of the impact of ARI has, appropriately, focused on mortality. In Ghana, for example, 94 percent of the estimated 52 days of life lost per case of ARI is due to mortality rather than morbidity (Ghana Health Assessment Project Team 1981). In more developed countries, where ARI mortality is relatively much rarer, more attention has been given to developmental issues. For example, in the United Kingdom, 1-2 weeks of schooling are lost per child per year (Crofton and Douglas 1975).

Malaria

Malaria is one of the most important parasitic diseases in terms of child mortality. Infection occurs worldwide, but 80 percent of clinical cases occur in tropical Africa. The infection is transmitted by mosquito vectors and involves four different species although, in the absence of complicating factors, acute severity and mortality occur almost exclusively in *Plasmodium falciparum* infections.

The risk of severe malaria is greatest in young children with poorly developed resistance to infection. In highly endemic areas severe malaria typically affects children older than 3-6 months, who have lost maternal protection, and children younger than 5 years, when survivors have developed some degree of resistance (figure 3). The effects of infection tend to be milder in young infants, with cerebral and severe malaria occurring most commonly after the age of 1 year. Malaria is increasingly seen in older children in Africa, however, perhaps because the development of immunity is delayed by personal protection or intermittent control. First infection at an older age is common in areas of low endemicity and in migrants, and it is the typical picture in much of Asia and South America.

The major focus of malaria research has, appropriately, been on mortality rather than morbidity. Where morbidity is examined, emphasis is typically on the acute contemporaneous consequences of cerebral and severe disease. Studies of the longer-term developmental consequences of malaria are lacking, although research exists on the effects of current disease on productivity and education (see later sections). Cerebral malaria results in neurological sequelae which are detectable in survivors 6-12 months afterward and which resolve in some cases (Bondi 1992; Schmutzhard and Gerstenbrand 1984). While anemia commonly complicates acute infection, much of the burden of anemia is associated with chronic infection, particularly when this occurs with other concurrent infections and nutritional deficits (Cardoso and others 1994; Mizushima and others 1994).

Intestinal Parasitic Worm Infections

In common with the infections listed above, parasitic worm infections occur throughout the developing world and are among the most prevalent infections of humans; the most common three species are each estimated to infect 1 billion people (Chan and others 1994). Unlike the other infections, however, they are rarely life-threatening and are typically chronic, with a process of infection and reinfection starting in early childhood and persisting throughout life. The largest mean worm burdens of the roundworm (*Ascaris*) and whipworm (*Trichuris*) tend to occur in children at the upper age limit of early childhood (figure 3), while the hookworms (*Necator* and *Ancylostoma*) reach peak incidence in adults, although first infection occurs soon after birth.

The majority of studies have focused on children at the boundary between early childhood and school age. These studies indicate that where the diet is poor and infection is at least moderately intense, infection with single or multiple species is associated with growth deficits, and treatment to remove worms is followed by catch-up growth (Stephenson 1987; Stephenson and others 1993a; Thein-Hlaing and others 1991). Anorexia appears to be an important factor in growth deficits, at least for some species (Stephenson and others 1993b). Hookworm infection, in particular, is associated with iron-deficiency anemia, and increasing evidence shows that infection is a major contributor to childhood anemia in endemic foci.

Fewer studies have examined the effects of infection on very young children. The dysentery syndrome associated with intense whipworm has been associated with growth stunting in children as young as 3 years. Figure 5 shows, however, that treatment for this infection results in remarkable rates of catch-up growth. In this study of 63 Jamaican children averaging 4.5 years, the growth velocities of height and weight were measured over a half-year following treatment. The ages shown on the figure are the midpoint of the interval for calculating velocities. On graph *B*, height-age refers to the age of the median reference child who is the same height as the subject; the graph shows weight growth related to height, indicating a change in the leanness or stoutness (body habitus) of the subject.

The same syndrome was associated with significantly lowered development quotients in a case-control study of children averaging 4 years, but only locomotor skills showed significant improvement after anthelmintic therapy (Callender and others 1992). Treatment of mixed infections results in growth improvement in children in the 1-5 year age range (Nabarro and others 1988; Stephenson 1987).

Figure 5. Growth Velocities of Height and Weight for Jamaican Children with Trichuris Dysentery Syndrome

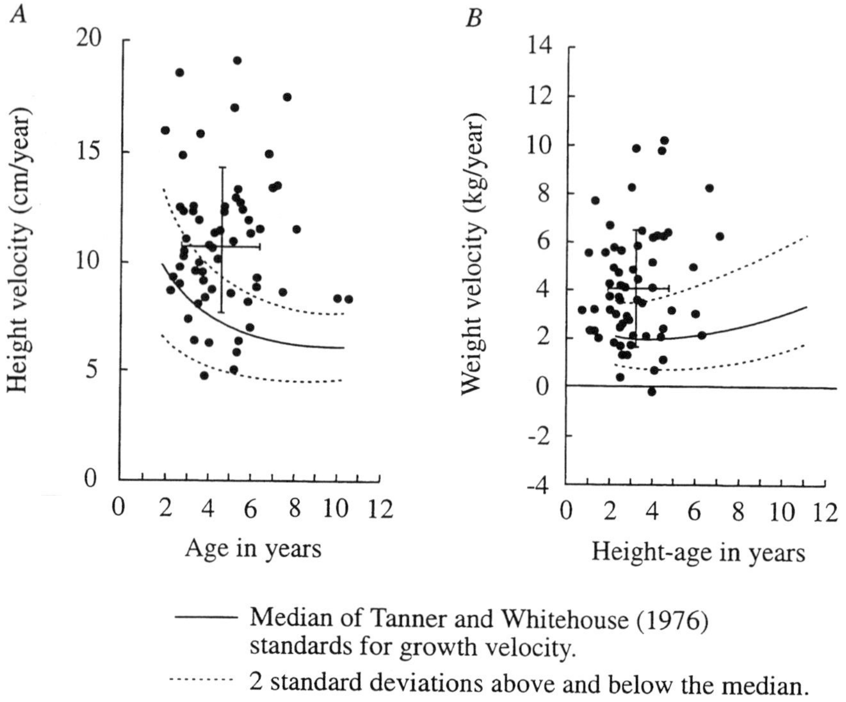

Source: Cooper and others 1990; Tanner and Whitehouse 1976.

A general conclusion is that the effects of worms on development are markedly different from those of the acute infections considered above. Instead of a clinically apparent acute episode accompanied by a rapid failure of growth, worms present an insidious, often clinically unapparent infection which appears to chronically constrain growth (Cooper and Bundy, 1988). Worm infections do not appear to contribute to classical growth faltering during the first year of life, but can affect growth at all stages of childhood thereafter.

Other Conditions

The diseases considered above are presented as examples of highly prevalent infections of early childhood which have contrasting modes of transmission and different developmental effects and which involve a variety of differing approaches to prevention or management. This list is not intended to be exhaustive, and good arguments might be made for including other important conditions, such as human immunodeficiency virus infection and acquired immunodeficiency syndrome, especially those with well-understood control approaches such as hepatitis B immunization.

Disability of infectious or noncommunicable etiology is also an important cause of developmental constraint. Asthma is now recognized to be of worldwide importance in children throughout the early childhood years. Disability as a result of accident, violence, abuse, neglect, or exploitation is also very common, but perhaps less well recognized (World Bank 1993). Blindness affects some 1.5 million children, approximately 85 percent of whom live in Africa or Asia. It is estimated that up to 70 percent of childhood blindness in developing societies is preventable or treatable, with vitamin A deficiency and measles making a major contribution to this pathology (Gilbert 1993).

The effects of these health conditions on early child development should not be viewed in isolation from other factors not considered in this review. Nutritional deficits, such as PEM and specific micronutrient deficiencies, can potentiate the ill effects of infection (as discussed for diarrhea and measles). Socioeconomic factors at the community level, such as political instability, and in the household, such as unemployment or parental ill health, can profoundly influence the quality of care children receive and thus their susceptibility to and recovery from infection (Rosenfield, Golladay, and Davidson 1984). Health should be viewed in the context of an overall strategy that also promotes nutritional status and social well-being.

Health and Cognitive and Mental Development

Before leaving the issue of the developmental consequences of ill health, the potential importance of ill health for mental and cognitive development is perhaps worth reemphasizing (see also the chapter by Sternberg, Grigorenko, and Nokes, this volume). It has long been recognized that about 70 percent of brain development occurs in utero and that the final stages of dendritic growth and synaptic branching to achieve what is effectively the adult brain are completed within 18-24 months of birth (Dobbing and Smart 1974). The latter fact indicates temporal coincidence between the final stages of brain development and the period of most severe somatic growth failure, but evidence for a direct effect of health on the brain is sparse. A study of children in Chile who experienced severe marasmus before 6 months of age suggests a negative effect on brain size and development (Winick 1970), and cerebral malaria in early life is known to induce significant changes in brain structure and function (Newton and others 1994).

Much more evidence exists for a correlation between physical growth and cognitive development, as classically shown for school-age children in Guatemala. A more recent study in the same country indicates that children on a high-protein and high-calorie supplement perform better on motor development scales at 24 months and on a general cognitive test battery at 48 and 60 months than children receiving a low-calorie supplement (Engle and others 1992). These observations may indicate that mild-to-moderate PEM in early life, whether a result of inadequate diet or infection, can result in impaired cognitive ability. But it has been argued that none of the studies exclude the possibility that iron deficiency is the primary lesion (Pollitt 1995). Iron deficiency in early life has been shown to have reversible effects on mental and motor development among infants in Indonesia (Idjradinata and Pollitt 1993) and to be a major contributory factor to cognitive deficits observed in middle childhood in Costa Rica (Lozoff, Jimenez, and Wolf 1991).

These studies indicate the potentially very large effect of health on mental development. They also illustrate the difficulties in quantifying this burden and in attributing causation.

Potential Long-term Consequences of Ill Health in Early Childhood

The previous sections focused largely on the contemporaneous effects of ill health. This section examines the potential longer-term consequences if ill health in early childhood is not prevented or if recovery does not occur. In terms of human capital development this issue is arguably the most important. But this area is also the one where it is most difficult to show convincing results because of the difficulty of relating early insults to effects that become apparent many years later. Here again the traditional approach is to use attained physical development as a proxy for earlier experience of ill health.

Health and Education

The definition of early childhood used in this volume (0-8 years) covers the first 6 years before entering school and the first 2 years of formal education. In considering the educational benefits of an ECD strategy, these two periods might be viewed as preparing a child for education and as sustaining a child during education. These aims are separate and require different programmatic approaches. Preparing a child for schooling—promoting development during the preschool years—seems intuitively sensible. Providing support during the first 2 years of school only seems much less satisfactory and perhaps indicates the weakness of setting an arbitrary upper limit to early childhood.

An approach that can help resolve this difficulty, at least intellectually, is to perceive the 6-8 year age class as a transitional period during which a significant, although declining, number of children remain out of school (figure 1) and still require the support of an ECD strategy. This approach is still not entirely satisfactory, however, as it begs the question as to why children should be unsupported after they have entered school. The following sections consider the effects of ill health on education variables during the preschool years and during the first years of education.

School Enrollment

A central issue is whether early development has consequences for the age at which children first enroll in school. This issue has been examined indirectly using school-based studies. In China, short stature was a predictor of "grades behind" (that is, the difference between expected and observed grade at a particular age), which was interpreted as showing that children with growth deficits enroll later or make less progress through school (Jamison 1986). Rather different study designs obtained a similar result in Nepal and Guatemala, and in both cases low height for age was a significant predictor of late enrollment even when socioeconomic variables were removed (Moock and Leslie 1986; Balderston 1981).

Recent studies have tended to be community-based and to make direct comparison between children in and out of school. Figure 6A shows that children in rural Tanzania in general were below NCHS standards and that nonenrolled children were even shorter on average than those in school. This pattern was found in every year class from 7 to 12 years of age (Tanzania Partnership for Child Development, cited in Beasley 1995). Furthermore, if children in any single year class are considered separately, those in the age-appropriate grade are taller on average than those who are old for their grade (figure 6B), which again suggests that late enrollment or progression is related to stunting. Comparison of the health of enrolled and nonenrolled 6-7 year olds in two dissimilar regions of Ghana also indicated a trend for shorter stature in children not in school, but few other significant health differences in this young age class (Ghana Partnership for Child Development 1995; UNICEF 1996).

The overall consistency of these results strongly suggests that children who experience early growth failure as a result of inadequate diet or of infection are more likely to delay enrollment. However, even in studies where the height effect remained after controlling for socioeconomic variables, socioeconomic factors were still a strong predictor of enrollment age. This finding is unsurprising given the multiplicity of factors that may determine whether a child attends school (UNESCO 1993; UNICEF 1996), but offers a caution against any simplistic view that improved health or stature will itself significantly improve enrollment.

Disability as a cause of nonenrollment does not appear to have been assessed in developing societies, but appears to have a relatively small quantitative effect, even if the qualitative consequences for an individual may be profound. For example, about 1 percent of 6-year-old children in Bangladesh are estimated to experience visual impairment from vitamin A deficiency at a level that precludes school enrollment (Pollitt 1990, based on data from Cohen and others 1985).

Absenteeism

Current illness may prevent a young child, at least temporarily, from attending school. Malaria, guinea worm infection, schistosomiasis, and asthma have all been identified as

Figure 6. Short Stature and School Enrollment in Tanzania

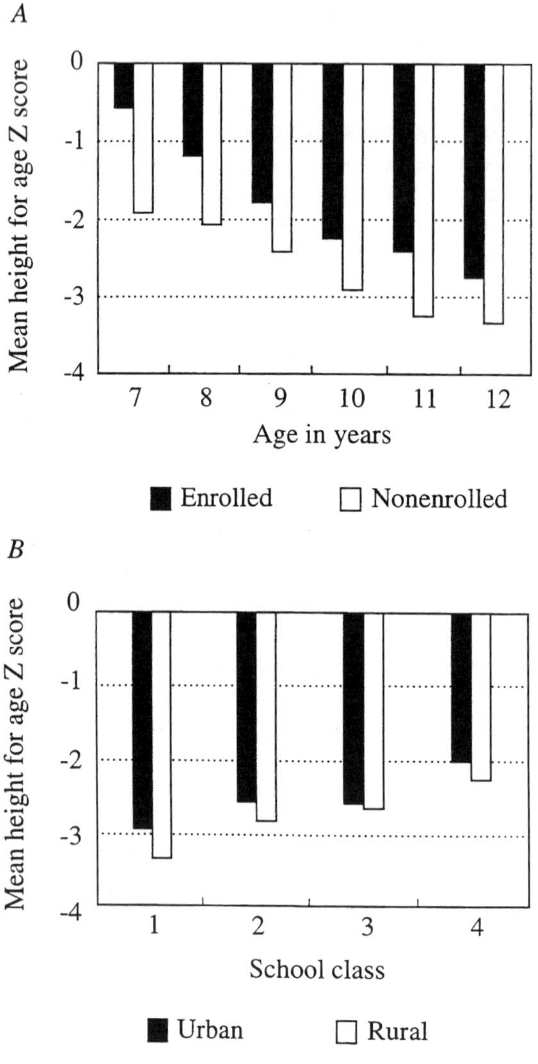

Source: Beasley 1995.

recurring reasons for nonattendance because of ill health (Bundy and Guyatt 1995b). A controlled intervention study in Africa showed that reduction in malaria incidence is accompanied by a significant decrease in absenteeism (Ogutu and others 1992). These diseases have acute clinical manifestations which might be expected to comprise attendance. More surprising is the systematic association between intestinal worm infection and proportion of time absent from school which has been shown in Jamaica

(Nokes and Bundy 1993). Whether infection is causally related to absenteeism, or is covariant with other, perhaps socioeconomic reasons for nonattendance is unclear. A subsequent controlled trial, however, showed that treatment of moderate whipworm infection enhances school attendance in the more stunted children, lending support to the causal hypothesis (Simeon and others 1995b).

Absenteeism is perhaps the least-studied educational variable in developing societies even though it is a ubiquitous problem and, together with enrollment, determines the available time-on-task. Well-documented evidence shows that absenteeism is negatively related to school performance (Weitzman 1987), and it is self evident that reduction in acute disease, at least, will remove a potential cause of absence.

Educational Achievement

The two main issues are: whether insults early in development have long-term consequences, and whether current ill health affects current performance. The nutritional aspects of these issues have been reviewed extensively (Pollitt 1990; Pollitt, Garza, and Leibel 1984; Simeon and Grantham-McGregor 1990; Grantham-McGregor 1990). There are many difficulties in interpreting the extant studies because of the variability, and often inadequacy, of design. But a cautious interpretation suggests that severe PEM and severe iodine-deficiency disorders have long-term consequences for mental function and educational achievement and that chronic mild-to-moderate undernutrition and iron deficiency can lead to developmental lags that may affect school performance. Primary prevention would be the preferred intervention, which implies early attention to feeding, and where necessary, supplementation. Evidence of the value of general nutritional intervention at school age is equivocal, but there can be benefits (Grantham-McGregor, Powell, and Walker 1989). Specific interventions at school age, such as alleviation of short-term hunger or iron deficiency, can result in remarkable improvements (Grantham-McGregor and others 1991; Soemantri, Pollitt, and Kim 1985).

These findings from nutritional studies also have broad relevance to defining a role in ECD strategies for infectious disease prevention. Since infection may contribute to PEM, undernutrition, and micronutrient deficiency a justification can be made for preventing infection during early childhood with the aim of promoting educational development, as has been argued for physical development outcomes. Furthermore, the contribution of malaria, intestinal nematode infections, and schistosomiasis to iron deficiency at school age suggests a need for intervention to alleviate this deficiency in this age group.

More direct evidence also shows the value of treating helminth infection in school-age children. Infection with some of the most prevalent species is associated with cognitive deficits, some of which may be at least partially reversed by anthelmintic therapy (Nokes and Bundy 1994; Kvalsvig, Cooppan, and Connolly 1991). Carefully conducted clinical trials of moderate whipworm infection suggest that undernourished children are more likely to benefit from treatment (Simeon, Grantham-McGregor, and Wong 1995; Simeon and others 1995). But there is an almost complete absence of studies of the effects on educational achievement of other common infections.

The contribution of disability to underachievement in education may be significant. Estimates vary as to the prevalence of disability in school-age children, but up to 7 percent may suffer some degree of visual, auditory, motor, or communication deficit. A study in the Philippines found that 13.5 percent of primary schoolchildren had some degree of hearing impairment and 2 percent were visually impaired.

Health, Productivity, and Employment

From a pragmatic viewpoint the most important effect of early ill health on human capital development is its potential impact on subsequent productivity and employment. Demonstrating such an impact, however, is complicated by two major factors: (a) the long time delay between early insult and measurement of an effect in adults, and (b) the confounding effects of socioeconomic circumstances (poorer communities are both more susceptible to ill health and have the most limited employment prospects). Studies in this area are therefore readily criticized as being narrowly unrealistic, because they cannot capture the full range of incident effects, or as being too reliant on inference, because they cannot reliably describe the full range of insults throughout the life cycle. Unequivocal evidence may therefore never be available, but an effect of ill health on productivity has been shown in a majority of studies where it has been sought.

Work Output and Growth

There is a consistent relationship between measures of nutritional status and maximal physical work capacity as measured by maximal oxygen consumption ($VO_{2\ max}$). For example, a study of groups of adults in Guatemala with progressively more severe malnutrition (based on anthropometrics and blood chemistry) showed a systematic reduction in $VO_{2\ max}$, which in the severely malnourished group was only partially reversible by dietary repletion (Barac-Nieto and others 1978, 1980). The potential importance of this relationship is that $VO_{2\ max}$ is positively correlated with output in actual work settings, as has been shown for sugar workers in East Africa, Sudan, and Colombia (Spurr, 1988). That this is a developmental relationship is suggested by the correlation between $VO_{2\ max}$ and both height and weight for Colombian boys in every year class from ages 7 to 15 (Spurr, Reina, and Barac-Nieto 1983).

Further evidence for a developmental relationship is offered by a study of the heart rate and work capacity relationships of boys 14-17 years old in rural India (Satyanarayana, Nadamuni Naidu, and Narasinga Rao 1979). The height and weight of children at age 5 correlated with their current physical work capacity and explained 64 percent of the variance. Importantly, only 10 percent of the variance could be attributed to the levels of current habitual physical activity.

These studies indicate that growth deficits attributed to early ill health result in a reduced level of work output that cannot be significantly reversed by subsequent physical activity in adolescence or nutritional rehabilitation in adulthood. A follow-up study in Guatemala, conducted by the Institute of Nutrition of Central America and Panama, suggests, however, that early nutritional intervention can have a significant effect (Martorell 1995a). Supplementation of mothers during pregnancy and of children during preschool years resulted in a higher $VO_{2\ max}$ at 14-19 years of age in the group that had received the higher-quality supplement. No comparable studies have examined the benefits of early disease prevention. But since the essential correlation appears to be between attained size and work output, and early infection is a recognized contributor to growth failure, the avoidance of early infectious insults probably would benefit productivity.

Work Output and Current Ill Health

Unsurprisingly, strong evidence exists for a relationship between current acute illness and reduced work output. This relationship has been particularly well demonstrated for malaria, where 5-20 days of disability may be associated with an acute episode, resulting in reductions in, for example, farming effort and in such secondary losses as the need to hire replacement labor (Barlow and Grobar 1986). Perhaps less obviously, chronic ill health caused by intestinal nematode infection, schistosomiasis, and anemia can also result in significant effects on productivity (Wolgemuth and others 1982; Basta and others 1979). Intestinal worms can also reduce the physical fitness of children at school age, and this effect is reversible by anthelmintic therapy (Stephenson and others 1993b). The importance of these findings in the present context is that they indicate that good health must be maintained if the benefits of early child development are to be fully realized.

Employment Prospects

An estimated 54 percent of the actively employed male population of South America is engaged in work that can be classified as requiring moderate to heavy physical activity (Spurr 1988). Selection of individuals to perform these tasks may be based on criteria reported from rural India where "better nourished boys were sought after by farmers and were assigned the more demanding jobs and were paid higher wages that went with these jobs" (Satyanarayana, Naidu, and Rao 1980: 282). The same study also suggests that men and women with better nutritional anthropometry earned 30 to 50 percent additional incentive money (over and above the uniform basic pay) in factories with work output incentive schemes. It has been suggested that stunting leads to a poverty trap whereby stunted parents with poor employment prospects and low wage earning capacity have children who suffer the same fate (Gopalan 1988).

Growth deficits have also been associated with educational underachievement, which may affect employment prospects through lack of skills and qualifications. More indirect effects may also occur: taller children are likely to enroll in school earlier, enter the workforce earlier, and enjoy greater opportunity to create wealth (Glewwe and Jacoby 1995).

The arguments presented above are consistent with an effect of early health on subsequent productivity and employment prospects. They might all be challenged, however, on the basis of the remarkable adaptability of people. For example, although stunted individuals have a lower capacity to perform external work, their maintenance costs are relatively unaffected, and a stunted person may approach a task in a way that maximizes the latter component (Ashworth 1968). It has also been suggested that stunting is irrelevant to work output since $VO_{2\,max}$ per kg for small individuals is similar to, or even greater than, that of larger individuals. These arguments have been dismissed as cynical (Gopalan 1988), not least because they suggest an expectation of the highest levels of adaptability and innovation from the most disadvantaged segment of the population.

Intervention

The previous sections reviewed the consequences of ill health in childhood for developmental outcomes. This section focuses on the opportunities for intervening against the conditions described earlier. These conditions are examples of those that have effects throughout early childhood, from birth to 8 years, and for which there is extensive programmatic experience of community intervention at scale. The interventions are sufficiently well understood to inform initial efforts to develop an ECD strategy.

Diarrhea

Individual episodes of diarrhea can be treated by oral rehydration with electrolyte solutions. It was recognized in the 1960s that the addition of glucose had important physiological consequences for fluid transport across the gastrointestinal tract (Nalin and others 1968). This understanding led to the development of highly effective oral rehydration solutions (ORS) which, in turn, became the central intervention in global efforts by UNICEF and WHO to extend oral rehydration therapy (ORT) to communities. ORS are now widely, but not universally, available; they are used in an estimated 20 percent of diarrheal episodes (Elliott and Attwell 1990). The costs involved are not negligible (World Bank 1993) because this palliative, rather than preventive, intervention must be repeatedly employed for each of the sequential episodes of diarrhea during early life. To address this issue, current ORT efforts promote home-made solutions, including those which are cereal-based (Elliott and Attwell 1990).

The effects of diarrhea appear to be most severe from the second semester of life, when breast milk alone may be nutritionally insufficient and when weaning foods may be inadequate and themselves serve as a vehicle for enteric pathogens. This observation indicates a need for ORT to be promoted in the context of a broad-based strategy (Keusch and Scrimshaw 1986) that also promotes breastfeeding, continued feeding during infection, development of adequate weaning foods from locally available commodities, specific nutrient fortification when required, and perhaps growth monitoring to identify the need for intervention.

Measles

Measles infection is preventable using readily available low-cost vaccines. Measles vaccination is a component of the package of six vaccines promoted globally by the UNICEF/WHO Expanded Programme of Immunization (EPI). The coverage of EPI is least effective in Africa where the "childhood cluster" of vaccine-preventable diseases remains a major source of childhood mortality and morbidity (World Bank 1993).

A problem with the use of measles vaccination is that 20 to 45 percent of measles cases occur in infants before 9 months of age, when immunization is recommended. The effectiveness of earlier vaccination is constrained by the presence of maternal antibody, and attempts to use high-titer vaccines to overcome this problem have been suspended because of evidence for an associated increase in late mortality (Garenne and others 1991). Delivery of current vaccines at both 6 and 9 months is used in some high-risk communities, such as overcrowded urban areas and refugee camps, in an attempt to enhance protection at a younger age.

Vitamin A supplementation offers remarkable benefits in terms of reduced childhood mortality in general (Sommer and others 1983; Sommer 1992). Clinical trials in Africa demonstrated that vitamin A supplementation also reduces severe morbidity and mortality among children who have acute measles in particular (Semba 1994). The supplements are widely available at low cost, and the benefit is achieved by a single intervention.

ARI

Current efforts to reduce the incidence of ARI advocate a combination of primary prevention and case management (WHO/ARI, 1991a). Prevention largely involves the promotion of EPI vaccine uptake (see above). It is estimated that deaths due to the four vaccine-preventable respiratory diseases (measles, diphtheria, pertussis, and tuberculosis) may account for up to 25 percent of total mortality in children under 5 years old in developing societies. Pneumococcal and, to a lesser extent, *Haemophilus influenzae* type b vaccines are under investigation as possible means of preventing pneumonia in developing societies, but they are not part of current programmatic practice. Promotion of breastfeeding is a more controversial part of the preventative strategy since the estimated reduction in ARI-specific mortality achievable by this approach is only about 2 to 3 percent and only in children under 12 months. Given the much greater value of breastfeeding to nutritional improvement and diarrhea reduction, its promotion may be viewed as an overall contributor to child development rather than part of a specific ARI control strategy.

The WHO/ARI case management strategy has the primary objective of reducing mortality due to acute lower respiratory tract infection. The approach involves the development of practical guidelines and algorithms for standard diagnosis and treatment (principally with antibiotics) at peripheral and referral health facilities and at the community level. Case management practices have been developed for children under 2 months of age and from 2 months to 5 years (WHO/ARI, 1991b). Multicenter operational research studies provide strong evidence of the effectiveness of this approach in achieving ARI-specific mortality reduction (WHO/ARI, 1988), and there is now programmatic experience in more than 50 countries. Some evidence indicates that case management of pneumonia with antibiotics also offers a subsidiary benefit of reducing diarrhea mortality.

Malaria

With some exceptions, control measures for malaria have become increasingly ineffective over the past decade, and efforts are increasing to develop more effective strategies (Nájera, Liese, and Hammer 1993). Mass chemoprophylaxis and medication of children with chloroquine were advocated as a control measure in Africa, but this proved ineffective and undoubtedly contributed to the widespread emergence of parasites resistant to antimalaria drugs. The alternative strategy of targeting therapy at those actually suffering from malaria involves a more-or-less sophisticated process of screening, not least to differentiate malaria from ARI, and today often involves more toxic and less affordable drugs because of the emergence of resistant parasites. Use of volunteer networks to support case detection and treatment has proven useful in Latin America (Ruebush and Godoy 1992).

Although treatment continues to be the main defense against severe disease and death from malaria, disease prevention is assuming a more important role. The use of bed nets impregnated with insecticide has recently been shown to significantly reduce infant mortality, malaria infection, and some morbidity measures, such as anemia (Premji and others 1995; Kroeger and others 1995; Greenwood and Pickering 1993). The initial efficacy trial in Gambia showed a 63 percent reduction in all-cause mortality in children 1-4 years of age. A recent evaluation of the National Bednet Programme in the same country showed a 25 to 38 percent reduction in all-cause mortality in children 1-9 years of age, the degree of protection varying with coverage and compliance (Olliaro, Cattani, and Wirth 1996; D'Alessandro and others 1995; Binka and others 1996; Nevill and others 1996). Results to date suggest that the benefit will be greatest for young children in high transmission areas and for children throughout the early childhood years in areas of lower endemicity.

This successful new development of an old idea is particularly attractive because it combines remarkable effectiveness with operational simplicity at the community level. Growing evidence shows that children and schools can play a central role in program promotion and implementation (Marsh and others 1996; Ogutu and others 1992).

Intestinal Parasitic Worm Infections

Anthelmintic treatments are safe, cheap, and widely available, and with broad spectrum drugs can remove all the major species simultaneously. Experience with using anthelmintic treatments in large-scale programs is considerable. Treatment is recommended as a component of community nutrition programs (Tomkins and Watson 1989) and, where infections are endemic, is typically given on a mass basis without the costly complication of individual diagnostic screening (Savioli, Bundy, and Tomkins 1992; Bundy and Guyatt 1995a). Targeting of mass treatment at the segment of the population with the most intense infection with roundworms and whipworms (children aged 5-14 years) has been shown to reduce transmission in the community as a whole (Bundy and others 1990) and may help prevent infection in earlier childhood. Regular, individual treatment is recommended for children under 5 years of age by the WHO Sick Child initiative. Because endemic infection is chronic and there appears to be little resistance to reinfection, the treatment must be repeated at regular intervals (WHO 1995a). If this is done on a mass basis then the intervals may be of the order of 12 months in areas of moderate transmission. Management of anemia requires both treatment for worms and iron supplementation.

Combining Interventions

Table 1 and figure 7 show how the interventions reviewed above relate to the period of early child development from birth to 8 years. The table indicates that multiple benefits can be expected for many of the interventions, and the figure illustrates the need for a continuum of overlapping interventions throughout childhood. It is assumed that all these interventions would be supported by community-wide education and communication. Achieving a coordinated approach is the central aim of the WHO/UNICEF initative for the Integrated Management of Childhood Illness (WHO 1995b).

The interventions presented in table 1 and figure 7 have a known effect on at least one of the health conditions considered in this chapter. The inclusion of nutritional interventions as measures to help combat infection serves to emphasize the central importance of good nutrition for child development. Nutritional issues per se are not

Table 1. Health Effects of Age-specific Interventions

Age range (months/years)	Intervention	Health effects on: Diarrhea	Measles	ARI	Malaria	Worms
0–2m	ARI case management I	+	+++	+++	–	–
0–6m	Breastfeeding	+++	+	+	?	–
2m–5y	ARI case management II	+	+++	+++	–	–
6m–3y	Vitamin A supplement	+	++	+	?	?
	Weaning foods	++	+	+	?	?
6m–8y	ORT and feeding	+++	–	–	–	–
	Case detection, treatment					
	Malaria	–	–	–	+++	–
	Worms	+	–	–	–	+++
9m–3y	EPI vaccines	+	+++	++	–	–
6y–8y plus	School-based promotion					
	Sanitation and hygiene	++	–	–	–	++
	Impregnated bed nets	?	–	?	+++	–
	Targeted mass anthelmintics	+	–	–	–	+++

\+ Number of +'s defines strength of evidence.
? Probable benefit.
– Unlikely benefit.

considered here (see the chapter by Martorell, this volume), but it would be expected that supplementary feeding, particularly at an early age, would also help consolidate the developmental benefits of controlling infection.

The prevention or treatment of infection might be viewed as providing an opportunity for physical development which can only be fully achieved if nutrition is adequate. By the same reasoning, mental and cognitive development may be promoted by good health, but the achievement of practical benefits in terms of social and educational outcomes may require additional inputs, such as good parenting practices, psychosocial stimulation, and adequate quality of education.

From a programming perspective preschool interventions present few difficulties because they build on existing experience in health delivery to this age group. However, extension of the early childhood period to include the first 2 years of schooling presents both a problem and an opportunity. The problem is that intervention only during the first 2 years at school is unlikely to result in significant benefits and will present major programmatic difficulties. The opportunity is that school-based interventions, if extended throughout the primary school-age range, can provide benefits to other age groups including preschool-age children.

Conclusion

Evidence shows that ill health in early childhood can constrain physical and mental development, educational achievement, and employment prospects. Evidence also shows

Figure 7. Timing of Age-specific Interventions During Early Childhood

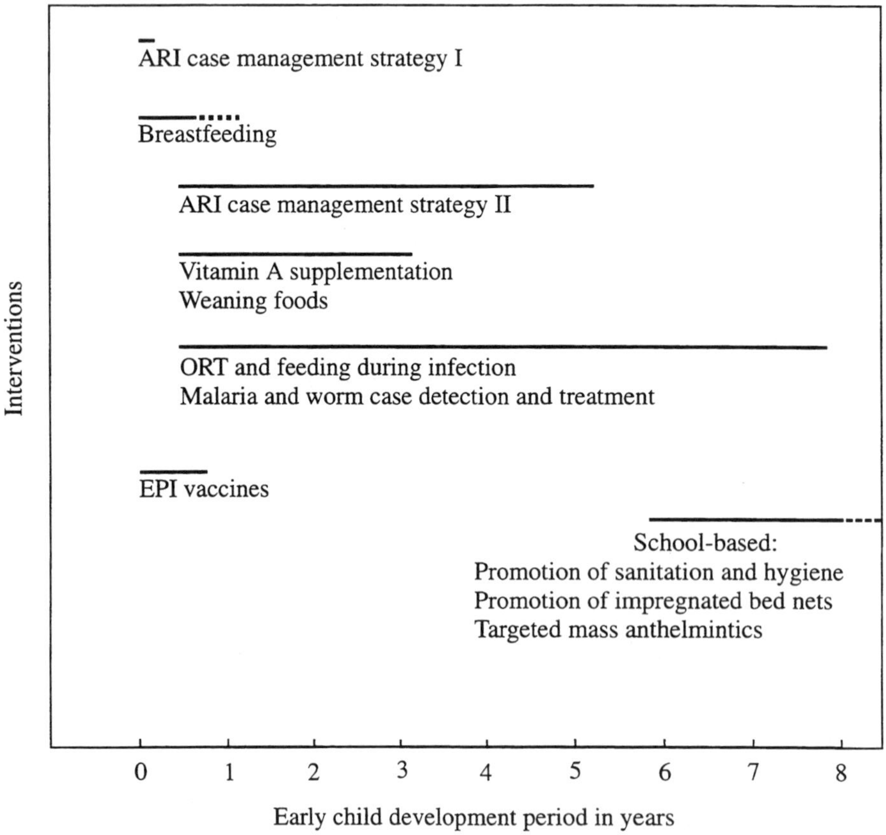

that health interventions at appropriate ages throughout early childhood can contribute to removing this constraint. The interventions are well understood and form part of the existing experience of health programs for preschool and school-age children. To realize the full developmental benefit, however, health interventions should form part of an ECD strategy that also provides nutritional, social, and educational inputs.

References

Ashworth, A. 1968. An Investigation of Very Low Calorie Intakes Reported in Jamaica. *British Journal of Nutrition* 22:341-55.

Balderston, J. B. 1981. Determinants of Children's School Participation. In J. B. Balderston, A. B. Wilson, M. E. Freire, and M. S. Simonen, eds., *Malnourished Children of the Rural Poor*. Boston, Mass.: Auburn House Publishing Co.

Barac-Nieto, M., G. B. Spurr, H. W. Dahners, and M. G. Maksud. 1980. Aerobic Work Capacity and Endurance during Nutritional Repletion of Severely Undernourished Men. *American Journal of Clinical Nutrition* 33:2268-75.

Barac-Nieto, M., G. B. Spurr, M. G. Maksud, and H. Lotero. 1978. Aerobic Work Capacity in Chronically Undernourished Adult Males. *Journal of Applied Physiology* 44:209-15.

Barlow, R., and L. M. Grobar. 1986. *Cost and Benefits of Controlling Parasitic Diseases*. PHN Technical Note 85-17. Washington D.C.: World Bank, Population, Health and Nutrition Department.

Basta, S. S., M. S. Soekirman, D. Karyadi, and N. S. Scrimshaw. 1979. Iron Deficiency Anaemia and the Productivity of Adult Males in Indonesia. *American Journal of Clinical Nutrition* 32:916-25.

Beasley, N. M. R. 1995. A Study of Parasitic Helminth Infection and Iron Deficiency in School Age Children: Population Distribution and Dynamics of Interaction. Doctor of Philosophy thesis, University of Oxford, Centre for the Epidemiology of Infectious Disease, England.

Beaton, G., A. Kelly, J. Kevany, R. Martorell, and J. Mason. December 1990. *Appropriate Uses of Anthropometric Indices in Children*. ACC/SCN State-of-the-Art Series, Nutrition Policy Discussion Paper No. 7. Geneva: United Nations, Administrative Committee on Coordination/Subcommittee on Nutrition.

Berman, S., and K. McIntosh. 1985. Selective Primary Health Care: Strategies for Control of Disease in the Developing World. XXI. Acute Respiratory Infections. *Reviews of Infectious Diseases* 71(5):674-91.

Binka, F., S. Morris, D. Ross, P. Arthur, and M. Aryeetey. 1996. Patterns of Malaria Morbidity and Mortality in Children in Northern Ghana. *Transactions of the Royal Society of Tropical Medicine and Hygiene* 88:381-5.

Black, R. 1993. Persistent Diarrhoea in Children in Developing Countries. *Pediatric Infectious Disease Journal* 12:751-61.

Black, R. E., K. H. Brown, and S. Becker. 1984. Malnutrition is a Determining Factor in Diarrheal Duration, but Not Incidence, among Young Children in a Longitudinal Study in Rural Bangladesh. *American Journal of Clinical Nutrition* 39:87-94.

Bondi, F. S. 1992. The Incidence and Outcomes of Neurological Abnormalities in Childhood Cerebral Malaria: A Long-term Follow-up of 62 Survivors. *Transactions of the Royal Society of Tropical Medicine and Hygiene* 86(1):17-19.

Briend, A. 1990. Is Diarrhoea a Major Cause of Malnutrition among Under Five Children in Developing Countries? *European Journal of Clinical Nutrition* 44:611-28.

Bundy, D. A. P., E. S. Cooper, D. E. Thompson, J. M. Didier, and I. Simmons. 1987. Epidemiology and Population Dynamics of *Ascaris lumbricoides* and *Trichuris trichuria* Infection in the Same Community. *Transactions of the Royal Society of Tropical Medicine and Hygiene* 81:987-93.

Bundy, D. A. P., and H. L. Guyatt. 1995a. Anthelmintic Chemotherapy: The Individual and the Community. *Current Opinion in Infectious Diseases* 8:466-72.

———. 1995b. The Health of School-age Children: Report of a Workshop. *Parasitology Today* 11(5):166-67.

Bundy, D. A. P., M. S. Wong, L. L. Lewis, and J. Horton. 1990. Control of Geohelminths by Delivery of Targeted Chemotherapy through Schools. *Transactions of the Royal Society of Tropical Medicine and Hygiene* 84:115-20.

Callender, J. E. M., S. Grantham-McGregor, S. Walker, and E. S. Cooper. 1992. *Trichuris* Infection and Mental Development in Children. *Lancet* 339:181.

Cardoso, M. A., M. U. Ferreria, L. M. A. Camargo, and S. C. Szarfarc. 1994. Anaemia, Iron-deficiency and Malaria in a Rural-Community in Brazilian Amazon. *European Journal of Clinical Nutrition* 48(5):326-32.

Chan, M. S., G. F. Medley, D. Jamison, and D. A. P. Bundy. 1994. The Evaluation of Potential Global Morbidity Attributable to Intestinal Nematode Infections. *Parasitology* 109:373-87.

Chen, R. T., R. Weierbach, Z. Bisoffi, F. Cutts, P. Rhodes, S. Ramaroson, C. Ntembagara, and F. Bizimana. 1994. A 'Post-honeymoon Period' Measles Outbreak in Muyinga Sector, Burundi. *International Journal of Epidemiology* 23(1):185-93.

Chowdhury, M. K., V. M. Gupta, R. Bairagi, and B. N. Bhattacharya. 1990. Does Malnutrition Predispose to Diarrhoea during Childhood? Evidence from a Longitudinal Study in Matlab, Bangladesh. *European Journal of Clinical Nutrition* 44:515-25.

Cohen, N., H. Rahman, J. Sprague, E. Jalil, L. de Regt, and M. Mitra. 1985. Prevalence and Determinants of Nutritional Blindness in Bangladeshi Children. *World Health Statistical Quarterly* 38:318-30.

Cooper, E. S., and D. A. P. Bundy. 1988. *Trichuris* Is Not Trivial. *Parasitology Today* 4(11):301-06.

Crofton, J., and A. Douglas. 1975. *Respiratory Diseases*. Oxford: Blackwell.

D'Alessandro, U., B. O. Olaleye, W. McGuire, M. C. Thomson, P. Langerock, B. M. Greenwood, and S. Bennett. 1995. Mortality and Morbidity from Malaria in Gambian Children after Introduction of an Impregnated Bed-net Programme. *Lancet* 345:479-83.

Dobbing, J., and J. L. Smart. 1974. Vulnerability of Developing Brain and Behaviour. *British Medical Bulletin* 30:164-68.

Elliott, K., and K. Attwell, eds. 1990. *Cereal-based Oral Rehydration Therapy for Diarrhoea*. Columbia, Md.: Aga Khan Foundation, Geneva and International Child Health Foundation.

Engle, P. L., K. Gorman, R. Martorell, and E. Pollitt. 1992. Infant and Preschool Psychological Development. *Food and Nutrition Bulletin* 14(3):201-14.

Filteau, S., S. S. Morris, J. G. Raynes, P. Arthur, D. A. Ross, B. R. Kirkwood, A. M. Tomkins, and J. O. Gyapong. 1995. Vitamin A Supplementation, Morbidity and Serum Acute Phase Proteins in Young Ghanaian Children. *American Journal of Clinical Nutrition* 62:434-38.

Foster, S. O., D. A. McFarland, and A. Meredith John. 1993. Measles. In D. T. Jamison, W. H. Mosley, A. R. Measham, and J. L. Bobadilla, eds., *Disease Control Priorities in Developing Countries*. Oxford: Oxford University Press.

Garenne, M., O. Leroy, J-P. Beau, and I. Sene. 1991. Child Mortality after High-titre Measles Vaccines: Prospective Study in Senegal. *Lancet* 338(2):903-06.

Ghana Health Assessment Project Team. 1981. A Quantitative Method of Assessing the Health Impact of Different Diseases in Less Developed Countries. *International Journal of Epidemiology* 10:73-80.

Ghana Partnership for Child Development. 1995. *Social, Economic and Cultural Factors Influencing Enrolment in School by Females in Ghana and the Health of Children in and out of School.* A Report for the Overseas Development Administration, United Kingdom.

Gilbert, C. 1993. Childhood Blindness: Major Causes and Strategies for Prevention. *Community Eye Health* 6:3-6.

Glewwe, P., and H. G. Jacoby. 1995. An Economic Analysis of Delayed Primary School Enrolment in a Low Income Country: The Role of Early Childhood Nutrition. *Review of Economics and Statistics* 77(1):156-69.

Golden, M. H. N. 1994. Is Complete Catch Up Possible for Stunted Malnourished Children? *European Journal of Clinical Nutrition* 48(suppl. 1):S58-S71.

Gopalan, C. 1988. Stunting: Significance and Implications for Public Health Policy. In J. C. Waterlow, ed., *Linear Growth Retardation in Less Developed Countries*. Nestlé Nutrition Workshop Series 14. New York: Raven Press.

Grantham-McGregor, S. M. 1990. Malnutrition, Mental Function and Development. In R. M. Suskind and L. Lewinter-Suskind, eds., *The Malnourished Child.* Nestlé Nutrition Workshop Series 19. New York: Raven Press.

Grantham-McGregor, S., C. Powell, and S. Walker. 1989. Nutritional Supplements, Stunting and Child Development. *Lancet* ii:809-10.

Grantham-McGregor, S. M., C. A. Powell, S. P. Walker, and J. H. Himes. 1991. Nutritional Supplementation, Psychosocial Stimulation, and Mental Development of Stunted Children: The Jamaican Study. *Lancet* 338:1-5.

Greenwood, B. M., and H. Pickering. 1993. A Malaria Control Trial Using Insecticide-treated Bed Nets and Targeted Chemoprophylaxis in a Rural Area of the Gambia, West-Africa. *Transactions of the Royal Society of Tropical Medicine and Hygiene* 87(S2):3-11.

Guerrant, R. L., L. V. Kirchoff, D. S. Shields, M. K. Nations, J. Leslie, M. A. de Sousa, J. G. Araujo, L. L. Correia, K. T. Suaer, and K. E. McClelland. 1983. Prospective Study of Diarrhoeal Illnesses in North-eastern Brazil: Patterns of Disease, Nutritional Impact, Etiologies, and Risk Factors. *Journal of Infectious Disease* 148:986-97.

Hill, A. V. S., C. E. M. Allsopp, D. Kwiatkowski, N. M. Anstey, P. Twumasi, P. A. Rowe, S. Bennet, D. Brewster, A. J. McMichael, and B. M. Greenwood. 1991. Common West African HLA Antigens Are Associated with Protection from Severe Malaria. *Nature* 352:595-600.

Idjradinata, P., and E. Pollitt. 1993. Reversal of Developmental Delays in Iron-deficient Anaemic Infants Treated with Iron. *Lancet* 341:1-4.
Jamison, D. 1986. Child Malnutrition and School Performance in China. *Journal of Development Economics* 20:299-309.
Keusch, G. T., and N. S. Scrimshaw. 1986. Selective Primary Health Care: Strategies for Control of Disease in the Developing World. XXIII. Control of Infection to Reduce the Prevalence of Infantile and Childhood Malnutrition. *Review of Infectious Diseases* 8(2):273-87.
Kroeger, A., M. Mancheno, J. Alarcon, and K. Pesse. 1995. Insecticide Impregnated Bed Nets for Malaria Control—Varying Experiences from Ecuador, Colombia and Peru Concerning Acceptability and Effectiveness. *American Journal of Tropical Medicine and Hygiene* 53(4):313-23.
Kvalsvig, J. D., R. M. Cooppan, and K. J. Connolly. 1991. The Effects of Parasite Infections on Cognitive Processes in Children. *Annals of Tropical Medicine and Parasitology* 85(5):551-68.
Lozoff, B., E. Jimenez, and A. W. Wolf. 1991. Long-term Developmental Outcome of Infants with Iron Deficiency. *New England Journal of Medicine* 325:687-94.
Marsh, V. M., W. Mutemi, E. S. Some, A. Haaland, and R. W. Snow. 1996 (forthcoming). Methods and Evaluation of a Community Education Programme during a Randomised Controlled Trial of Insecticide-treated Bed Nets on the Kenyan Coast. *Health Policy and Planning.*
Martorell, R. 1989. Body-size, Adaptation and Function. *Human Organizations* 48:15-20.
———. 1995a. Results and Implications of the INCAP Follow-up Study. *Journal of Nutrition* 125:1127S-38S.
———. 1995b. Promoting Health Growth: Rationale and Benefits. In P. Pinstrup-Andersen, D. Pelletier, and H. Alderman, eds., *Child Growth and Nutrition in Developing Countries. Priorities for Action.* New York: Cornell University Press.
Martorell, R., J-P. Habicht, C. Yarborough, A. Lechtig, R. E. Klein, and K. A. Western. 1975. Acute Morbidity and Physical Growth in Rural Guatemalan Children. *American Journal of Diseases of Children* 129:1296-1301.
Martorell, R., L. K. Khan, and D. G. Schroeder. 1994. Reversibility of Stunting: Epidemiological Findings in Children from Developing Countries. *European Journal of Clinical Nutrition* 48(suppl. 1):S45-S57.
Martorell, R., D. G. Schroeder, J. A. Rivera, and H. J. Kaplowitz. 1995. Patterns of Linear Growth in Rural Guatemalan Adolescents and Children. *Journal of Nutrition* 125(4 suppl.):1090S-96S.
Martorell, R., C. Yarborough, S. Yarborough, and R. E. Klein. 1980. The Impact of Ordinary Illness on the Dietary Intakes of Malnourished Children. *American Journal of Clinical Nutrition* 33:345-54.
Mata, L. J., R. A. Kromal, J. J. Urrutia, and B. Garcia. 1977. Effect of Infection on Food Intake and the Nutritional State: Perspectives as Viewed from the Village. *American Journal of Clinical Nutrition* 30:1215-27.
Mizushima, Y., H. Kato, H. Ohmae, T. Tanaka, A. Bobogare, and A. Ishii. 1994. Prevalence of Malaria and Its Relationship to Anaemia, Blood-glucose Levels, Serum Somatomedin-C (UGF-1) Levels in the Solomon Islands. *Acta Tropica* 58(3-4):207-20.
Moock, P., and J. Leslie. 1986. Childhood Malnutrition and Schooling in the Terai Region of Nepal. *Journal of Development Economics* 20:33-52.
Nabarro, D., P. Howard, C. Cassels, M. Pant, A. Wijga, and N. Padfield. 1988. The Importance of Infections and Environmental Factors as Possible Determinants of Growth Retardation in Children. In J. C. Waterlow, ed., *Linear Growth Retardation in Less Developed Countries.* Nestlé Nutrition Workshop Series 14. New York: Raven Press.
Nájera, J. A., B. H. Liese, and J. Hammer. 1993. Malaria. In D. T. Jamison, W. H. Mosley, A. R. Measham, and J. L. Bobadilla, eds., *Disease Control Priorities in Developing Countries.* Oxford: Oxford University Press.
Nalin, D. R., R. A. Cash, R. Islam, M. Molla, and R. A. Phillips. 1968. Oral Maintenance Therapy for Cholera in Adults. *Lancet* 2:370-73.
Nevill, C., E. Some, V. Mung'ala, W. Mutemi, L. New, and R. Snow. 1996 (forthcoming). A Randomised Controlled Trial of Permethrin-treated Bednets in the Reduction of Severe, Life-threatening Malaria and Mortality among Kenyan Children. *Tropical Medicine and International Health* 1.

Newton, C. R. J. C., N. Peshu, B. Kendall, F. J. Kirkham, A. Sowunmi, C. Waruiru, I. Mwangi, S. A. Murphy, and K. Marsh. 1994. Brain Swelling and Ischaemia in Kenyans with Cerebral Malaria. *Archives of Disease in Childhood* 70(4):281-87.

Nokes, C., and D. A. P. Bundy. 1993. Compliance and Absenteeism in School Children: Implications for Helminth Control. *Transactions of the Royal Society of Tropical Medicine and Hygiene* 87:148-52.

———. 1994. Does Helminth Infection Affect Mental Processing and Educational Achievement? *Parasitology Today* 10(1):14-18.

Ogutu, R. O., A. J. Oloo, W. S. Ekissa, I. O. Genga, N. Mulaya, and J. I. Githure. 1992. The Effect of Participatory School Health Programme on the Control of Malaria. *East African Medical Journal* 69(6):298-301.

Olliaro, P., J. Cattani, and D. Wirth. 1996. Malaria, the Submerged Disease. *Journal of the American Medical Association* 275(3):230-33.

Pollitt, E. 1990. *Malnutrition and Infection in the Classroom.* Paris: United Nations Educational, Scientific, and Cultural Organization.

———. 1995. The Relationship between Undernutrition and Behavioral Development in Children: Functional Significance of the Covariance between Protein Energy Malnutrition and Iron Deficiency Anaemia. *Journal of Nutrition* 125:2272S-77S.

Pollitt, E., C. Garza, and R. L. Leibel. 1984. Nutrition and Public Policy. In H. Stevenson and A. Seigel, eds., *Child Development and Public Policy.* Chicago: University of Chicago Press.

Premji, Z., P. Lubega, Y. Hamisi, E. Mchopa, J. Minjas, W. Checkley, and C. Shiff. 1995. Changes in Malaria Associated Morbidity in Children Using Insecticide Treated Mosquito Nets in the Bagamoyo District of Coastal Tanzania. *Tropical Medicine and Parasitology* 46(3):147-53.

Rhode, J. 1988. Beyond Survival: Promoting Healthy Growth. *Indian Journal of Paediatrics* 55:S3-58.

Roche, A. F., and J. H. Himes. 1980. Incremental Growth Charts. *American Journal of Clinical Nutrition* 33:2041-52.

Rondo, P., and A. Tomkins. 1993. Risk Factors for Intra-uterine Growth Retardation in Campinas, Brazil. *Proceedings of the Nutrition Society* 52:65.

Rosenfield, P. L., F. Golladay, and R. K. Davidson. 1984. The Economics of Parasitic Diseases: Research Priorities. *Social Sciences and Medicine* 19:1117-26.

Ruebush, T. K., and H. A. Godoy. 1992. Community Participation in Malaria Surveillance and Treatment. 1. The Volunteer Collaborator Network of Guatemala. *American Journal of Tropical Medicine and Hygiene* 46(3):248-60.

Satyanarayana, M. B., A. Nadamuni Naidu, and S. Narasinga Rao. 1979. Nutritional Deprivation in Childhood and the Body Size, Activity, and Physical Work Capacity of Young Boys. *American Journal of Clinical Nutrition* 32:1769-75.

———. 1980. Agricultural Employment, Wage Earnings and Nutritional Status of Teenage Rural Hyderabad Boys. *Indian Journal of Nutrition and Diet* 17:281-86.

Savioli, L., D. A. P. Bundy, and A. Tomkins. 1992. Intestinal Parasitic Infections: A Soluble Public Health Problem. *Transactions of the Royal Society of Tropical Medicine and Hygiene* 86:353-54.

Schmutzhard, E., and F. Gerstenbrand. 1984. Cerebral Malaria in Tanzania. Its Epidemiology, Clinical Symptoms and Neurological Long Term Sequelae in the Light of 66 Cases. *Transactions of the Royal Society of Tropical Medicine and Hygiene* 78(3):351-53.

Schorling, J. B., and R. L. Guerrant. 1990. Diarrhoea and Catch-up Growth. *Lancet* 335:599-600.

Semba, R. D. 1994. Vitamin A, Immunity and Infection. *Clinical Infectious Diseases* 19:489-99.

Sepulveda, J., W. Willett, and A. Munoz. 1988. Malnutrition and Diarrhoea: A Longitudinal Study among Urban Mexican Children. *American Journal of Epidemiology* 127:365-76.

Simeon, D. T., and S. M. Grantham-McGregor. 1990. Nutritional Deficiencies and Children's Behaviour and Mental Development. *Research Review* 3:1-24.

Simeon, D. T., S. M. Grantham-McGregor, J. E. Callender, and M. S. Wong. 1995. Growth, School Achievement and School Attendance in Children after the Treatment of *Trichuris trichuria. Journal of Nutrition* 125:1875-83.

Simeon, D. T., S. M. Grantham-McGregor, and M. S. Wong. 1995. *Trichuris trichuria* Infection and Cognition in Children: Results of a Randomized Clinical Trial. *Parasitology* 110:457-64.

Soemantri, A., E. Pollitt, and I. Kim. 1985. Iron Deficiency Anemia and Educational Achievement. *American Journal of Clinical Nutrition* 42:1221-28.

Sommer A. 1992. Vitamin A Deficiency and Childhood Mortality. *Lancet* 339:864.

Sommer, A., I. Tarwotjo, G. Hussaini, and D. Susanto. 1983. Increased Mortality in Children with Mild Vitamin A Deficiency. *Lancet* 298:585-88.

Spurr, G. B. 1988. Body Size, Physical Work Capacity, and Productivity in Hard Work: Is Bigger Better? In J. C. Waterlow, ed., *Linear Growth Retardation in Less Developed Countries*. Nestlé Nutrition Workshop Series 14. New York: Raven Press.

Spurr, G. B., J. C. Reina, and M. Barac-Nieto. 1983. Marginal Malnutrition in School-aged Colombian Boys: Anthropometry and Maturation. *American Journal of Clinical Nutrition* 37:119-32.

Stansfield, S. K., and D. S. Shepard. 1993. Acute Respiratory Infection. In D. T. Jamison, W. H. Mosley, A. R. Measham, and J. L. Bobadilla, eds., *Disease Control Priorities in Developing Countries*. Oxford: Oxford University Press.

Stephenson, L. S. 1987. *Impact of Helminth Infections on Human Nutrition*. London: Taylor & Francis.

Stephenson, L. S., M. C. Latham, E. J. Adams, S. N. Kinoti, and A. Pertet. 1993a. Weight Gain of Kenyan School Children Infected with Hookworm, *Trichuris trichuria* and *Ascaris lumbricoides* Is Improved Following Once- or Twice-yearly Treatment with Albendazole. *Journal of Nutrition* 123(4):656-65.

———. 1993b. Physical Fitness, Growth and Appetite of Kenyan School Boys with Hookworm, *Trichuris trichuria* and *Ascaris lumbricoides* Infections Are Improved Four Months after a Single Dose of Albendazole. *Journal of Nutrition* 123(6):1036-46.

Thein-Hlaing, Thane-Toe, Than-Saw, Myat-Lay-Kyin, and Myint-Lwin. 1991. A Controlled Chemotherapeutic Intervention Trial on the Relationship between *Ascaris lumbricoides* Infection and Malnutrition in Children. *Transactions of the Royal Society of Tropical Medicine and Hygiene* 85:523-28.

Tomkins, A. 1981. Nutritional Status and Severity of Diarrhoea among Preschool Children in Rural Nigeria. *Lancet* 294:860-62.

———. 1992. Nutrition and Infection. In J. C. Waterlow, ed., *Protein Energy Malnutrition*. London: Edward Arnold.

Tomkins, A., R. Behrens, and A. Roy. 1993. The Role of Zinc and Vitamin A Deficiency in Diarrhoeal Syndromes in Developing Countries. *Proceedings of the Nutrition Society* 52:131-42.

Tomkins, A., and F. Watson. 1989. *Malnutrition and Infection: A Review*. ACC/SCN State-of-the-Art Series Nutrition Policy Discussion Paper No. 5. Geneva: United Nations, Administrative Committee on Coordination/Subcommittee on Nutrition.

UNESCO (United Nations Educational, Scientific, and Cultural Organization). 1993. *World Education Report*. Paris.

UNICEF (United Nations Children's Fund). 1995. *State of the World's Children*. New York.

———. 1996. *Factors Influencing Female School Enrollment and Attendance*. Ghana.

Van Lerberghe, W. 1990. Growth, Infection and Mortality: Is Growth Monitoring an Efficient Screening Instrument? In J. M. Tanner, ed., *Auxology 88. Perspectives in the Science of Growth and Development*. Nishimura and London: Smith-Gordon.

Weitzman, M. 1987. Excessive School Absences. *Advances in Developmental and Behavioural Paediatrics* 8:151-78.

WHO (World Health Organization). 1984. A Programme for Controlling Acute Respiratory Infection in Children: Memorandum from a WHO Meeting. *Bulletin of the World Health Organization* 62:47-58.

———. 1995a. *Health of School Children. Treatment of Intestinal Helminths and Schistosomiasis*. WHO/CDS/95.1. Geneva.

———. 1995b. Integrated Management of the Sick Child. *Bulletin of the World Health Organization* 73(6):735-40.

WHO/ARI (World Health Organization/Programme for Control of Acute Respiratory Infections). 1988. *Case Management of Acute Respiratory Infection in Children: Intervention Studies*. Publication 88-2. Geneva.

———. 1991a. *Programme for Control of Acute Respiratory Infections: Interim Programme Report*. Publication 91-19. Geneva.

———. 1991b. *Technical Bases for the WHO Recommendations on the Management of Pneumonia in Children at First-level Health Facilities.* Publication 91-20. Geneva.

Winick, M. 1970. Biological Correlations. *Nutrition, Growth and Mental Development* 120:416-18.

Wolgemuth, J. C., M. C. Latham, A. Hall, A. Chesher, and D. W. T. Crompton. 1982. Worker Productivity and the Nutritional Status of Kenyan Road Construction Laborers. *American Journal of Clinical Nutrition* 36:68-78.

World Bank. 1993. *Investing in Health: World Development Report.* Oxford: Oxford University Press.

Young, M. E. 1995. *Investing in Young Children.* Washington, D.C.: World Bank.

Early Child Development: Investing in our Children's Future
M.E. Young, editor.

Undernutrition During Pregnancy and Early Childhood: Consequences for Cognitive and Behavioral Development

Reynaldo Martorell

Nutrition is vital to cognitive development, an important aspect of human capital. Studies show that undernutrition, specifically during pregnancy and early childhood, can have profound effects on cognition and behavior throughout life. Particularly influential are intrauterine growth retardation, severe and moderate protein-energy malnutrition, and iodine and iron deficiencies. These conditions affect many of the world's children today and partly determine the extent to which they will become productive individuals in their societies. The legacy of their early undernutrition can be long term, resulting in poor educational achievement, reduced work capacity, and poor reproductive health, all of which lead to social and economic consequences for societies.

This chapter addresses the full range of potential effects of undernutrition during pregnancy and early childhood. These effects are explored in an in-depth, comprehensive review of the rich and diverse literature on this subject, from both developing and industrial countries. Attention is given to the specific conditions mentioned above, as well as to interventions to ameliorate these conditions. Such interventions include improving the home environment, food and nutrition supplementation, psychosocial stimulation and support, and preschool and early school programs. Critical questions include: What are the effects of undernutrition on cognition and behavior? When in a child's life are effects more likely to be expressed? Are the deleterious effects of undernutrition magnified in poverty settings? Are effects reversible, and if so, to what extent?

Additional findings on the effects of nutrition and nutritional interventions are reported in two related chapters in this volume: Bundy addresses ill health and nutrition in relation to physical development, and Sternberg and colleagues consider ill health and nutrition in relation to cognitive development. For cognitive and behavioral development, as for ill health and physical development, timing and poverty are critical, associated factors. Earlier occurrences of undernutrition (for example, in utero and the first 3 years of life) appear to have greater effects on cognition and behavior than later occurrences, just as earlier interventions appear to result in better outcomes than later interventions. Timing of undernutrition and interventions, whether early or late, along with poverty, has long-term effects on the development of human capital (for example, income, education, and employment levels). The economic effects of these relationships are significant and indicate many opportunities for improving early child development globally.

This chapter opens by considering the definition and concepts of undernutrition and cognitive and behavioral development. The effects of undernutrition on cognition and behavior are then explored in nine categories. The chapter concludes with a brief description of the functional consequences of undernutrition and requirements for nutrition programs.

Definitions and Concepts

The Nature of Undernutrition

In much of the literature on nutrition and cognitive and behavioral development, the term "protein-energy malnutrition," or PEM, designates both the increasingly rare forms of severe clinical malnutrition (for example, kwashiorkor and marasmus) and the more common forms of growth failure (often called mild and moderate PEM). The syndrome, however, has a complex etiology and can be caused by deficiencies in many nutrients, not just protein and energy; for example, deficiencies in iron, zinc, and vitamin A generally coexist with deficiencies in protein and energy. "Sindrome pluricarencial" (multiple deficiency syndrome) was used some years ago in the Spanish literature and is a more appropriate designation.

In addition to nutrient deficiencies, many nondietary factors may be involved in causing general undernutrition. For example, infections, particularly of the respiratory and gastrointestinal tracts, and deficiencies in childcare are important causes of undernutrition. The causal model of undernutrition used by United Nations Children's Fund (UNICEF), which gives equal weight to three factors (food, health, and care), is well known.

Many of the studies on growth failure or nutrition interventions reviewed in this chapter offer information on the possible role of nutrition in general rather than only on the value of improving protein-energy status. Even in the case of micronutrients, attributing effects to a specific nutrient may be difficult because of the multiple, rather than single, deficiencies that generally occur. For example, studies of anemic and nonanemic children also show contrasting degrees of other deficiencies (for example, protein-energy, vitamin A, and zinc).

Undernutrition also is intertwined with poverty. The poor are more undernourished than the wealthy, and they are less educated, have poorer houses, more illnesses, larger families, and many other disadvantages. Because the relationship between poor nutrition and poverty is so strong, understanding the effects of undernutrition on development must take place within a context that includes them both. In summary, the multifactorial causes of undernutrition (food, health, and care) and the setting of poverty are relevant when interpreting the possible effects of undernutrition on cognitive and behavioral development.

Age-specific Undernutrition

Focusing on achieved size as a marker of undernutrition obscures the fact that growth fails almost exclusively during intrauterine life and the first few years of life (Beaton 1989; Beaton and others 1990; Martorell, Kettel Khan, and Schroeder 1994). The literature abounds with references to children who are chronically malnourished, even applying this to schoolchildren whose diets and growth rates may be adequate at the time of measurement but who failed to grow in early childhood. Even in poor countries, children generally grow adequately after 2 or 3 years of age, neither catching up nor falling further behind.

Demonstrating the importance of adequate early growth, Martorell, Kettel Khan, and Schroeder (1994) assessed the extent to which stunted growth, a phenomenon of early childhood, can be reversed in later childhood and adolescence. Their review of the literature shows that the potential for catch-up growth increases with delayed maturation and a prolonged growth period. However, maturational delays in developing countries are usually less than 2 years, which is enough only to compensate for a small fraction of the growth retardation of early childhood. Martorell, Kettel Khan, and Schroeder (1994) also relate that follow-up studies of subjects continuing in the setting where their growth was stunted reveal little or no catch-up growth in later life. By interpretation, most early failure in growth is irreversible.

Iron deficiency also occurs most often during early childhood, the period of maximum growth failure. Iron deficiency is most prevalent at 6-24 months of age (Lozoff 1990). Incidence of severe vitamin A deficiency (xerophthalmia and keratomalacia) peaks at ages 2-5 years (McLaren 1986), but retinol liver reserves become depleted at greatly accelerated rates during the first 2 years of life (Wallingford and Underwood 1986).

Small children are at greater risk of becoming undernourished and suffering from growth failure, anemia, or vitamin A deficiency than older children for several reasons (Martorell 1995). In part the higher risk arises from their greater relative nutritional needs (that is, needs per kilogram of bodyweight), resulting from more rapid rates of growth and higher metabolism than older children. For example, for each kilogram, a 1-year-old child needs more than twice as much protein of higher quality than a schoolchild needs (World Health Organization 1985). The greater relative nutritional needs of small children may be neglected through infrequency and inadequacy (low energy and nutrient concentration) of typical complementary foods and family diet.

Young children also are at higher risk than older children for undernourishment because of their developing immune systems. Young children fall prey to many respiratory and gastrointestinal tract infections; by school age, survivors have acquired considerable immunity and suffer from fewer infections of these types.

Finally, young children suffer from undernutrition because they are more susceptible to the effects of poor care and are less able to express or satisfy their needs. In developing countries, denial of breastfeeding is an example of poor care that has tremendous effects on the nourishment and health of small children.

Measures of Cognitive and Behavioral Development

The literature on effects of undernutrition is vast, but most studies only emphasize cognitive development. This chapter explores the greater breadth of effects from undernutrition by considering both cognitive and behavioral development because the two are intertwined. For example, aspects of behavioral development such as socioemotional development, motor development, and physical activity are recognized increasingly for helping shape intellectual functioning (Pollitt and Gorman 1989).

Although intellectual functioning appears to be affected by factors such as behavioral development, the dominant measures of cognition or intelligence are psychometric. They measure certain linguistic, logical, and spatial abilities but exclude other forms of intelligence such as wisdom, creativity, practical knowledge, and social skills (Neisser and others 1995).

Studies reviewed in this chapter used various general and single-dimension psychometric tests to measure intelligence. General tests, such as the Weschsler and Stanford Binet tests, include verbal and nonverbal items, yielding subscores as well as an overall score (that is, a general factor, g, or intelligence quotient, IQ). General tests may involve defining words, completing a series of pictures, or identifying words that do not belong in a set (Neisser and others 1995). Single-dimension tests include the Peabody Picture Vocabulary Test, which measures verbal intelligence in children, and the Raven's Progressive Matrices, a nonverbal, untimed test that requires inductive reasoning about perceptual patterns (Neisser and others 1995).

General and single-dimension tests are each limited in terms of what they do and do not measure. Although performance may be correlated across general tests and between subscores, the limitations make generalizing difficult across studies that use different tests. These tests also contain bias, which means that cross-cultural equivalency of psychometric performance should not be assumed. However, intracultural relationships between performance and undernutrition, which this chapter emphasizes, may be less subject to bias.

Effects of Undernutrition on Cognition and Behavior

The literature on the relationship among nutrition, cognition, and behavior addresses a broad range of topics that can be organized into several categories: (a) follow-up studies of severely malnourished children, (b) response of severely malnourished children to improvements in the home environment, (c) undernutrition in industrialized countries, (d) low birthweight, (e) correlational studies, (f) food supplementation and stimulation trials, (g) breastfeeding and development, (h) micronutrients, and (i) mechanisms. Each of these categories is explored below. An overview of all the findings concludes this section.

Follow-up Studies of Severely Malnourished Children

Studies show that severe malnutrition affects cognitive development. For example, survivors of severe PEM almost always have deficits in cognitive functioning and school achievements compared to matched neighborhood children, classmates, or siblings (Pollitt and Thomson 1977; Galler 1984; Grantham-McGregor 1995). The degree of deficit varies, but many studies show a difference of 15 or more IQ points. Differences appear to be more consistent when survivors are compared to matched controls rather than to siblings (Grantham-McGregor 1995), and recent reviews are less certain that marasmus leads to greater deficits than kwashiorkor (Galler 1984; Grantham-McGregor 1995). All reviews agree that the data do not permit unequivocal testing of whether outcome is affected by age of onset of the severe episode during the first or second years of life.

As well as affecting cognitive functioning, the acute stage of severe malnutrition leads to marked behavioral abnormalities, such as apathy, reduced activity, and reduced exploration of the environment. These effects are greater in severely undernourished children than in children with other diseases. Recuperation, however, quickly leads to general improvement in the gross behavioral abnormalities (Grantham-McGregor 1995).

The Barbados study of Galler and colleagues (Galler and others 1983; Galler, Ramsey, and Forde 1986) and that of Richardson, Birch, and Ragbeer (1975) in Jamaica demonstrate that severe malnutrition affects the behavioral as well as cognitive development of children. Jamaican school boys who were severely malnourished in infancy were less liked by siblings and more unhappy at school than classmates of the same age and sex. Affected children also behaved immaturely more often and were more clumsy than those not suffering from undernutrition. Children with a history of malnutrition were either more highly active or lethargic than their classmates and were more often withdrawn, solitary, or unsociable (Richardson, Birch, and Ragbeer 1975). Previously severely malnourished children in both Barbados and Jamaica had poorer relationships with classmates and teachers, exhibited a greater degree of attention deficits, and received poorer grades.

The Barbados study, one of the most comprehensive studies of the long-term cognitive and behavioral effects of severe malnutrition, also showed an effect of undernutrition on physical development. Children with marasmus weighed less than 75 percent of normal weight for age during infancy, a liberal definition since marasmus is defined as less than 60 percent weight for age in many other studies. Although it was the extreme in Barbados, weighing less than 75 percent of the normal weight for age is common for children in many parts of the world, such as rural India.

Despite indications from the various studies, it is difficult to unequivocally attribute cognitive, behavioral, or physical effects to severe malnutrition. According to Grantham-McGregor (1995), wide-ranging disadvantages in the homes and families of undernourished children make it nearly impossible to match index and comparison children. Also, with the exception of one prospective study (Cravioto and DeLicardie 1976), it has been impossible in cases and controls to compare conditions existing before malnutrition.

Just as these factors may cause both malnutrition and poor development, other factors associated with malnutrition may directly influence cognition or behavior. For example, although not controlled for in most studies, severe malnutrition often leads to hospitalization, which could itself influence cognition (Grantham-McGregor 1995).

Also, recent work by Grantham-McGregor and others (1989) suggests that growth failure, rather than the clinical definition of marasmus or the presence of edema, is the most important factor in cognitive and behavioral development. They compared twenty-nine children 6-24 months old who had recently recovered from severe malnutrition with twenty-nine children who had not been admitted for nutritional recuperation, matched for age and level of stunted growth, from a similar socioeconomic background. Development of children in these two groups, and in a third group without stunted growth, was measured by the Griffiths Test. Performance was best in the nonstunted group and equally poor in the group with a history of severe malnutrition and in the group with stunted growth.

Showing the importance of family environment as a factor in child development, the Barbados study suggests that the mother of a child who develops severe malnutrition may be less likely to establish healthy maternal-child interaction. Cravioto and DeLicardie (1976) found that families of malnourished children were deficient in social stimulation, and mothers were passive and lethargic before the onset of malnutrition. Comparison to siblings, rather than to matched controls, may narrow down some of the outside factors of causation by controlling for factors constant to the family. However, "development of undernutrition in one child in an environment where a sibling is well-nourished indicates either differential treatment, differential response to treatment, or a combination of both conditions. Thus the apparent control is deceptive" (Pollitt and Thomson 1977: 273). However, using siblings or classmates as controls (studies in Barbados and Jamaica) probably understates nutritional effects on development because comparison children invariably suffer, although to a lesser degree, from undernutrition. Caution must be exercised when interpreting all the findings mentioned in this chapter as evidence of a direct causal link between early severe malnutrition and subsequent mental functioning because "the particular socioenvironmental factors which led to the development of early clinical malnutrition in some children and not in others in the same family or in the same community may also have contributed directly to the reduced intellectual performance observed" (Ricciuti 1981: 117).

The Barbados Study

Methods

Two groups of schoolchildren with a history of moderate to severe malnutrition in the first year of life were studied from 5 to 18 years of age and compared to classmates without any history of malnutrition. The malnourished group was composed of 129 children weighing less than 75 percent of the normal weight for age. These cases were selected after excluding children with low birthweight and other health problems likely to affect development. The control group comprised 129 children matched on the basis of age, sex, and socioeconomic status. The index children were hospitalized for an average of 37 days and received medical care, including home visits, nutritional counseling, and subsidized milk to 11 years of age. Assessments were made of both cognitive function and behavioral performance at school and home.

Results

The formerly malnourished group had significantly lower scores than the comparison group on verbal, performance, and full-scale IQ scores, as measured by the Wechsler's Intelligence Scale for Children-Revised (WISC-R); on average, differences were around 12 IQ points for both boys and girls ages 8-15 (Galler, Ramsey, and Forde 1986). Fine motor skills, as assessed by the Purdue Pegboard Test, also were affected (Galler, Ramsey, and Solimano 1985). Teachers evaluated classroom behavior and found a 4-fold increase in the frequency of attention deficit disorder among the formerly malnourished (Galler 1986). They also found greater frequency of reduced social skills, poorer physical appearance, and emotional instability (Galler and others 1983). Children with a history of malnutrition performed more poorly on eight of nine academic subject areas (Galler, Ramsey, and Solimano 1984). Despite matching by socioconomic status, some differences in home background characteristics were demonstrated during the follow-up period, but these factors were not strongly related to intellectual performance. Finally, depressive symptoms, especially feelings of hopelessness, occurred more often among mothers of previously malnourished children than among mothers of control children; this was examined when the children were 5-11 years old. Maternal depression may have led to the malnutrition episode or exacerbated its effects or may have resulted from having a malnourished child (Salt, Galler, and Ramsey 1988).

Response to Improving Stimulation in the Home Environment of Severely Malnourished Children

Even after recuperating nutritionally, severely malnourished children discharged into their original home environments lag behind classmates in intellectual performance and school achievement, as shown above. What if the level of stimulation in the home environment were enhanced? Would performance be improved, and if so, to what extent?

A few important and relevant studies show the response of formerly malnourished children to an improved home environment. One study deals with the long-term effects of a home intervention designed to stimulate cognitive development (Grantham-McGregor and others 1994), and the others show the effects of adoption on child development (Winick, Meyer, and Harris 1975; My Lien, Meyer, and Winick 1977; Colombo, de la Parra, and Lopez 1992).

In the first long-term follow-up of severely malnourished children who participated in a program to stimulate cognitive development, Grantham-McGregor and colleagues (1994) controlled for hospitalization by selecting three groups of children for the study: eighteen nonintervened, severely malnourished children (NIM); twenty-one intervened, severely malnourished children (IM); and twenty-one nonmalnourished children with acute diseases, the control group (C). All children had birthweights of more than 2.5 kilograms, and all were patients in the University Hospital of the West Indies in Kingston, Jamaica, between 6 and 24 months of age.

The children were tested up to 14 years after their discharge from the hospital using the Griffiths Test (up to 6 years after discharge), Stanford-Binet Test (7, 8 and 9 years), and the WISC (14 years) (figure 1). Although the children in C performed low in comparison with children from industrial countries, they were clearly superior to children from NIM and IM, the two formerly malnourished groups. Children in IM, who had participated in a stimulation program, showed performance levels between children in C and NIM. Similar differences showed up in reading, spelling, arithmetic, and global scores on the Wide Range Achievement Test (WRAT) and in the Peabody Picture Vocabulary Test (PPVT).

This Jamaican study demonstrates that an intervention using psychosocial stimulation during home visits every 1 or 2 weeks for 3 years improves intellectual performance and school achievement. Stimulation included toy demonstrations and encouragement to mothers to increase verbal interaction. However, although the previously malnourished children receiving psychosocial stimulation performed better than those in NIM, why did they fall short of the performance by children in C? One possibility is the effect of having been severely malnourished; for example, organic brain lesions may have limited performance. Differences in socioeconomic status and maternal cognitive performance at the time of hospitalization between the control and malnourished groups suggest that other factors, which caused both malnutrition and poor intellectual performance, also could be important.

Two studies of Korean orphans adopted by U.S. families also illustrate that survivors of malnutrition perform better if their fortunes improve (Winick, Meyer, and Harris 1975; My Lien, Meyer, and Winick 1977). The definition of malnutrition in these studies was solely anthropometric. The height and weight of girls (boys were excluded from the study because fewer were available) were compared to Korean reference data, and three study

Figure 1. Mean Standard Scores of Two Groups of Children with a History of Malnutrition

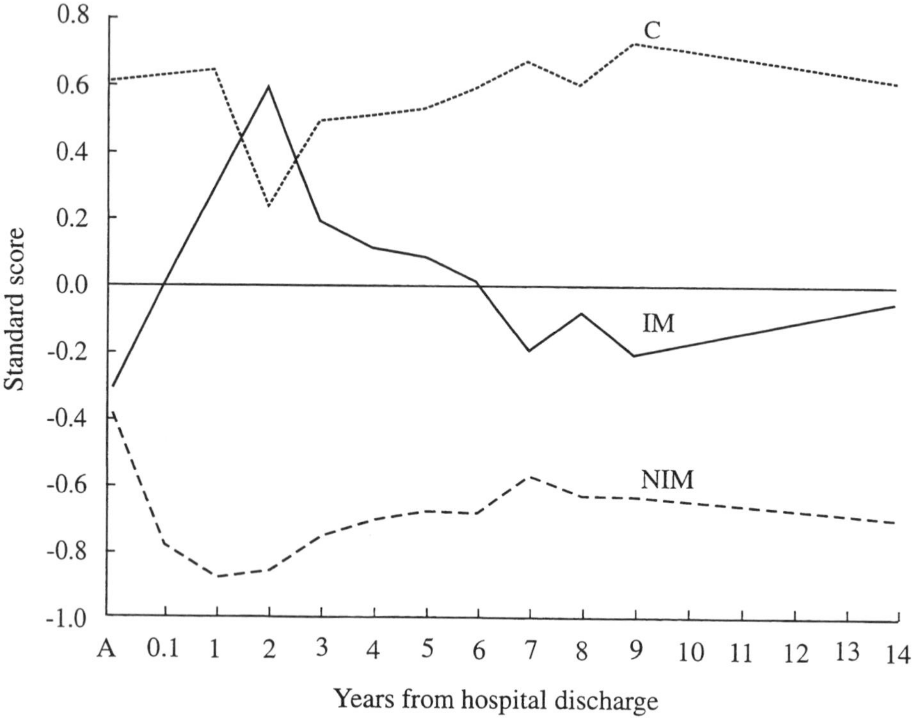

Source: Grantham-McGregor and others 1994.

groups were formed: malnourished (below the 3rd percentile), moderately malnourished (3rd through the 24th percentile), and well nourished (at or above the 25th percentile). Both height and weight had to agree in classification for the children to be considered.

The first study included children who were adopted before the age of 2 years, and the second study focused on children adopted between 2 and 5 years of age. All of the children were tested at school age (grades 1-8) several years after adoption. The results, shown in figure 2, indicate that adopted children performed better as a group than the general U.S. population on standardized tests of intelligence. This finding shows that severe growth failure in early childhood, indicated by height and weight data, did not necessarily lead to irreversible low performance. In both studies, performance was a function of former nutritional status; for example, the difference between malnourished and well-nourished girls, the extreme nutrition groups, was 10 IQ points in both studies. Performance also depended on the child's age at adoption; for example, children adopted at younger ages performed 6 IQ points better than children adopted at ages 2-5 years. Overall, these two studies suggest that (a) adoption leads to performance improvements, despite severe growth failure; (b) early malnutrition has an important residual effect on performance; and (c) the earlier adoption occurs, the better the results will be.

Figure 2. School-age IQ of Adopted Korean Children

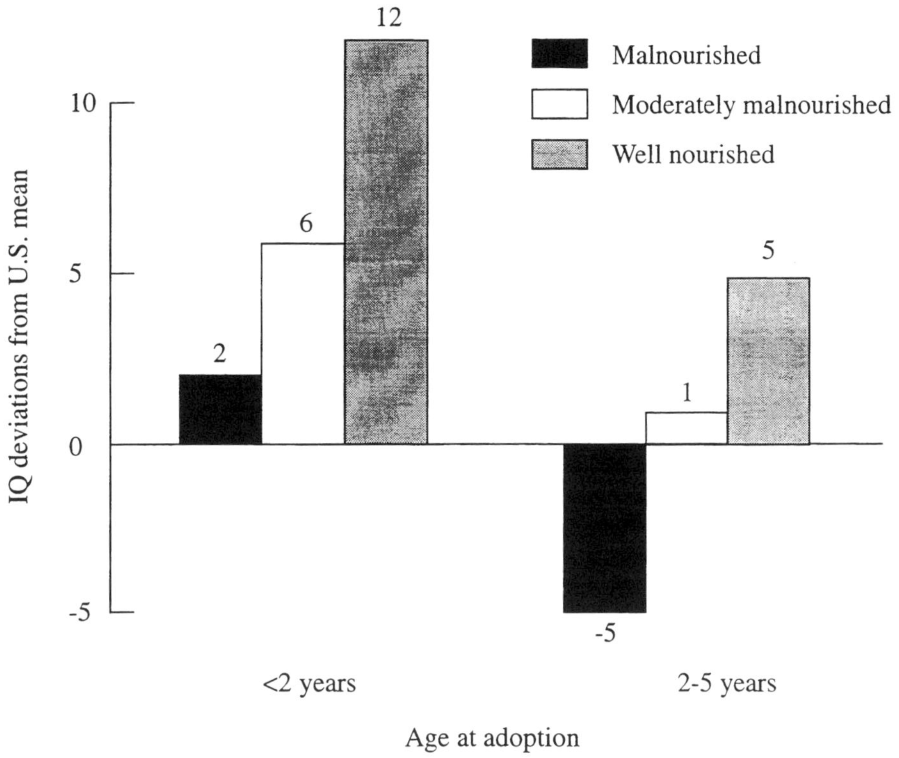

Source: Winick, Meyer, and Harris 1975; My Lien, Meyer, and Winick 1977.

A small study in Chile confirms that adoption leads to substantial gains in performance for children who were severely malnourished at an early age (Colombo, de la Parra, and López 1992). At 8-9 years of age, previously malnourished children who were adopted, mostly by middle-class families, had an IQ of 97 compared to values of 81 in children who remained institutionalized and 83 in children who were returned to their biological families. Differences were consistent across WISC subscales. Years earlier, the developmental quotient had been similar across groups at admission and discharge from a nutritional recuperation center.

Undernutrition in Industrial Countries

Does undernutrition in industrial countries lead to poor development? Many persons expect favorable settings, particularly the absence of abject poverty, to ameliorate the effects of undernutrition on intellectual development. One approach to this issue is studying the effects of potential causes of undernutrition, such as famine and disease, in industrial countries.

Stein and colleagues (1972) examined results of the famine during the "hongerwinter" of 1944-45 in the Netherlands. As a result of a transport embargo by the Nazis and a severe winter that froze the barges in the canals, very little food reached the cities of western Holland. From December 1944 to May 1945, the average ration provided only around 700 calories a day, nearly one-half of what was previously provided. Using data collected at about age 19 by the army, Stein and colleagues (1972) examined the frequency of mental retardation and intellectual ability (Raven's Progressive Matrices) among 125,000 males born in selected famine and control cities. They found no relationship between exposure to the famine and these outcomes.

However, the data show that the famine did reduce birthweights at one point by as much as 250 grams. Mean birthweights were about 3,000 grams, the current average birthweight in many developing countries. The literature on low birthweight (LBW) and development in industrialized nations suggests a small, but lingering, effect on intellectual ability and performance (see below), but this would have been detected only in the portion of males studied with LBW. If an effect were present, it may have been obscured by comparing the entire exposed and control cohorts.

Perhaps there was no effect at all. The famine may not have affected development of the males studied because the mothers most likely were not malnourished before acute exposure to famine. Most were taller and heavier than women from poorer areas of developing countries. Also, micronutrient reserves may have been adequate in many women before the famine, and these levels may not have been depleted enough to cause severe deficiency. Under these circumstances, the fetus may have been protected from an extreme, acute famine better than is generally the case during famine in developing countries. Finally, parental behavior toward the Dutch children, many living outside the culture of poverty, may have been a buffer against the effects of undernutrition.

Other studies in industrial countries address the effects of disease on mental development in children from middle-class families. A number of diseases cause PEM in children, including congenital heart disease, inflammatory bowel disease, cystic fibrosis, and chronic liver disease (Fuchs 1990), and these conditions occur independently of socioeconomic status (SES).

One condition, cystic fibrosis, generally is associated with exocrine pancreatic insufficiency and malabsorption as well as with chronic, obstructive lung disease (Fuchs 1990). In the past, problems with malabsorption of fat were compounded by efforts to restrict fat consumption in patients (Ramsey and others 1992). Dietary energy consumption is quite low because many patients have reduced appetites (Ramsey and others 1992).

To determine some effects of the condition, an assessment of thirty-six children with cystic fibrosis at 7-10 years of age was carried out in Toronto (Ellis and Hill 1975). The group was subdivided into children who reached 80 percent or less of the normal weight for age before 12 months of age (n=22; malnourished) and those who did not (n=16; control group). However, data show that most of the children in the control group weighed near the 3rd percentile in infancy. Children in the control group, then, experienced growth retardation as well, although not as severely as the malnourished children.

At later ages, children in both the malnourished and control groups had normal weights and heights, indicating that nutritional conditions improved dramatically after infancy. Only one statistically significant difference was found between the two groups in twelve comparisons using the WISC and the WRAT. However, the differences were systematic and always favored the control group. For the full-scale IQ of the WISC, the values were 104.1 for the control group and 99.3 for the malnourished group, but the differences were not statistically significant. Although not included in the study, a comparison group of nonhospitalized, noncystic fibrosis children of similar SES would have enabled better interpretation of these results; IQ may have been depressed in the malnourished and control groups of children studied.

Pyloric stenosis, another congenital anomaly unrelated to SES, involves a period of brief starvation in early infancy (usually 0-3 months of age) and is easily corrected (Klein and others 1975). A study and follow-up were done to determine the effects of pyloric stenosis. A group of fifty subjects, 5-14 years of age, who had been treated for pyloric stenosis in infancy were compared to a control group of fifty subjects matched for age, sex, and father's level of education as well as to forty-four siblings, 5-15 years old, and a variety of tests were administered (PPVT, WISC, Raven's, and achievement tests in reading and arithmetic) (Klein and others 1975). No differences were found between siblings and subjects in the control group on any of the tests.

At follow-up, body size was evaluated. The index group was divided into three categories depending on the degree of weight-for-age deficit in early infancy: low (0 to 10 percent), moderate (11 to 20 percent), and high (greater than 21 percent). No differences were found in body size between any of these index groups or with respect to siblings or the control group, indicating that the growth failure resulting from a brief episode of starvation in early infancy was completely made up.

However, all tests and comparisons showed that greater degrees of weight-for-age deficit in infancy were related to poorer performance. Comparisons of the index group to the control group revealed consistent and statistically significant differences, particularly for index groups with high and moderate degrees of growth deficit. The authors concluded that "our data . . . reveal that even a brief period of severe starvation in early infancy, uncontaminated by socioeconomic conditions, has a long lasting effect on learning abilities and general adjustment as measured at 5 to 14 years of age" (Klein and others 1975: 12). General adjustment refers to findings indicating a relationship between weight deficit and parental evaluation of the subjects' intellectual development and educational potential.

Besides studying the effects of potential causes of malnutrition, another approach to understanding the developmental effects of malnutrition in industrial countries is examining the performance of children who fail to thrive. A study by Skuse and others (1994) compared forty-seven children with serious faltering in growth, but otherwise healthy, with forty-seven children in a control group matched by sex, age, ethnic origin, birthweight, birth order, and SES from a cohort of about 1,500 potential subjects. All children had been full-term singletons. Growth failure was defined as a weight-for-age Z score of −1.88 or less before 12 months of age and sustained for 3 months or more.

According to results of the study, the growth trajectory of infants 0-15 months with serious faltering in growth mirrors the growth trajectory usually seen in developing countries. At 15 months, the Z score for weight for age was −2.07 in the cases and 0.10 in the controls. Statistically significant differences between the two groups were found for the mental (98.2±19 for the cases and 108.5±14.4 for the controls) and motor components (96.7±17.3 and 103.6 respectively) of the Bayley Scales. Psychosocial variables, including cognitive stimulation received at home, did not modify the findings, indicating that growth failure and cognitive stimulation contribute independently to mental development.

Although this study matched cases and controls and adjusted for confounding, it showed no adequate explanation for why children in the case group failed to grow. The pattern of growth failure among these families from the inner city, who were ethnically diverse and generally poor, matched the pattern for developing countries. This type of setting may explain why growth failure had such a strong effect on development. However, because of the unclear etiology of failure to thrive in industrial countries, the value of this approach to studying the developmental effects of undernutrition is uncertain.

These studies of undernutrition in industrial countries indicate a tendency for events in infancy to be reflected in poorer performance years later. Although the Dutch famine suggests this may not be the case for prenatal undernutrition, considerably more information from studies of LBW and development in industrialized countries suggests otherwise (see below).

LBW

An estimated 19 percent of newborns in developing countries have LBW, defined as less than 2.5 kilograms, compared with only 6 percent of newborns in industrial countries (UNICEF 1993). Estimates of LBW vary greatly by region: Latin America and the Caribbean, 11 percent; East Asia and the Pacific, 11 percent; Sub-Saharan Africa, 16 percent; and South Asia, including India, Bangladesh, Nepal, and Pakistan, 34 percent. According to Villar and Belizán (1982), 55 percent of newborns with LBW in industrial countries are born prematurely at less than 37 weeks of gestation (overall rate of prematurity, 3.3 percent). Only about 25 percent of newborns with LBW in developing countries are premature (overall rate of prematurity, 6.7 percent), but developing countries have a greater number of full-term, small-for-date infants than industrial countries (17.0 and 2.6 percent respectively), indicating a larger prevalence of LBW overall.

In the studies reviewed below, full-term (greater than or equal to 37 weeks gestation), small-for-date infants are referred to as intrauterine growth-retarded (IUGR) newborns. The literature defines growth retardation in many ways: less than 2,500 grams, less than the 3rd or 10th percentile of the birthweight distribution, and more than 2 standard deviations below the mean. Most studies compare LBW newborns to term infants without growth retardation, who are referred to below as controls without specifying the exact criterion used in defining growth adequacy.

Prematurity and Mental Development

Premature infants in poor areas of developing countries often die. However, babies in industrialized nations who weigh as little as 500 grams often survive. Although an infant weighing 280 grams at birth after 26 weeks of gestation was reported to be developmentally normal at 2 years of age (Muraskas and others 1992), many survivors exhibit a range of serious problems. A meta-analysis of 111 studies focused on morbidity outcomes of very-low-birthweight infants (VLBW) weighing less than 1,500 grams. Analysis showed that the median incidence of cerebral palsy among VLBW infants was 7.7 percent and the median incidence of disability was 25 percent (Escobar, Littenberg, and Petitti 1991). Despite substantial improvements in the mortality of VLBW infants, poor outcomes are common among survivors. This observation raises important ethical questions. How small is too small to save and at what cost to newborns, families, and society?

Prematurity is related to learning impairment as well as physical disability, as shown by a meta-analysis of development in LBW infants that included eighty studies and more than 4,000 infants from North America, Europe, Australia, and New Zealand (Aylward and others 1989). Because these are industrialized countries, it is assumed that more infants were premature than IUGR. At follow-up from 1 to more than 10 years after birth, the average IQ or developmental quotient was 97.8 for LBW infants compared with 103.8 for infants in control cases. The difference of 6 IQ points represents about 0.4 of a standard deviation. When follow-up occurred 2 or more years after birth, differences were slightly larger, from 7 to 8 IQ points. Differences in IQ were small, but IQ is too gross a measure; substantial evidence exists for more subtle dysfunctions that indicate learning disabilities in LBW babies.

Recent studies continue to indicate that cognitive development is impaired in premature, LBW infants who survive (Saigal and others 1991; Stjernqvist and Svenningsen 1995; Smedler and others 1992; Hack and others 1994; Hille and others 1994).

Not much is known about the causes of prematurity. Low pregnancy weight is a causal factor, but little evidence otherwise suggests that poor maternal nutrition is a major cause of prematurity (Kramer 1987). For this reason, studies of prematurity and child development may not show the importance of nutrition for cognition and behavior.

IUGR and Mental Development in Industrial Countries

The etiology of IUGR is better defined than that of prematurity, and poor maternal nutrition, before and during pregnancy, is a predominant causal factor (Kramer 1987). A number of studies from industrialized countries report developmental outcomes in IUGR newborns, the common type of LBW in developing countries and the type more likely to survive. Table 1 shows key data from studies of births after 1960 with follow-up 6 or more years later reporting IQ and minor neurological problems. These and other relevant studies are reviewed below.

The effect of IUGR on intelligence varies by social class according to the Edinburgh prospective study of 600 infants born during 1953-55 and followed to secondary school age (Drillien 1970). In the middle and upper classes, the mean IQ of IUGR newborns was 110.9, similar to that of controls. In poor classes, the mean IQ was 93.4 for IUGR cases and 102.1 for controls, an IQ difference of 8.7.

An English study of 139 IUGR subjects and 183 controls partially supported these findings (Neligan and others 1976). A difference of 11.2 IQ points in the WISC at 6 years of age was found between IUGR cases and controls at the top of the social scale (classes I and II, 9 percent of the population). In the middle class (class III, 60 percent of the population), the corresponding difference was 3.3 points, and for the lower classes (classes IV and V, 30 percent of the population), the difference was 12.7 points. Comparing middle to lower classes indicates that poverty magnifies the effects of IUGR on intelligence. The difference between IUGR and control newborns in the upper classes (11.2 points) is puzzling; the estimate may be unstable because sample sizes were smaller in this group (thirteen IUGR and sixteen controls) than in the other classes.

Table 1. Follow-up Studies of IUGR and Controls

Authors	Birth	Number		Mean birthweight (g or %)		Mean gestational age (wk)		Follow-up (yr)	Minor neurological problems (%)$^{+}$		IQ and developmental quotients^{+}	
		IUGR	C	IUGR	C	IUGR	C		IUGR	C	IUGR	C
Neligan et al. 1976	1960-62	141	187	2,537	3,508	40.1	40.1	7	–	–	92.7	99.1
Hill et al. 1984	1964-65	33	13	–	–	>37	>37	12-14	9.0	0	104	121
Rubin, Rosenblatt, & Balow 1973	1960-64	46	85	≤2,500	>2,500	>37	>37	7	–	–	97.5	103.3
Fitzhardinge & Steven 1972	1960-66	96	60	2,144	>3%	40.0	≥38	5.6	25	1.7	95/101	106/102
Westwood et al. 1983	1960-64	33	33	2,188	25-75%	40.0	38-42	13-19	–	–	103.6	108.7
Low et al. 1982	early 1970s	76	88	2,302	3,485	39.1	40.3	6	23.0	17	106/105	103/106
Ounsted, Moar, & Scott 1984[a]	1970-74	138	138	2,180	3,380	≥33	≥33	7	6.5	7.2	36.8/39.2	38.2/41.6
Walther 1988	1976-77	24	24	2,372	3,433	39.5	39.7	7	50	4.2	–	–
Hadders-Algra et al. 1988	1977-78	166	206	2,706	>10%	>37	>37	6	24	15	–	–
Paz et al. 1995	1970-71	64	1,643	<3%		>37	>37	17	10/8.8^{+}	6.8/4.7^{+}	103.1/100.3	105.8/104.7

$^{+}$ Values for male and female respectively.
[a] This study included cases 33 weeks or greater in gestational age; most cases were IUGR.
— Not available.

Source: Teberg, Walther, and Peña 1988.

The effects of IUGR on neurological and intellectual characteristics were assessed in a prospective study from Montreal, Canada (Fitzhardinge and Steven 1972). The study compared ninety-six IUGR cases and sixty sibling controls in children up to 8 years old (table 1). The families were a cross-section of society, representing upper, middle, and lower class professions. Major neurological defects were uncommon, but evidence of minimal cerebral dysfunction was present in 25 percent of IUGR cases and only one individual in the control group. Speech defects were present in about one-third of IUGR cases, compared with about 6 percent occurrence in sibling controls and a population incidence of 1.5 percent. IQ for IUGR cases was within the normal range (95 for boys and 101 for girls), slightly less than in sibling controls (106 for boys and 102 for girls). However, IUGR children showed a higher incidence of poor school performance and failure; 50 percent of the boys and 36 percent of the girls were doing poorly compared to 5 percent of the sibling controls.

Westwood and others (1983) later studied thirty-three of these IUGR cases at ages 13-19 years, excluding cases with a history of asphyxia at birth. The IUGR cases were compared to thirty-three controls matched by sex, ethnicity, and SES. Small but consistent differences in the WISC favored the control children (108.7 compared with 103.6, p=0.050) as did differences in the WRAT (reading 105.9 in contrast to 99.7, p=0.062; spelling 99.0 and 94.5, p=0.098; and arithmetic 94.2 and 87.8, p=0.011). Cases with a history of asphyxia included in the study by Fitzhardinge and Steven (1972) had an IQ of 87.1 (n=11), suggesting that inclusion of these cases in the earlier study inflated the importance of IUGR.

A Minnesota study compared the effects of IUGR and prematurity on mental development (Rubin, Rosenblatt, and Balow 1973). Table 1 shows data for IUGR and control groups. IQ differences (among preterm, IUGR, and control groups) in WISC at 7 years were small (97.0, 97.5, and 103.3 respectively). However, school performance differed significantly. Out of twenty-nine preterm newborns, 17.2 percent had to repeat a grade, compared with 32.5 percent in the IUGR group (n=40) and 11.5 percent in the control group (n=78). Differences also existed in the percentage of infants who were later in special classes (6.8, 10.0, and 2.5 percent respectively).

A Dutch study also examined IUGR and prematurity. A greater incidence of neurological abnormalities was found in IUGR infants, preterm infants small for their gestational age, and preterm infants adequate for their gestational age than in controls as assessed at 6 years of age (Hadders-Algra, Huisjes, and Touwen 1988). No striking behavioral differences were found between the three LBW groups and the control group, but clumsiness was reported more often by parents and teachers of the LBW groups. Neither of the full-term groups (IUGR and controls) had children who attended a school for special learning disorders. Ratings for motor skills and cognitive development were significantly lower in the preterm groups than the full-term groups, but the full-term groups had similar ratings to each other. Ratings of social and emotional skills were similar in all groups.

Walther and Ramaekers (1982) examined the effects of IUGR on language development by comparing twenty-five IUGR children to twenty-five controls matched by age, birth rank, and social class at 3 years of age. Language development was delayed significantly in the IUGR group. Differences were found in verbal comprehension and in expressive language, particularly vocabulary. Using standard deviations of the raw scores of the control group, the effect sizes were 0.6 for both aspects of language development.

To find further developmental effects of IUGR, Walther (1988) followed twenty-four IUGR and twenty-four control children to age 7 (table 1). Twelve IUGR children and one control child had minor neurological problems. Teachers reported more behavior problems in the IUGR group than among controls, and hyperactivity, poor concentration, and clumsiness were more common in the IUGR group. Nine children in the IUGR group, in contrast to none from the control group, had behavioral scores greater than 7, which indicates serious problems.

Ounsted, Moar, and Scott (1984) also studied 138 IUGR and 138 control infants at 7 years of age (table 1). Out of these, five IUGR infants and two controls had major congenital abnormalities. However, the frequency of gross and fine motor coordination was similar (6.5 and 7.2 respectively). The groups showed no differences in the incidence of hearing, sight, and speech defects. Developmental scores were 36.8 and 39.2 for IUGR boys and girls respectively; the corresponding values in the control cases were only slightly greater, 38.2 and 41.6. Effect sizes were approximately 0.2 and 0.3 respectively for boys and girls.

According to studies that used ultrasound measurements to identify slow growth in biparietal diameter, effects of IUGR on development and school performance vary depending on the timing of intrauterine growth retardation (Parkinson, Wallis, and Harvey 1981; Harvey and others 1982; Parkinson and others 1986). In one study, teachers in London evaluated the school achievement and behavior at ages 5-9 of forty-five children who had been IUGR and nineteen control children (Parkinson, Wallis, and Harvey 1981). Overall achievement was greater for controls than for IUGR subjects; there was a clear gradient among the latter, depending on the timing of slow growth: at or below 26 weeks of gestation, between 27 and 34 weeks, after 35 weeks, or no slowing at all. Earlier growth failure was associated with lower scores in reading, writing, drawing, creative activities, imaginative activities, and reasoning ability. Earlier growth failure also was associated with behavior problems in boys; they were more clumsy, worried, fidgety, unhappy, and upset by new situations than boys experiencing later or no growth failure.

Another study from the same group compared fifty-one IUGR cases at 5 years of age with a control group; the IUGR group was further subdivided into growth failure before or after 26 weeks gestation (Harvey and others 1982). Early growth failure was associated with poorer performance on the McCarthy Scales of children's abilities (that is, in general cognitive index, perceptual-performance, and motor scales).

Parkinson and others (1986) compared the behavior patterns at age 7.7 of twenty-one IUGR infants whose growth failure began at or below 34 weeks with twenty-one controls matched for sex, social class, age, birth order, and race. Five sessions were held, and a child's behavior in different situations, with and without the mother, was videotaped and analyzed. The IUGR children were quieter, more compliant, and less active than the control group children, and their play behavior suggested that they were less advanced developmentally (Parkinson and others 1986).

Although the studies of these two groups of children suggest a timing effect, birthweight confounds the relationships. For example, in the IUGR infants with evidence of growth failure before 26 weeks, the mean birthweight was 1.8 kilograms compared with 2.4 kilograms for the IUGR infants without such evidence (Harvey and others 1982).

Table 1 gives details of a prospective follow-up study from Ontario, Canada, of seventy-six IUGR children and eighty-eight controls by Low and others (1982). They found no differences between IUGR and controls in motor and cognitive development or in school performance.

A different study was carried out later in Ontario, Canada, but it was a more general study of high-risk newborns (Low and others 1992). In this study, fetal growth retardation and the father's occupation were independently associated with learning deficits in reading, spelling, or mathematics for 218 high-risk newborns who were assessed at ages 9-11. The sample of high-risk newborns included seventy-seven infants small for their gestational age. Of these, thirty-nine were IUGR and thirty-eight were preterm. Because the incidence of learning deficits was 46 and 50 percent respectively, gestational age did not seem to confer risk beyond that carried by fetal growth retardation.

Although the study did not include controls from the school, the criteria used for defining learning deficits suggest that their incidence was several times greater in the IUGR group than in the general population. The study defined a major learning deficit as having one or more achievement measures that scored more than 2 standard deviations lower than expected (less than the 3rd percentile). A minor deficit was two or three achievement measures that scored between 1 and 2 standard deviations lower than expected (less than the 15th percentile).

A Finnish study compared 3,375 control children at 2 years of age with 488 IUGR cases (Tenovuo and others 1988). The sample was composed of infants small for their gestational age, but 94 percent of the cases were IUGR. IUGR infants had a greater frequency of developmental delays than controls. Also, abnormalities among IUGR cases were more frequent than in controls (3.1 and 0.08 percent respectively; p=<0.001), and statistically significant differences occurred in walking, manual performance, and comprehension.

Finally, neonatal data of 1,758 infants were matched to medical and intelligence assessments performed at 17 years of age by the Israeli army (Paz and others 1995), and children with IUGR were compared to controls. Controls had IQ scores significantly greater than IUGR cases, but the differences were small (108.9 and 104.8 for control and IUGR males and 107.6 and 102.5 for control and IUGR females). Adjustment for confounding attenuated the differences (105.8 and 103.1 in males and 104.7 and 100.3 in females), and differences ceased to be significant in males. A higher proportion of male IUGR cases than controls had low academic achievements (that is, less than 12 years of schooling or attendance at a vocational school); after controlling for possible confounders, the adjusted odds ratio for low academic achievement for IUGR males was 2.40 (95 percent confidence interval 1.07-5.39; p<0.03).

As table 1 shows, IUGR cases consistently tend to have more frequent neurological problems and lower IQ than controls. The order of magnitude of the differences appears the same as that found in a meta-analysis of the effects of prematurity—6 IQ points (Aylward and others 1989; see above). Some of the older studies discussed above identified a magnified significance of IUGR in environments of poverty, suggesting that IUGR in developing countries should have a more marked effect on behavioral outcomes than it does in industrial countries.

IUGR and Development in Developing Countries

Most studies of IUGR in developing countries, such as those done by the Institute of Nutrition of Central America and Panama (INCAP), involve young children. Lasky and others (1975) studied the relationship between birthweight and the Brazelton Assessment Scale at 2 weeks and the Composite Infant Scale (CIS) at 6 months in four Guatemalan villages. Birthweight was strongly related to three components of the Brazelton scale (motor fitness, tremors and startles, and habituation) and less strongly related to alertness. The CIS, consisting of ninety-one items drawn from four widely used scales, assessed psychomotor development in infancy and found a relationship between birthweight and the motor subscale. Controlling for confounding factors did not modify the relationship.

In another study, Villar and others (1984) assessed development at 3 years in three groups of children from the same four Guatemalan villages studied by Lasky and others (1975). The three groups of children included those with normal birthweight (controls), IUGR cases with low ponderal index (LPI), and IUGR cases with adequate ponderal index (API). In a manner similar to the three ultrasound studies described earlier, the ponderal index may distinguish IUGR cases with late fetal malnutrition (LPI) from IUGR cases with early and chronic fetal malnutrition (API). Because weight gain of the fetus is rapid at the later stages of pregnancy relative to growth in length, IUGR-LPI infants may represent acute undernutrition in late pregnancy. The IUGR-API infants, small but proportionate, may represent chronic undernutrition throughout the entire pregnancy. It should be noted that Kramer and others (1990) believe that disproportionality represents (as a proxy) severe IUGR and that it carries little or no risk above and beyond risk associated with the degree of IUGR. This view is based on studies in industrial countries and the conclusion may not hold for developing countries, where a different mix of IUGR predominates. For example, in developing countries, IUGR-API predominates in 67 to 79 percent of IUGR cases; in industrial countries, IUGR-LPI predominates in 60 to 80 percent of IUGR cases (Villar and others 1986).

Results evaluated at birth showed that the birthweight of the two IUGR groups were similar to each other, but the length and head circumference of the IUGR-API children were smaller. For these two variables, the IUGR-LPI cases had values similar to controls. The IUGR-LPI infants recuperated from their thinness within the first few months, but the IUGR-API infants remained lighter and shorter and had smaller head circumferences than infants in the other two groups. At 3 years of age, the IUGR-API children performed the lowest of children in the three groups on seven of eight developmental measures and on the CIS, and IUGR-LPI children had intermediate values. The adjusted mean values of the cognitive composite score at 3 years of age, similar to an overall IQ, were 63 for controls, 48 for the IUGR-LPI group, and 38 for the IUGR-API group. Values were adjusted for SES and other confounding variables.

Using the same Guatemalan population and incorporating growth in infancy as an additional factor, Gorman and Pollitt (1992) focused on performance at 3, 4, and 5 years. The effects of IUGR on behavior were found to interact with other characteristics. Growth in infancy and SES were related to performance among IUGR cases but not among controls. In other words, postnatal growth retardation and SES influenced behavioral performance only in the presence of IUGR. Pollitt, Gorman, and Metallinos-Katsaras (1991) extended this analysis to adolescence and found that growth during infancy, rather than birthweight, was related to performance on cognitive and achievement tests. Low statistical power may explain the waning explanatory power of IUGR at adolescence.

There are fewer studies of effects of IUGR on cognition and behavior in developing countries than in industrial countries. Yet, IUGR is more common in developing countries than in industrial countries, and these newborns, if they survive, are more likely to grow in poverty, a condition that probably magnifies the effects of IUGR on mental development. Also, development of infants in the proportionate IUGR-API, the predominant type of IUGR in developing countries, is more affected than development in the disproportionate IUGR-LPI. For these reasons, the more numerous studies from industrialized countries probably underestimate the deleterious effect of IUGR on mental development in developing countries.

Correlational Studies

The literature is full of studies on the association between anthropometric indicators of growth failure and development, but interpretation can create problems. In many studies, anthropometry is equated loosely with mild-to-moderate malnutrition, and many researchers interpret correlations between anthropometry and cognitive tests and school performance to mean that less severe forms of malnutrition also affect development. As discussed earlier, anthropometry in older children may measure malnutrition, but it measures the malnutrition that occurred at younger ages when there was active growth failure.

Another difficulty arises from correlating anthropometry with cognitive and behavioral development. The correlation may be spurious because poverty and associated factors also result in poor growth and poor development. Some researchers deal with this problem by controlling for SES. The well-known article, *Is Big Smart? The Relation of Growth to Cognition*, by Klein and others (1972) is an example. Even after controlling for SES, the authors showed an independent association between growth indicators and psychological performance.

A recent review of the literature reports that "many studies show that even when predictors such as socioeconomic status, family education level, literacy or duration of schooling are covaried out, indexes of suboptimal nutrition still contribute unique predictive variance" (Wachs 1995: 2249S). Indices of suboptimal nutrition mean anthropometric indicators such as height, weight, and head circumference (Wachs 1995). Wachs (1995) also reports that studying the interaction of growth with psychosocial-contextual factors results in the strongest predictions of developmental outcome.

Examining the correlation between early growth failure and intellectual development, the INCAP follow-up study reported on the performance of adults who experienced varying degrees of growth failure at 3 years (Martorell and others 1992). After controlling for family SES and maternal education, greater levels of slow growth in early childhood were associated with poorer school achievement and poorer performance on tests of intelligence, numeracy, knowledge, and literacy. For example, males whose growth was severely stunted at 3 years of age (more than 3 standard deviations below the reference mean) had 4.4 years of schooling; those whose growth was moderately stunted (between 2 and 3 standard deviations below the reference mean) had 5.8 years of schooling; and those without stunted growth (2 standard deviations or less below the reference mean) had 6.2 years of schooling. The corresponding values for females were 4.2, 5.2, and 5.2 years of schooling respectively.

Food Supplementation and Stimulation Trials

Investigators also have considered the effects of food supplementation on cognitive and behavioral development. Some studies emphasize understanding the combined effects of food supplementation and psychosocial stimulation (referred to herein as "stimulation") in promoting cognitive development. In particularly interesting studies from developing countries, investigators assess interactions between various combinations of supplementation and stimulation. The only studies available from industrial countries focus on stimulation in poor or high-risk children.

Studies from Industrial Countries

Researchers in industrial countries have studied the effects of early intervention on cognitive and behavioral development. Studies focus on different types of stimulation and different ages of high-risk children, from premature infants to school age. One type of intervention studied was the Head Start program, a comprehensive, U.S. federal program for preschool children and families living in poverty. During fiscal 1993, Head Start served an estimated 721,000 children and their families nationwide (Zigler, Piotrkowski, and Collins 1994). The program has four components: education, social services, parental involvement, and health. It focuses on preparing children 4 years old to enter kindergarten at age 5.

The conclusion from numerous evaluations of Head Start is that the program "has been highly successful in improving the physical well-being and school readiness of poor children" (Zigler 1995: 304). Although the difficulties of evaluating a service program, such as identifying an appropriate control group, make this conclusion controversial, a review of thirty-six U.S. studies that included large-scale public programs such as Head Start and smaller demonstration projects led to a similar conclusion: "Results indicate that early childhood programs can produce large short-term benefits for children on intelligence quotient (IQ) and sizable long-term effects on school achievement, grade retention, placement in special education, and social adjustment. Not all programs produce these benefits, perhaps because of differences in quality and funding across programs" (Barnett 1995: 25).

A few examples of controlled trials not included in the review by Barnett (1995) are discussed below along with a discussion of the Abecedarian Project, one of the model demonstration projects featured in Barnett's review (1995).

A well-designed study tested the effect on cognitive development of an early intervention program aimed at premature infants (less than 37 weeks gestation, less than 2,500 grams). The clinical trial conducted at eight sites studied 985 infants stratified by site and weight (less than or equal to 2,000 grams or 2,001-2,500 grams). Infants were assigned randomly to receive an educational curriculum focused on child development and family support activities in addition to pediatric follow-up or only pediatric follow-up. The program began in the neonatal nursery and continued until 36 months of age.

The educational curriculum in the early intervention program consisted of home visits, child attendance at a child development center, and parental attendance at group meetings. Home visits were weekly during the first year and biweekly thereafter. Home visitors provided health and developmental information and family support via two curricula. One emphasized cognitive, linguistic, and social development through a program of games and activities for the parent to use with the child, and the second helped parents manage self-identified problems. From 12 to 36 months, children attended a development center 5 days a week where the same home curricula were used by the teachers. At 12 months, information on childrearing, health, safety, and other parental concerns was provided along with social support at bimonthly group meetings for parents.

Table 2 shows the results of this intervention, determined by evaluating the children's performance on the Stanford-Binet Test at 3 years of age. Nonintervened controls performed about 15 IQ points below normal, representing the typical performance of children from disadvantaged families who survive LBW. The educational intervention had a marked effect that varied by birthweight. In the heavier group, the effect of 13.2 IQ points was twice the 6.6 effect found in the lightest group. A follow-up study in progress will assess maintenance of these gains. Other reports also suggest that this type of intervention benefits development in LBW babies (Achenbach and others 1993; Barrera, Cunningham, and Rosenbaum 1986).

Table 2. Performance on the Stanford-Binet

	Pediatric follow-up			Early intervention			Effect size
Birthweight group (g)	n	$\bar{x}$	S.D.	n	$\bar{x}$	S.D.	(*p*)
2,001-2,500 g	203	84.8	19.0	125	98.0	18.5	0.83 (<0.001)
≤2,000	358	84.4	20.5	222	91.0	19.0	0.41 (<0.001)

Source: The Infant Health and Development Program 1990.

In a randomized clinical trial, Black and others (1995) assessed whether a home intervention program could boost cognitive development in children with inorganic failure-to-thrive. The subjects were children younger than 25 months weighing less than the 5th percentile for their age at recruitment. For the most part, they were being raised by single, Black mothers. The 1-year trial included a group that received clinical services and a weekly home intervention (n=64) and a control group that received clinical services only (n=66). The groups were subdivided into children younger than 12 months at recruitment and older children. Home interventions were conducted by three part-time, trained lay home visitors supervised by a community health nurse. Efforts were made to provide social support and parenting advice as well as to increase mother-child interaction and play. The home visitors carried portable mats and toys to demonstrate activities, and frequently they made toys with the mothers from household items.

The outcomes were measured on the Bayley and Receptive/Expressive Emergence Language scales. Growth improved regardless of intervention status. Cognitive development declined in all groups by an average of 11 IQ points. However, the decline was least in the intervention group younger than 12 months at recruitment. Both younger and older intervention children declined less than controls in receptive language. No effects were found on motor development. These findings support "a cautious optimism regarding home intervention during the first year of life provided by trained lay home visitors" (Black and others 1995: 807).

The Abecedarian Project indicates substantial, long-term improvements in intellectual and academic achievement from early intervention (Campbell and Ramey 1994). Subjects for the project were infants recruited from low-income families and assigned randomly to an intervention of experimental preschool or to a control group of those entering school without preschool. Within each group, subjects were randomized to a school-age intervention program before entering school, generating four groups; children with 8 years of intervention (5 from preschool and 3 in school); children who received intervention only from preschool; children with school-age intervention but no preschool; and children with no intervention. Mean age at entry to the preschool program was 4.4 years; the curriculum was delivered at a day-care center for 8 hours a day, 5 days a week, 50 weeks a year. The curriculum was designed to enhance cognition, language, perceptual-motor development, and social development; later in the preschool years, emphasis was placed on language development and preliteracy skills. The school-age intervention was designed to increase family support for the child's learning by having a home school resource teacher provide individualized sets of educational activities to supplement treated children.

About twenty-one to twenty-five cases from each group were available for follow-up at 12 years of age. Follow-up was conducted 4 years after the school-age intervention ended, in part, to investigate whether effects persisted. Although the school-age intervention was not very effective, the preschool intervention resulted in gains in IQ and achievement scores. The groups receiving preschool education (n=47) had an IQ of 93.7 compared with 88.4 for the groups without preschool education (n=43), a difference of 5.3 points (significant at $p<0.05$ in multivariate analysis of variance for repeated measures on tests taken from 6 months to 12 years). Differences in achievement scores (Woodcock-Johnson Psychoeducational Battery) were statistically significant between groups attending preschool and those not attending. Reading scores were 91.3 and 86.0 respectively; mathematics scores were 91.3 and 86.0; written language scores were 95.6 and 89.5; and knowledge scores were 93.0 and 85.3.

A similar project (Project CARE) in a disadvantaged population also showed benefits of the center-based early intervention program used by the Abecedarian Project (Ramey and Ramey 1994). In addition, it showed that home visits without center-based support did not affect the intellectual performance of children at 5 years.

These studies from industrial countries show the effectiveness of early intervention programs on the cognitive and behavioral development of high-risk infants. They also show the importance of a child's age at the beginning of the program. Zigler (1994) calls for adding a 0-3 year component to the existing U.S. Head Start program to make the program have an even greater effect on development.

Studies from Developing Countries

Although studies from industrial countries show the developmental effects of stimulation only, the studies discussed below from developing countries show the effects of stimulation, food supplements, and a combination of the two.

Stimulation Only. The Jamaican study by Grantham-McGregor and others (1990) discussed earlier showed the effects of a stimulation program on severely malnourished young children. Benefits from stimulation were observed up to 14 years after discharge from the hospital (figure 1).

A randomized trial at four centers in Latin America showed whether psychosocial support during pregnancy affected pregnancy outcomes (Villar and others 1992). Women at high risk for adverse outcomes were assigned randomly to an intervention group (n=1,115) receiving four to six home visits from a nurse or social worker in addition to routine prenatal care or to a control group (n=1,120) receiving only routine prenatal care (a mean of eight prenatal visits). The intervention focused on increasing social support and reducing stress and anxiety. The intervention did not affect incidence of LBW, prematurity, or maternal and neonatal morbidity.

A meta-analysis also was done of ten studies providing data on preterm delivery and eleven including LBW and type of delivery as outcomes. The combined odds ratios and 95 percent confidence intervals were 0.93 (0.82-1.05) for preterm delivery, 0.93 (0.81-1.07) for LBW, and 0.96 (0.86-1.07) for forceps delivery or caesarean section. Findings from studies on stimulation in developing countries suggest that psychosocial support to pregnant women does not improve pregnancy outcomes.

Food Supplementation Only. Several studies from developing countries show the effects of food supplementation on development. For example, a 90-day intervention providing a supplement of 400 kilocalories and 5 grams of protein twice a day improved weight and motor development in children 6-20 months of age in West Java, Indonesia (Husaini and others 1991). Pollitt, Watkins, and Husaini (forthcoming) did a follow-up 8 years later of these children and children who were 21-60 months old during the original controlled trial. The follow-up tested a variety of areas, including cognitive ability, emotionality, vocabulary, and arithmetic. When the sample receiving intervention was compared with controls, no differences were found. However, when the analysis was limited to subjects who were 18 months old or younger before treatment, children receiving supplements performed better than controls on the Sternberg Test of working memory. In this study, timing was important to achieve the specific effects of the intervention.

Data from the Bacon Chow study in Taiwan were analyzed by Joos and others (1983) using the Bayley Scale to assess effects of supplementation on performance at 8 months. During the study mothers were supplemented during pregnancy and lactation with a liquid preparation that provided 800 kilocalories and 40 grams of protein and with a daily vitamin and mineral tablet. They were randomly assigned to treatment and control groups. Differences were found in the motor but not the mental subscale.

In a meta-analysis of trials that included a nutrition intervention, Pollitt and Oh (1994) found beneficial effects of supplementation on motor development in infants 8-19 months old and on both motor and mental development in older children. Of the six studies analyzed by Pollitt and Oh (1994), five are described here: the West Java and Taiwan study discussed above, the Bogotá study (Waber and others 1981) and the Jamaica study (Grantham-McGregor and others 1991) discussed in the next section, and a series of INCAP studies in four Guatemalan villages (Engle and others 1992; Pollitt and others 1993) described below.

The INCAP studies have taken place in four villages located in the "Ladino," or Spanish-speaking, eastern part of Guatemala (Martorell, Habicht, and Rivera 1995). In 1968, two pair of villages were selected from among dozens; one pair of villages each had about 900 people and the other about 500 each. The villages were paired and selected on the basis of similarities in sociocultural, anthropometric, dietary, and morbidity characteristics.

A longitudinal supplementation trial between 1969 and 1977 randomly assigned one large and one small village to receive a nutritious supplement; the other two villages received a low-energy drink. All four villages received medical care from auxiliary nurses under the supervision of a physician. The nutritious supplement was a high-protein, high-energy gruel called Atole. It was made with Incaparina, a vegetable-protein mix developed by INCAP, dry skim milk, sugar, and flavoring. Atole was served hot in cups containing 180 milliliters, which provided 163 kilocalories and 11.5 grams of high-quality protein. The Atole was available at the feeding center twice daily, in midmorning and midafternoon, not interfering with meal times. Anyone in the village could participate, but consumption, including additional servings and leftovers, was recorded carefully only for women who were pregnant or breastfeeding and for children 7 years or younger.

To investigate the effect of protein supplementation on mental development, it was necessary to control for the socialization effects of attending a feeding center. This involved duplicating the setting in the control villages down to the fastidious measurement of consumption. Control villages received a low-energy drink called Fresco that looked and tasted somewhat like Kool Aid™. It had no protein but contained sugar; a cup provided 59 kilocalories, about one-third of the Atole energy density. To create a greater protein contrast, a number of vitamins and minerals were added to the Fresco in equal concentration to the Atole.

The investigators recorded the household structure, composition, and socioeconomic status for every family involved in the longitudinal study. Women were monitored during pregnancy, and data were collected on maternal characteristics and pregnancy outcomes, including birthweight. Data were collected periodically from children on a variety of aspects including growth and maturation, home diet consumption, frequency and duration of illness, and psychological development. Data on psychological development included an infant battery based on items from the Bayley, Gessell, Psyche Cattell, and Merrill-Palmer scales, adapted for the Guatemalan population. Also, a preschool battery consisting of twenty separate tests was administered to children at 3, 4, 5, 6, and 7 years of age (Engle and others 1992).

A follow-up of participants in the longitudinal study was conducted during 1988-89 (Martorell, Habicht, and Rivera 1995). The subjects of the follow-up study were longitudinal participants who had been 7 years old or younger at any point during the feeding experiment. Out of 2,169 such subjects, 1,574, or 74 percent, were examined at ages ranging from 11 to 27 years. Of those examined, 89 percent were nonmigrants (n=1,278), and 41 percent were migrants (n=296). Data collection included social, economic, and demographic information about subjects and their families as well as subjects' body size and composition, skeletal maturation, hand strength, work capacity, school attendance history, and intellectual performance.

Many publications address the effects of supplementation on preschool development in these INCAP studies. Reviews of the publications and new analyses reveal helpful information (Engle and others 1992; Pollitt and others 1993). Children receiving Atole prenatally and up to 24 months old had significantly higher scores on the motor scale at 24 months than children receiving Fresco; no interactions with treatment were detected. A factor analysis applied to the preschool battery generated two factors, general and memory (Pollitt and others 1993). After adjustment for sex, attendance, and SES, Atole subjects performed better in the general factor at 4 and 5 years of age; no differences were observed in the memory factor. Atole had a greater effect on low-SES subjects.

Effects of supplementation on physical growth also were found. Severe failure in growth (height 3 or more standard deviations below the reference median) among children 3 years of age declined in Atole villages (n=451), from 45 percent in 1969 to 20 percent during 1976-77 when the supplementation program ended. In Fresco villages (n=429), the prevalence of severe failure in growth remained about 45 percent throughout the period (Martorell and others 1992). Multivariate analyses demonstrate that only Atole exposure and intake in the first 3 years of life improved growth rates. Supplementation after 3 years did not affect growth (Schroeder and others 1995). A possible reason for the different effects by age is that growth fails only in the first 3 years of life. After 3 years, children receiving no previous supplement grow as well as children in the U.S. reference population. At follow-up, the gains in growth were maintained, although with some attenuation (Rivera and others 1995).

In further evaluation, Atole supplementation showed positive effects in adolescence and young adulthood on the results of psychoeducational tests of knowledge, numeracy, reading, and vocabulary (Pollitt and others 1993). Exposure to Atole also was associated with a faster reaction time for information processing tasks. One of the most interesting findings of this review was the strong interaction between supplementation and SES and education. Figure 3 shows the interaction between supplementation treatments and SES for vocabulary (in percentiles of the standardized score). Figure 4 shows the interaction between supplementation treatments and primary school education for vocabulary (maximum grade percentiles; average schooling was 3.7±2.1 years). Atole had a greater impact than Fresco on low-SES children, and its benefits were magnified when children attended school.

Finally, the effect of Atole on the cohort with maximum exposure (pregnancy and up to at least 24 months; n=305) was clearer and stronger than effects on the cohort exposed after 24 months (n=103). However, subjects in the latter cohort were older (born before 1967) than subjects in the former (born during 1970-74). Sample sizes also were smaller for the older cohort, another factor that could have influenced the results.

An additional study in Mexico also suggests that food supplementation leads to better, long-term performance (Chávez, Martínez, and Soberanes 1995). Despite a weak design, small samples, and deficient analyses, the 24-year duration of the study and the breadth of the information collected are impressive. The study began in 1968 in the village of Tezonteopan. Unsupplemented women and newborns were recruited during the first year of the study, and the supplemented cases were women who became pregnant during the second and third years. A nutritious drink was given twice daily to mothers as the food supplement. Children were supplemented from 12 weeks to 10 years and the type of supplement changed with age; for example, milk was given to young children, and milk and sandwiches were given to children starting at 4 years. Supplementation benefited infant behavior, child IQ, behavior at school, school performance, and adult body size.

Stimulation and Food Supplementation. In Cali, Colombia, McKay and others (1978) performed one of the most important studies in developing countries that combined food supplementation and stimulation. The study was conducted with low-SES children showing poor growth. A preschool battery was used to assess development in the children, and an estimate of their general cognitive ability was obtained. Within neighborhood clusters, children were allocated to various combinations of education, nutritional supplementation, and health care (medical examination and treatment) interventions. The education intervention was designed to develop cognitive processes and language, social abilities, and psychomotor skills through an integrated curriculum model.

Figure 3. SES-by-treatment Interactions for Vocabulary

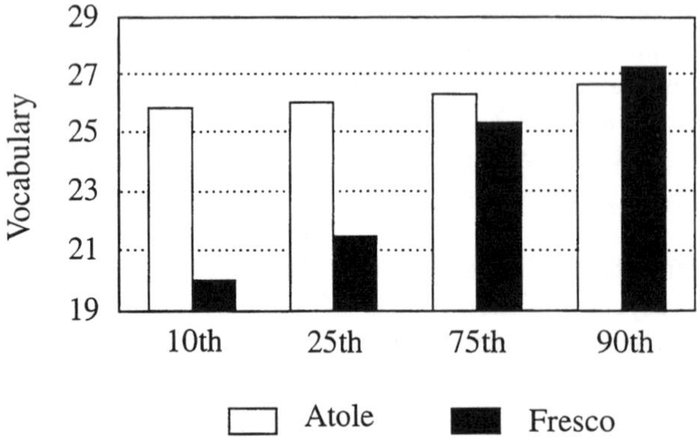

Source: Pollit and others 1995.

Figure 4. Maximum Grade-by-treatment Interactions for Vocabulary

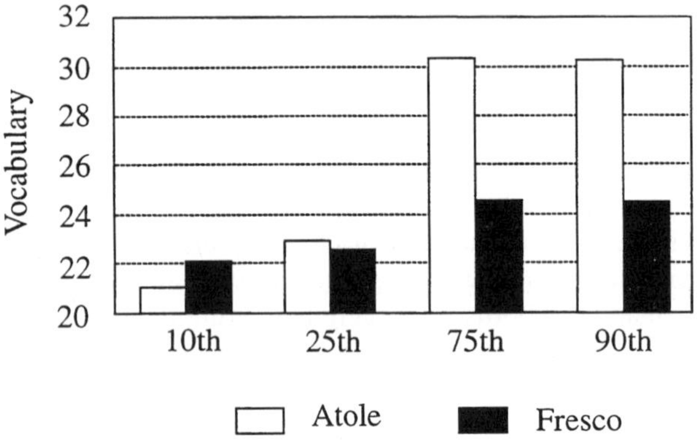

Source: Pollit and others 1995.

Figure 5 shows a schematic of the project design, indicating which groups received what types of intervention. The components of the interventions for groups T4-T1 were provided in a treatment center, but groups T1 (a, b, c) received nutritional supplements at home and health care at the center before receiving the combined intervention package. Group HS children, the upper-class comparison group, received no treatment, but they were measured periodically during the treatment years, which lasted about 9 months each.

The results of the project are presented in figure 6, which compares growth in the general cognitive ability of children from 43 to 87 months of age (the beginning of primary school) for each of five groups: HS (high SES), T4 (received four treatment

Figure 5. Schematic Presentation of the Cali Project Design

Experimental Design of Nutrition, Health, and Education Preschool Project, Cali, Colombia						
Groups	*Sample sizes in 1971*	*Treatment years*				*Sample sizes in 1974*
		1971	*1972*	*1973*	*1974*	
T4	60	enh	enh	enh	enh	53
T3	60		enh	enh	enh	50
T2	60			enh	enh	
T1	60				enh	50
HS	60					52
T1 (a)	20	nh	nh	nh	enh	16
T1 (b)	20		nh	nh	enh	17
T1 (c)	20			nh	enh	16
Total	360					315

Note: *e*, education; *n*, nutritional supplementation; *h*, health care.

Source: Sinisterra and others 1979.

periods), T3 (received three treatment periods), T2 (received two treatment periods), and T1 (received one treatment period). In figure 6, T1 combines the groups in figure 5 designated as T1 proper and T1 (a, b, c). This was done because no differences in cognitive performance were found between children who did or did not receive food supplementation before receiving 1 year of education.

As shown in figure 6, nutrition combined with stimulation had a clear effect, and a clear dose response is evident. Initial response to the intervention package varies by age; younger children seem to respond to a greater extent. Ability scores are scaled sums of correct test items, and solid lines represent periods of treatment. Brackets to the right of each curve indicate plus or minus 1 standard deviation for values at the end of the study. The pooled standard deviation of the general cognitive ability score at 87 months was 1.16 units, and the difference between T4 and T1 is estimated to be 0.93, equivalent to an effect size of 0.8. T1 is not a true control because children received one treatment period, although at older ages.

Sinisterra and others (1979) followed the children's performance in school through 112 months (9.3 years). Some attenuation occurred in the differences among groups, but the gradient with duration of treatment was still evident. A conclusion is that "contrary to the evidence from other studies, the effect of intervention does not disappear in the absence of continued treatment, although it is reduced" (Sinisterra 1979: 235). Long-term treatment

Figure 6. Growth of General Cognitive Ability in the Cali Study

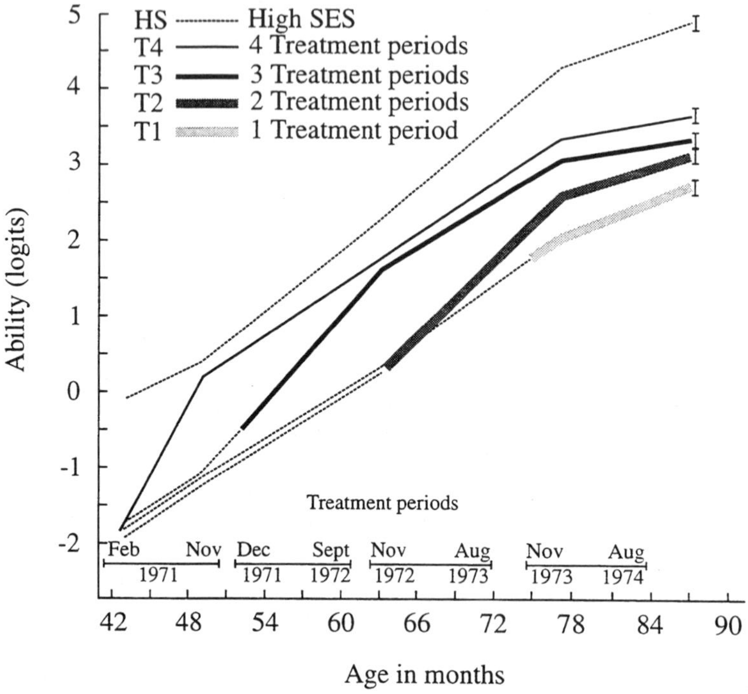

Source: McKay and others 1978.

effects varied by scale and remained very strong for five subtests of the WISC that test logical processes (that is, arithmetic, mazes, similarities, block design, and picture arrangement).

Another study of simulation and food supplementation, in Bogotá, Colombia, involved randomly assigning families to one of six experimental groups (Super and others 1990; Waber and others 1981). Four of the six groups formed a 2×2 factorial design: nonintervened control, supplementation only, home visit only, and combined supplementation and home visit. The two other groups were designed to test the effects of timing the supplementation; although neither group received stimulation, one received supplements during pregnancy and up to 6 months postpartum, and the other received supplements from 6 to 36 months postpartum. Supplementation for all groups receiving it included a package of foods delivered to the home as well as direct micronutrient supplements. Foods were provided from week 26 of pregnancy to when the child turned 3 years old, depending on the group. Home visits were twice weekly for the first 3 years. The home visitor provided intensive tutoring to increase the level of cognition and social stimulation.

Waber and others (1981) reported the effects of stimulation and supplementation on motor and mental development assessed by the Griffiths Test. Supplementation had a clear effect on five of the subscales, particularly on motoric components, and on the general quotient. The effect of stimulation was weaker than supplementation and evident only on language performance, showing no evidence of an interaction with supplementation. Food supplements during pregnancy and the first 6 months did not appear to be as important as supplementation from 6 to 36 months of age.

Findings of the effects of stimulation and supplementation on growth were reported by Super, Herrera, and Mora (1990). At 3 years of age, children who had received food supplementation were 2.6 centimeters and 642 grams larger than controls. Home stimulation, by itself, had no effect, but home stimulation combined with supplements had a greater effect than the supplement alone. The intervention ended at 3 years of age, but a follow-up through 6 years was done. The effects of supplementation remained, but the effects of home visits increased over time, strengthening the interaction with supplementation. At 6 years, the mean height of the controls was 105.1 centimeters, which was less than the mean height (107.1 centimeters) of the group with home visits and less than that of the group with supplementation (107.7 centimeters). The tallest group (109.2 centimeters) had received both supplements and home visits. The increased effect of home stimulation after the interventions ended suggests that enduring changes were established in caring behaviors (Super, Herrera, and Mora 1990).

The benefits from nutritional supplementation, with or without psychosocial stimulation, on the growth and development of stunted children were reported by Grantham-McGregor and others (1991) and Walker and others (1991). The subjects were 129 Jamaican children aged 9-24 months with lengths less than 2 standard deviations of the U.S. National Center for Health Statistics reference curves at enrollment. Assignment was random to one of four groups: supplement only, stimulation only, both treatments combined, or no treatment (controls). The supplement was 1 kilogram of a milk-based formula each week, intended for the child, and 1 kilogram each of skimmed-milk powder and cornmeal, provided for other household members to reduce sharing of the child's ration. The stimulation program consisted of structured play sessions with mothers and children at 1-hour weekly visits. Mothers were taught how to promote development through play, and toys were left in the home to promote playing between visits.

Performance was measured by the Griffiths Test. Figure 7 shows the results of these interventions for 2 years. Mean developmental quotients (DQs) shown for the four groups of children with stunted growth were adjusted by age and initial score at enrollment. Mean DQs for children without stunted growth (comparison group) were adjusted for age only. Stimulation and supplementation had significant but independent effects (that is, they were not interactive). Children who received both supplement and stimulation had DQs higher than the controls by 13.4 and nearly equal to DQs of children in the comparison group. Groups receiving treatment improved in all of the subscales, but children receiving supplements showed strikingly greater effects in the locomotor subscale.

Analysis of the effects on growth in height and weight showed that supplementation, not stimulation, improved growth after 1 year of intervention (Walker and others 1991). Significant interactions were found between supplement and growth. Thinner and younger children benefited more from effects of supplementation, which only occurred in the first 6 months of the study. The failure of supplementation to effect growth during the second 6 months of this study may be explained by the older age of the children, who were about 24 months old at the start of the second 6 months of the study. As was found in Guatemala, older children may not respond to supplementation (Schroeder and others 1995).

Figure 7. Mean Developmental Quotients of Children with Stunted Growth

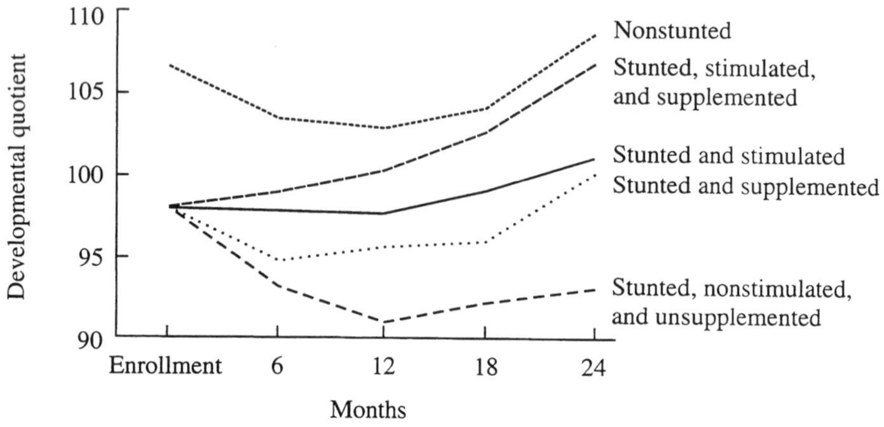

Source: Grantham-McGregor 1992.

Breastfeeding

Reports from industrialized countries link breastfeeding and cognitive development (Pollock 1994). The best studies control carefully for two things: confounding, because women who breastfeed are likely to be wealthier and better educated and have better parenting skills than those who do not breastfeed; and reverse causality, because for example, a serious illness may interrupt breastfeeding and lead to bottle feeding. Although well-controlled cohort studies consistently indicate that effects of breastfeeding attenuate with adjustment for confounding, they show small, but significant, differences in favor of breastfeeding (Morrow-Tlucak and others 1988; Rogan and Gladen 1993; Lanting and others 1994; Pollock 1994). However, uncontrolled self-selection factors, such as maternal differences or differences in the home environment, may account for the findings (Morrow-Tlucak and others 1988; Jacobson and Jacobson 1992).

One study of the effects of breastfeeding on cognitive development showed assessments of IQ at 7.5-8 years of age in two groups of children born prematurely (Lucas and others 1992). Both groups had been fed by gastric tube, but one received breastmilk and the other formula. After adjusting for differences in mothers' education and social class, the breastmilk group had an 8.3 IQ point advantage (over one-half a standard deviation). In the breastmilk group, a correlation was shown between IQ and the amount of breastmilk consumed, suggesting that breastmilk contributes to development. However, the issue of confounding remains because the decision whether to provide breastmilk was made by mothers. Children whose mothers chose to provide breastmilk but failed to do so had the same IQ as children whose mothers elected not to provide breastmilk. A better design would be to randomize breastmilk and formula feedings, perhaps for cases where mothers elect not to provide breastmilk but do not object if it is provided.

Assuming that breastfeeding rather than self-selection explains the positive effects on cognitive development, what are the possible mechanisms? Several mechanisms have been suggested: (a) the psychosocial act of breastfeeding may improve the mother-child interaction; (b) maternal hormones, such as thyroid-stimulating hormone and thyroid hormones, and other biologically active peptides that might reach the infant via breastmilk may cause the effects; and (c) some components of breastmilk may have a beneficial effect on brain development (Lanting and others 1994; Uauy and de Andraca 1995). Candidates for (c) are long-chained polyunsaturated fatty acids, particularly arachidonic and docosahexaenoic acid because of their role as structural lipids in brain and nervous tissue.

Micronutrients

The effects of iodine, iron, and zinc on human development have been studied. Findings from studies of these micronutrients are reviewed below.

Iodine

The hallmark of endemic cretinism is serious and irreversible mental retardation (Hetzel, Dunn, and Stanbury 1987). More important from a public health perspective is whether the noncretinous population, the apparently healthy group in an iodine-deficient area, also shows mental abnormalities (Bleichrodt and Born 1994).

Bleichrodt and Born (1994) have undertaken a meta-analysis of eighteen studies with relevant objectives and adequate designs. Children, adolescents, and adults were included in these studies. Most studies compared subjects from iodine-deficient regions to subjects from noniodine-deficient regions, but a few were controlled trials of iodine administration. However, the meta-analysis made no distinction among types of studies. Without exception, all eighteen studies linked poor performance with the iodine-deficient or untreated groups. The average effect size was 0.9 of a standard deviation, or 13.5 IQ points. Despite the need for a more selective meta-analysis, it is clear that improvement in the iodine status of the noncretinous population would bring substantial increases in cognitive development and great economic benefits (Pandav 1994).

Iron

Iron deficiency is most prevalent among children 6-24 months old (Lozoff 1990). This period is also the time marked by development of fundamental motor and cognitive abilities, completion of the brain growth spurt, and occurrence of physical growth failure and high rates of infectious disease.

Several studies of behavior in infants and toddlers show that iron deficiency severe enough to cause anemia is associated with impaired performance on mental and motor scores of the Bayley or similar scales (Lozoff 1990). The results came from comparing carefully defined anemic and nonanemic control groups at baseline, or before treatment.

In a recent study, Idjradinata and Pollitt (1993) found baseline values of 90.6 for mental scores of anemic subjects 12-18 months old; scores of 102.1 for nonanemic, iron-deficient children; and scores of 105.1 for iron-sufficient children. Corresponding values for motor scores were 90.5, 103.2, and 105.6 respectively. Clearly, iron-deficiency anemia, or as Lozoff (1990) notes, some unidentified but closely linked condition, alters human behavior. Because risk factors for anemia, a condition that takes a long time to develop, are like those that apply to stunted growth, interpreting associations between anemia and development is as difficult as interpreting associations between stunting and development.

Double-blind, randomized trials possible for micronutrients are a powerful type of research design and have proven very useful in unraveling the effects of iron. Pollitt (1995) divides the intervention trials into two groups, depending on which of two hypotheses they address. One group includes short-term trials, 7-10 days in duration, that test the hypothesis that depletion of cellular iron in the brain alters mental and motor test performance. The other group includes trials that assess effects up to 4 months after treatment and test whether improved hematological status influences performance. The trials also can be further divided into those that use severely affected subjects (anemic children) or more moderately affected children (iron-deficient, nonanemic children).

Several reviews are available of studies on iron and development (Pollitt and Metallinos-Katsaras 1990; Lozoff 1990). Also, proceedings were published from a major conference held on the subject in 1988 (Haas and Fairchild 1989). Conference participants concluded that "new studies using randomized designs with appropriate controls, many of which were presented at this conference, have shown that iron therapy in preschool and school-aged children with IDA (iron-deficiency anemia) results in improvements in certain behavioral tests" (Haas and Fairchild 1989). Long-term studies, in contrast to short-term studies, have shown improvements in anemic subjects. However, there is no consistent evidence of long- or short-term behavioral gains after treatment in nonanemic, iron-deficient subjects.

At least one additional study using a double-blind randomized design has appeared since the conference (Idjradinata and Pollitt 1993). The study involved three groups of children: iron-deficient and anemic (n=50), iron-deficient and nonanemic (n=29), and iron-replete (n=47). The children were assigned randomly to receive dietary ferrous sulphate or placebo for 4 months. Only the iron-deficient, anemic children showed an effect in performance on the Bayley Scales. The effects of the supplement were large, reversing the initial disadvantage between anemic and nonanemic children. The evidence supports the view that iron-deficiency anemia, not less severe forms of iron deficiency, causes impairment in development.

Zinc

Zinc has multiple roles in brain function, and zinc deficiency has been linked to poor development in studies using animal models, primarily rats and rhesus monkeys. These studies show that zinc deficiency leads to reduced activity and responsiveness and to deficiencies in learning, attention, and memory (Golub and others 1995).

Although no studies have examined zinc supplementation and mental development in preschool children, two double-blind, randomized trials assessed attention and short-term memory in children 5-7 years of age in Canada (Gibson and others 1989) and Guatemala (Cavan and others 1993). The Canadian children were short (less than the 15th percentile), and the Guatemalan children were from a disadvantaged, peri-urban background. Children were treated with 10 milligrams of zinc a day (as $ZnSo_4$) for 12 months in Canada and 25 weeks in Guatemala. Zinc supplementation showed no effects on cognitive tests in either study. More research is needed, particularly in young children, to clarify the possible role of zinc in human development.

Mechanisms

Figure 8 depicts the old and new theories regarding the mechanisms through which malnutrition leads to developmental delays. In the mid-1960s, many scientists believed in sensitive periods during early development when malnutrition could damage the growing and evolving brain permanently, resulting in irreversible, impaired function (Levitsky and Strupp 1995). As a result of this view, early models of malnutrition showed that cognitive deficiencies resulted only from brain damage. Now a less deterministic view recognizes that there can be partial recovery in many brain structures although effects on others, such as the hippocampus and cerebellum, may be permanent. Also, it is widely recognized that long-lasting, if not permanent, changes in brain neural receptor function follow an early episode of malnutrition (Levitsky and Strupp 1995).

Timing is the critical element in determining whether malnutrition has permanent effects. The literature from animal and human studies strongly indicates that the earlier the deprivation, the greater the behavioral effects and the greater the probability that these effects will be permanent. Also, the earlier rehabilitation begins, whether nutritional or stimulatory in nature or both, the more favorable the prognosis will be (Morgan and Gibson 1991; Smart 1991; Bedi 1987). Effects of malnutrition on major areas of the brain, such as the cerebellum, may help explain consistent reports of effects on motor coordination and development as measured by the Bayley and similar scales.

As Brown and Pollitt (1996) imply in figure 8, malnutrition hinders cognitive abilities through several interacting routes. For example, malnutrition may alter cognitive development by interfering with overall health or the child's energy level or by limiting physical activity and interaction with other people and the environment. In some cases, psychosocial stimulation may reverse the effects of undernutrition. Other routes that malnutrition may take are through delaying development of motor skills and physical growth, in part because of adults' lowered expectations caused by a child's younger appearance. In addition, figure 8 shows that low economic status can exacerbate all of these factors, implying that effects of malnutrition on behavior depend on the environment and place impoverished children at particular risk for cognitive impairment in later life.

A consideration of mechanisms is included in this chapter to reinforce the view that *timing is critical* for most, if not all, current mechanisms. Malnutrition is highly age-specific; most nutritional deficiencies and failure in growth are at their peak during intrauterine life and the first few years of life. Whether caused by diet, infection, or both, apathy and withdrawal are problems more during weaning, roughly in children 6-24 months old. Delayed motor development and growth failure are similarly highly age-specific, appearing during early childhood. The child who survives this early period but remains small is likely to provoke lower expectations from parents, neighbors, and teachers throughout all of childhood, not just early in life. Age is clearly important. To address the effects and conditions that cause delayed development and growth failure, the interventions must be initiated early in life.

Overview of Findings

The studies reviewed above lead to nine generalizations about the relationship of undernutrition to cognitive and behavioral development. Answers given to the questions below summarize the findings.

Figure 8. How Malnutrition Hinders Cognitive Abilities

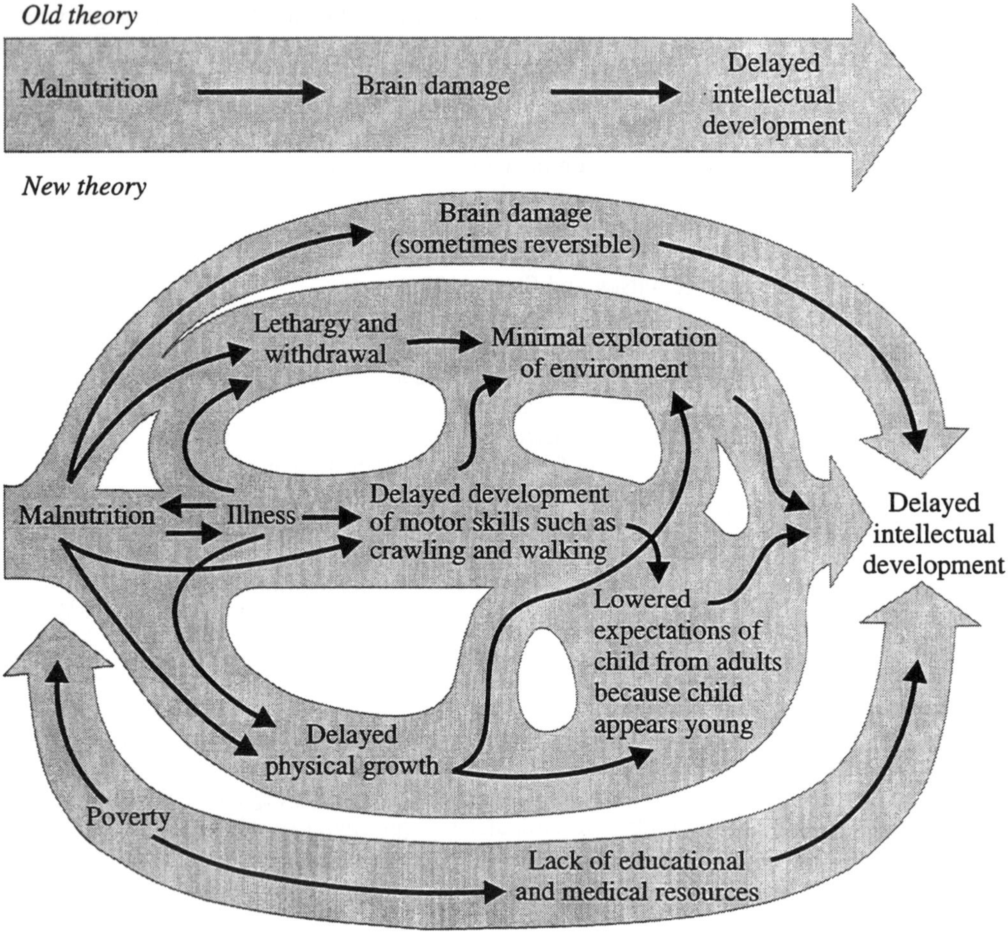

Source: Brown and Pollit 1996.

1. *Does undernutrition impair behavioral development?*

   Poor nutrition during intrauterine life and early years leads to profound and varied effects including:

   - Delayed physical growth and motor development
   - General effects on cognitive development resulting in lower IQs (lower by 15 points or more in the severely malnourished)
   - Greater degree of behavioral problems and deficient social skills at school age
   - Decreased attention, deficient learning, and lower educational achievement.

2. *Are these effects found only in the severely malnourished?*

   No. The effects of undernutrition on cognition occur as well in children without clinical signs of undernutrition but who are retarded in growth. Most of the food supplementation experiments in developing countries, for example, were aimed at the nonseverely malnourished population.

3. *What are mechanisms for the effects of undernutrition on behavior?*

   A definite answer is uncertain, but several mechanisms have been proposed: organic-based mechanisms, such as damage to the brain, and more subtle mechanisms, such as reduced exploration of the environment and lack of interest in novel stimuli by the malnourished child. Because these and many other mechanisms are not mutually exclusive, it is almost certain that varied and multiple pathways lead to poor development.

4. *Who is more affected by undernutrition?*

   Undernutrition and the socioeconomic context in which it occurs appear to be related. Undernutrition has a greater effect on development in children living in poverty, whether in industrialized or in developing countries, than on children who are not poor. Some evidence suggests that nutrition interventions benefit cognition and behavior to a greater extent among the poorer segment of society.

5. *Which nutrients are responsible for cognitive and behavioral impairments?*

   Because nutrient deficiencies tend to cluster in individuals, isolating the specific contributions of single nutrients is difficult from nonintervention studies. Iodine deficiency and iron-deficiency anemia are easier to study than macronutrient deficiencies, and relevant research has shown that both of these micronutrients are involved specifically in causing impairments. Less severe forms of iron deficiency do not appear to affect behavior. This degree of certainty is not possible in studies of protein-energy deficiency because the food supplements provide protein and energy as well as other nutrients. However, no evidence indicates that deficiencies in protein and energy are unimportant. The safest course for ensuring cognitive and behavioral development is to meet all nutrient needs with natural or fortified foods prepared appropriately for young children. The benefits of breastfeeding also must be considered in fostering growth and development.

6. *When in life are nutrition interventions more likely to be effective?*

   Strong evidence suggests that the earlier children begin benefiting from nutrition interventions the greater the improvement on behavioral development. In the case of physical growth, nutrition interventions may be effective only during pregnancy and the first 2-3 years of life. For behavioral development, nutrition intervention may have a benefit, although much reduced, at later ages.

7. *Are the effects of undernutrition irreversible?*

   Considerable evidence indicates that substantial improvements can be achieved, even in severely malnourished children, if appropriate steps are taken at a young age to satisfy nutritional and psychosocial needs. The longer the developmental delays remain uncorrected, the greater the chance of permanent effects. In developing countries, where few children live to see their situation improve, once the effects of undernutrition are established in early childhood, they typically become permanent. The intellectual potential of such children at school entry most likely is already damaged irrevocably.

8. *Are the effects of improved nutrition long lasting?*

   Yes. Long-term studies indicate that nutrition interventions aimed at preschool children in the first few years of life lead to measurable improvements in adolescence and adulthood.

9. *Do early interventions to stimulate cognitive development interact with nutrition interventions?*

   Early intervention programs to stimulate cognition have improved cognition and perhaps physical growth. Similar to nutrition interventions, the earlier the program is started, the better the results tend to be. Although current evidence is not conclusive regarding whether the effects of stimulation are additive or interactive, children who receive combined nutrition and stimulation programs perform better than those who receive either type of intervention alone.

Other Functional Consequences of Undernutrition

Early nutrition affects, directly or indirectly, many other functional outcomes besides cognitive and behavioral development. Consider, for example, the effects of nutrition on intellectual development and school achievement noted above. Undoubtedly, these effects influence an individual's choice of occupation, future earning power, and the survival and quality of life of the next generation. Recognition of these effects has led international agencies, for example, to promote female education as a child survival measure.

Two additional examples of domains influenced by nutrition in early childhood are considered briefly below: work capacity and productivity, and reproductive health.

Work Capacity and Productivity

Work capacity, measured in the laboratory by maximal oxygen consumption, is partly determined by lean body mass; for example, taller men will have greater lean body mass and greater work capacity than shorter men (Spurr 1983). Field research in developing countries suggests a relationship between body size and productivity in agriculture, particularly for demanding tasks (Haddad and Bouis 1990). The INCAP follow-up study also showed smaller lean body mass, less strength, and reduced work capacity in adolescents and adults whose growth in early childhood was stunted (Martorell and others 1992). Because growth failure in early childhood is important in determining reduced adult stature (Martorell, Kettel Khan, and Schroeder 1994), these studies imply a link between childhood undernutrition and adult productivity.

In Guatemala, food supplementation during early childhood resulted in taller adults with greater lean body mass (Rivera and others 1995) and work capacity (Haas and others 1995) than adults not given supplements when they were children. However, the possible repercussions of reduced work capacity on productivity have not been studied in this population.

Reproductive Health

About 500,000 women die each year in childbirth, and 99 percent of these deaths occur in developing countries (Koblinsky 1995). Anemia, common among women in developing countries, is a complicating factor "which may shift a pregnant woman's balance toward death, particularly when joined by an obstetrical complication (e.g., hemorrhage, eclampsia)" (Koblinsky 1995: 528). Major causes of maternal death in developing countries are hemorrhage, obstructed labor, sepsis, eclampsia, and septic abortion. In some cases of obstructed labor, mother and child may die unless a cesarean section is done.

A well-known risk factor for cephalopelvic disproportion and obstructed labor is short maternal stature or stunted growth (Aitken and Walls 1986). The INCAP follow-up study provides information about repercussions of growth failure on reproductive health (Martorell and others, forthcoming). Almost 40 percent of the women studied who were more than 18 years old were shorter than 149 centimeters, a widely used cutoff point for obstetric risk to the mother and LBW.

Results showed that among women with severely stunted growth (more than 3 standard deviations below the reference mean) at 3 years of age, nearly 67 percent were short adults (less than 149 centimeters). Among women with moderately stunted growth at 3 years of age (between 3 and 2 standard deviations below the reference mean), 34 percent were short, and in the last group (2 standard deviations or less below the reference mean, or approximately to the right of the 3rd percentile of the reference curves), only 5 percent were short. Women with a greater degree than others of stunted growth in childhood also had smaller body frames, including reduced external pelvic dimensions and hip circumference. These findings link growth failure in early childhood to obstetric risk for obstructed labor.

Short women also have a reduced muscle mass and tend to have smaller newborns than taller women (Kramer 1987), perpetuating the sequelae of malnutrition across generations. Preliminary data from the INCAP follow-up study indicate that the prevalence of LBW (less than 2,500 grams) is nearly doubled in women whose growth was severely stunted at 3 years of age (more than 3 standard deviations below the reference mean) compared with women whose growth was not stunted (2 standard deviations or less below the reference mean) (Martorell and others 1996).

Nutrition Programs: Required Features

Programs that effectively reduce undernutrition will have certain features in common. Some successful programs, such as the Tamil Nadu Integrated Nutrition Project, which was funded partly by the World Bank (Balachander 1993), and the Iringa Nutrition Program of Tanzania (Jonsson, Ljungqvist, and Yambi 1993) excel in terms of quality of design, implementation, and management (Jennings and others 1991).

Other lessons can be learned from problems faced in current nutrition programs. To do this, Musgrove (1991) analyzed food programs in Latin America, many of them designed to combat undernutrition in young children. Because these programs are deficient in design and poorly targeted, they do not always reach the poor, and they very often miss young children. Although few evaluations are available, these programs probably are not preventing undernutrition despite vast allocations of money; some US$1.6 billion a year, or roughly $20 for each beneficiary, are spent in Latin America on food programs. Musgrove (1991) concludes that redirecting the investment toward programs that are designed better could benefit nutrition in Latin America enormously.

To be effective, nutrition programs should reach women and children less than 3 years of age. The needs of other population groups are less compelling when preventing undernutrition. Nutrition efforts should be integrated with health services, offering prenatal and postnatal care to mothers and children; building targeted, supplementary feeding where necessary and a strong nutrition education around the promotion of healthy growth; and making micronutrient interventions available for mothers and children.

Psychosocial stimulation, also shown to affect cognitive and behavioral development, should be incorporated into integrated nutrition and health interventions for optimal outcomes. As discussed above, stimulation appears to augment the effects of nutrition. Heaver and Hunt (1995: 27) call for programs that include all three types of intervention, referring to them as programs of early childhood development and stating that the aim "is not only to promote survival but also to promote the physical, intellectual, social, and emotional development of those who survive, recognizing that children cannot develop fully as personalities or contribute fully to society unless attention is paid to all these aspects of development."

The need is urgent for applied research on how to incorporate psychosocial stimulation activities into integrated nutrition and health programs. Center-based activities seem impractical for children less than 3 years of age and also would be costly. For years, the Integrated Child Development Services (ICDS) program in India has focused on promoting cognitive development in children 3-5 years of age. As with Head Start in the United States, judging the program's success is difficult based on existing evaluation studies. Observations of India's program suggest that children spend much of the time sitting or sleeping, crowded into a dark and gloomy room. Although this may provide childcare, it probably does not promote cognitive development. Perhaps a better approach would be training home visitors to promote what UNICEF understands as childcare. This cadre of workers, perhaps linked to women's groups and schools, could assist nutrition and health personnel in promoting the best ways to meet nutritional and health needs while fostering psychosocial development.

In examining the costs of nutrition programs, the Administrative Committee on Coordination/Subcommittee on Nutrition (ACC/SCN) has concluded that US$10-$30 are needed per beneficiary each year to support an effective, integrated program. These amounts are not unlike those currently being spent in Latin America (Musgrove 1991). Food costs often are a large component and create the need for targeting by socioeconomic status and age or for developing alternative, more sustainable strategies to improve diets.

Although the benefits of improving nutrition are not yet quantified, they are presumed to be substantial, certainly worth many times the investment.

Conclusion

Programs that help families meet the nutritional, health, and psychosocial needs of young children will substantially improve human capital, understood as the physical and behavioral development necessary for becoming a productive member of society. Even when approached with a limited focus, the scientific literature supports the beneficial effects of such programs on the development of human capital. For this reason, early child development programs, as defined by Heaver and Hunt (1995), should be viewed as long-term, economic development strategies. Because poverty compounds the effects of deficient nutrition and psychosocial deprivation, the programs are needed most desperately in developing nations and underprivileged sectors of society. Compelling scientific findings and considerable programmatic experience indicate the need to promote widespread and energetic support for early child development programs.

Notes

This work was funded in part by grants from the National Institutes of Health (NIH-1 RO1 HD22440 and NIH-1 RO1 HD29927). Comments and suggestions from Ernesto Pollitt are gratefully acknowledged.

References

Achenbach T. M., C. T. Howell, M. F. Aoki, and V. A. Rauh. 1993. Nine-year Outcome of the Vermont Intervention Program for Low Birth Weight Infants. *Pediatrics* 91:45-55.

Aitken I. W., and B. Walls. 1986. Maternal Height and Cephalopelvic Disproportion in Sierra Leone. *Tropical Doctor* 16:132-34.

Aylward G. P., S. I. Pfeiffer, A. Wright, and S. J. Verhulst. 1989. Outcome Studies of Low Birth Weight Infants Published in the Last Decade: A Metaanalysis. *Journal of Pediatrics* 115:515-20.

Balachander, J. 1993. Tamil Nadu's Successful Nutrition Effort. In J. Rohde, M. Chatterjee, and D. Morley, eds., *Reaching Health for All.* Delhi: Oxford University Press.

Barnett, W. S. 1995. Long-term Effects of Early Childhood Programs on Cognitive and School Outcomes. *The Future of Children. Long-Term Outcomes of Early Childhood Programs* 5(3):25-50.

Barrera, M. E., C. E. Cunningham, and P. L. Rosenbaum. 1986. Low Birth Weight and Home Intervention Strategies: Preterm Infants. *Journal of Developmental and Behavioral Pediatrics* 7:361-66.

Beaton, G. 1989. Small But Healthy? Are We Asking the Right Questions? *Human Organization* 48(1):30-39.

Beaton, G., A. Kelly, J. Kevany, R. Martorell, and J. Mason. December 1990. *Appropriate Uses of Anthropometric Indices in Children.* ACC/SCN State-of-the-Art-Series Nutrition Policy Discussion Paper No. 7. Geneva: United Nations, Administrative Committee on Coordination/Subcommittee on Nutrition.

Bedi, K. S. 1987. *Lasting Neuroanatomical Changes Following Undernutrition During Early Life.* London: Academic Press, Inc.

Black, M. M., H. Dubowitz, J. Hutcheson, J. Berenson-Howard, R. H. Starr. 1995. A Randomized Clinical Trial of Home Intervention for Children with Failure to Thrive. *Pediatrics* 95(6):807-14.

Bleichrodt, N., and M. P. Born. 1994. A Metaanalysis of Research on Iodine and Its Relationship to Cognitive Development. In J. B. Stanbury, ed., *The Damaged Brain of Iodine Deficiency: Neuromotor, Cognitive, Behavioral, and Educative Aspects.* New York: Cognizant Communication Corp.

Brown. J. L., and E. Pollitt. 1996. Malnutrition, Poverty and Intellectual Development. *Scientific American* 274:38-43.

Campbell, F. A., and C. T. Ramey. 1994. Effects of Early Intervention on Intellectual and Academic Achievement: A Follow-up Study of Children from Low-income Families. *Child Development* 65:684-98.

Cavan, K. R., R. S. Gibson, C. F. Grazioso, A. M. Isalgue, M. Ruz, and N. W. Solomons. 1993. Growth and Body Composition of Periurban Guatemalan Children in Relation to Zinc Status: A Longitudinal Zinc Intervention Trial. *American Journal of Clinical Nutrition* 57:344-52.

Chávez, A., C. Martínez, and B. Soberanes. 1995. The Effect of Malnutrition on Human Development. A 24-year Study of Well-nourished and Malnourished Children Living in a Poor Mexican Village. In N. S. Scrimshaw, ed., *Community-Based Longitudinal Nutrition and Health Studies: Classical Examples from Guatemala, Haiti and Mexico.* Boston: International Nutrition Foundation for Developing Countries.

Colombo, M., A. de la Parra, and I. López. 1992. Intellectual and Physical Outcome of Children Undernourished in Early Life Is Influenced by Later Environmental Conditions. *Developmental Medicine and Child Neurology* 34:611-22.

Cravioto, J., and E. R. DeLicardie. 1976. Microenvironmental Factors in Severe Protein-energy Malnutrition. In N. S. Scrimshaw and M. Behar, eds., *Nutrition and Agricultural Development: Significance and Potential for the Tropics.* New York: Plenum Press.

Drillien, C. M. 1970. The Small-for-Date Infant: Etiology and Prognosis. *Pediatric Clinics of North America* 17(1):9-23.

Ellis, C. E., and D. E. Hill. 1975. Growth, Intelligence, and School Performance in Children with Cystic Fibrosis Who Have Had an Episode of Malnutrition during Infancy. *Journal of Pediatrics* 87(4):565-68.

Engle, P. L., K. Gorman, R. Martorell, and E. Pollitt. 1992. Infant and Preschool Psychological Development. *Food and Nutrition Bulletin* 14(3):201-14.

Escobar, G. J., B. Littenberg, and D. B. Petitti. 1991. Outcome among Surviving Very Low Birthweight Infants: A Meta-analysis. *Archives of Disease in Childhood* 66:204-11.

Fitzhardinge, P. M., and E. M. Steven. 1972. The Small-for-Date Infant. II. Neurological and Intellectual Sequelae. *Pediatrics* 50(1):50-57.

Fuchs, G. J. 1990. Secondary Malnutrition in Children. In R. M. Suskind and L. Lewinter-Suskind, eds., *The Malnourished Child.* New York: Raven Press.

Galler, J. R. 1984. Behavioral Consequences of Malnutrition in Early Life. In J. R. Galler, ed., *Nutrition and Behavior.* New York: Plenum Press.

———. 1986. Malnutrition—A Neglected Cause of Learning Failure. *Malnutrition* 80(5):225-30.

Galler, J. R., F. Ramsey, and V. Forde. 1986. A Follow-up Study of the Influence of Early Malnutrition on Subsequent Development: 4. Intellectual Performance during Adolescence. *Nutrition and Behavior* 3:211-22.

Galler, J. R., F. Ramsey, and G. Solimano. 1984. The Influence of Early Malnutrition on Subsequent Behavioral Development. III. Learning Disabilities as a Sequel to Malnutrition. *Pediatric Research* 18(4):309-13.

———. 1985. A Follow-up Study of the Effects of Early Malnutrition on Subsequent Development. II. Fine Motor Skills in Adolescence. *Pediatric Research* 19(6):524-27.

Galler, J. R., F. Ramsey, G. Solimano, and W. E. Lowell. 1983. The Influence of Early Malnutrition on Subsequent Behavioral Development. II. Classroom Behavior. *Journal of the American Academy of Child Psychology* 22(1):16-22.

Gibson, R. S., P. D. Smit Vanderkooy, A. C. MacDonald, A. Goldman, B. A. Ryan, and M. Berry. 1989. A Growth-limiting, Mild Zinc-deficiency Syndrome in Some Southern Ontario Boys with Low Height Percentiles. *American Journal of Clinical Nutrition* 49:1266-73.

Golub, M. S., C. L. Keen, E. Gershwin, and A. G. Hendrickx. 1995. Developmental Zinc Deficiency and Behavior. *Journal of Nutrition* 125:2263S-71S.

Gorman, K.S., and E. Pollitt. 1992. Relationship between Weight and Body Proportionality at Birth, Growth during the First Year of Life, and Cognitive Development at 36, 48, and 60 Months. *Infant Behavior and Development* 15:279-96.

Grantham-McGregor, S. M. 1992. The Effect of Malnutrition on Mental Development. In J. C. Waterlow, ed., *Protein Energy Malnutrition*. London: Edward Arnold (a division of Hoddere & Stoughton).

———. 1995. A Review of Studies of the Effect of Severe Malnutrition on Mental Development. *Journal of Nutrition* 125(8S):2233S-38S.

Grantham-McGregor S., C. Powell, and P. Fletcher. 1989. Stunting, Severe Malnutrition and Mental Development in Young Children. *European Journal of Clinical Nutrition* 43:403-09.

Grantham-McGregor, S., C. Powell, S. Walker, S. Chang, and P. Fletcher. 1994. The Long-term Follow-up of Severely Malnourished Children Who Participated in an Intervention Program. *Child Development* 65:428-39.

Grantham-McGregor, S., C. Powell, S. Walker, and J. H. Himes. 1991. Nutritional Supplementation, Psychosocial Stimulation, and Mental Development of Stunted Children: the Jamaican Study. *Lancet* 338:1-5.

Haas, J. D., and M. W. Fairchild. 1989. Summary and Conclusions of the International Conference on Iron Deficiency and Behavioral Development, October 10-12, 1988. *American Journal of Clinical Nutrition* 50:703-05.

Haas, J. D., E. J. Martinez, S. Murdoch, E. Conlisk, J. A. Rivera, and R. Martorell. 1995. Nutritional Supplementation during the Preschool Years and Physical Work Capacity in Adolescent and Young Adult Guatemalans. *Journal of Nutrition* 125(4S):1078S-89S.

Hack, M., G. Taylor, N. Klein, R. Eiben, C. Schatschneider, and N. Mercuri-Minich. 1994. School-age Outcomes in Children with Birth Weights under 750 g. *New England Journal of Medicine* 331(12):753-59.

Haddad, L. J., and H. E. Bouis. 1990. The Impact of Nutritional Status on Agricultural Productivity: Wage Evidence from the Philippines. *Oxford Bulletin of Economics and Statistics* 53(1):45-68.

Hadders-Algra, M., H. J. Huisjes, and C. L. Touwen. 1988. Preterm or Small-for-Gestational-Age Infants. Neurological and Behavioural Development at the Age of 6 Years. *European Journal of Pediatrics* 147:460-67.

Harvey, D., J. Prince, J. Bunton, C. Parkinson, and S. Campbell. 1982. Abilities of Children Who Were Small-for-Gestational-Age Babies. *Pediatrics* 69(3):296-300.

Heaver, R. A., and J. M. Hunt. 1995. *Improving Early Childhood Development. An Integrated Program for the Philippines*. Washington, D.C.: World Bank.

Hetzel, B. S., J. T. Dunn, and J. B. Stanbury, eds. 1987. *The Prevention and Control of Iodine Deficiency Disorders*. Amsterdam: Elsevier.

Hill, R. M., W. M. Verniaud, R. L. Deter, L. M. Tennyson, G. M. Rettig, T. E. Zion, A. L. Varderman, P. G. Helms, L. B. McCulley, and L. L. Hill. 1984. The Effect of Intrauterine Malnutrition on the Term Infant. A 14-year Progressive Study. *Acta Paediatrica Scandinavica* 73:482-87.

Hille, E. T. M., A. L. Den Ouden, L. Bauer, C. van den Oudenrijn, R. Brand, and S. P. Verloove-Vanhorick. 1994. School Performance at Nine Years of Age in Very Premature and Very Low Birth Weight Infants: Perinatal Risk Factors and Predictors at Five Years of Age. *Journal of Pediatrics* 125:426-34.

Husaini, M. A., L. Karyadi, Y. K. Husaini, Sandjaja, Karyadi D., and E. Pollitt. 1991. Developmental Effects of Short-term Supplementary Feeding in Nutritionally-at-Risk Indonesian Infants. *American Journal of Clinical Nutrition* 54:799-804.

Idjradinata, P., and E. Pollitt. 1993. Reversal of Development Delays in Iron-deficient Anaemic Infants Treated with Iron. *Lancet* 341(8836):1-4.

Jacobson, S. W., and J. L. Jacobson. 1992. Breastfeeding and Intelligence. *Lancet* 339:926.

Jennings, J., S. Gillespie, J. Mason, M. Lotfi, and T. Scialfa. September 1991. *Managing Successful Nutrition Programmes*. ACC/SCN State-of-the-Art-Series Nutrition Policy Discussion Paper No. 8. Geneva: United Nations, Administrative Committee on Coordination/Subcommittee on Nutrition.

Jonsson, U., B. Ljungqvist, and O. Yambi. 1993. Mobilization for Nutrition in Tanzania. In J. Rohde, M. Chatterjee, and D. Morley, eds., *Reaching Health for All*. Delhi: Oxford University Press.

Joos, S. K., E. Pollitt, W. H. Mueller, and D. L. Albright. 1983. The Bacon Chow Study: Maternal Nutritional Supplementation and Infant Behavioral Development. *Child Development* 54:669-76.

Klein, P. S., G. B. Forbes, and P. R. Nader. 1975. Effects of Starvation in Infancy (Pyloric Stenosis) on Subsequent Learning Abilities. *Pediatrics* 87:8-15.

Klein, R. E., H. E. Freeman, J. Kagan, C. Yarbrough, and J-P Habicht. 1972. Is Big Smart? The Relation of Growth to Cognition. *Journal of Health and Social Behavior* 13:219-25.

Koblinsky, M. A. 1995. Beyond Maternal Mortality—Magnitude, Interrelationship, and Consequences of Women's Health, Pregnancy Related Complications and Nutritional Status on Pregnancy Outcomes. *International Journal of Gynecology and Obstetrics* 48(suppl):S21-32.

Kramer, M. S. 1987. Intrauterine Growth and Gestational Duration Determinants. *Pediatrics* 80(4):502-11.

Kramer, M. S., M. Olivier, F. H. McLean, D. M. Willis, and R. H. Usher. 1990. Impact of Intrauterine Growth Retardation and Body Proportionality on Fetal and Neonatal Outcome. *Pediatrics* 86(5):707-13.

Lanting, C. I., V. Fidler, M. Huisman, B. C. L. Touwen, and E. R. Boersma. 1994. Neurological Differences Between 9-year-old Children Fed Breast-milk or Formula-milk as Babies. *Lancet* 344:1319-22.

Lasky, R. E., A. Lechtig, H. Delgado, R. E. Klein, P. Engle, C. Yarbrough, and R. Martorell. 1975. Birth Weight and Psychomotor Performance in Rural Guatemala. *American Journal of Diseases of Children* 129:566-69.

Levitsky, D. A., and B. J. Strupp. 1995. Malnutrition and the Brain: Changing Concepts, Changing Concerns. *Journal of Nutrition* 125:2212S-20S.

Low, J. A., R. S. Galbraith, D. Muir, H. Killen, B. Pater, and J. Karchmar. 1982. Intrauterine Growth Retardation: A Study of Long-term Morbidity. *American Journal of Obstetrics and Gynecology* 142:670-77.

Low, J. A., M. H. Handley-Derry, S. O. Burke, R. D. Peters, E. A. Pater, H. L. Killen, and E. J. Derrick. 1992. Association of Intrauterine Fetal Growth Retardation and Learning Deficits at Age 9 to 11 Years. *American Journal of Obstetrics and Gynecology* 167:1499-1505.

Lozoff, B. 1990. Has Iron Deficiency Been Shown to Cause Altered Behavior in Infants? In J. Dobbing, ed., *Brain, Behaviour, and Iron in the Infant Diet.* London: Springer-Verlag.

Lucas, A., R. Morley, T. J. Cole, G. Lister, and C. Leeson-Payne. 1992. Breast Milk and Subsequent Intelligence Quotient in Children Born Preterm. *Lancet* 339:261-64.

Martorell, R. 1995. Promoting Healthy Growth: Rationale and Benefits. In P. Pinstrup-Andersen, D. Pelletier, and H. Alderman, eds., *Child Growth and Nutrition in Developing Countries. Priorities for Action.* Ithaca: Cornell University Press.

Martorell, R., J-P Habicht, and J. A. Rivera. 1995. History and Design of the INCAP Longitudinal Study (1969-77) and its Follow-up (1988-89). *Journal of Nutrition* 125:1027S-41S.

Martorell, R., L. Kettel Khan, and D. G. Schroeder. 1994. Reversibility of Stunting: Epidemiological Findings in Children from Developing Countries. *European Journal of Clinical Nutrition* 48(1):S45-S57.

Martorell, R., U. Ramakrishnan, J. A. Rivera, and P. Melgar. 1996. Stunting at 3 Years of Age in Guatemalan Girls and Birthweight of their Children. Abstract. Federation of American Societies for Experimental Biology (FASEB) meeting, Washington, D.C. Bethesda, Md.: FASEB.

Martorell, R., J. A. Rivera, H. Kaplowitz, and E. Pollitt. 1992. Long-term Consequences of Growth Retardation During Early Childhood. Proceedings of the Vlth International Congress of Auxology, Madrid, Spain, 15-19 September 1991. In M. Hernández and J. Argente, eds., *Human Growth: Basic and Clinical Aspects.* Amsterdam: Elsevier.

Martorell, R., J. A. Rivera, D. G. Schroeder, U. Ramakrishnan, E. Pollitt, and M. T. Ruel. n.d. Consecuencias a Largo Plazo del Retardo en el Crecimiento Durante la Niñez. *Archivos Latinoamericanos de Nutrición.* Forthcoming.

McKay, H., L. Sinisterra, A. McKay, H. Gomez, and P. Lloreda. 1978. Improving Cognitive Ability in Chronically Deprived Children. *Science* 200(21):270-78.

McLaren, D. S. 1986. Pathogenesis of Vitamin A Deficiency. In J. C. Bauernfeind, ed., *Vitamin A Deficiency and Its Control.* Orlando: Academic Press, Inc.

Morgan, B., and K. R. Gibson. 1991. Nutritional and Environmental Interactions in Brain Development. In K. R. Gibson and A. C. Petersen, eds., *Brain Maturation and Cognitive Development: Comparative and Cross-Cultural Perspectives.* New York: De Gruyter.

Morrow-Tlucak, M., R. H. Haude, and C. B. Ernhart. 1988. Breastfeeding and Cognitive Development in the First 2 Years of Life. *Social Science and Medicine* 26:635-39.

Muraskas, J. K., T. F. Myers, G. H. Lambert, and C. L. Anderson. 1992. Intact Survival of a 280 g Infant: An Extreme Case of Growth Retardation with Normal Cognitive Development at Two Years of Age. *Acta Paediatrica* 382:16-20.

Musgrove, P. 1991. Feeding Latin America's Children: An Analytical Study of Food Programs. World Bank, Latin America and the Caribbean Technical Department, Regional Studies Program Report 11. Washington, D.C.: World Bank.

My Lien, N., K. K. Meyer, and M. Winick. 1977. Early Malnutrition and "Late" Adoption: A Study of Their Effects on the Development of Korean Orphans Adopted into American Families. *American Journal of Clinical Nutrition* 30:1734-39.

Neisser, U., G. Boodoo, T. J. Bouchard Jr., A. W. Boykin, N. Brody, S. Ceci, D. F. Halpern, J. C. Loehlin, R. Perloff, R. J. Sternberg, and S. Ubina. 1995. Intelligence: Knowns and Unknowns. Report of a Task Force established by the Board of Scientific Affairs of the American Psychological Association. Washington D.C.: Science Directorate.

Neligan, G. A., I. Kolvin, D. M. Scott, and R. F. Garside. 1976. Born Too Soon or Born Too Small. A Follow-up Study to Seven Years of Age. *Clinics in Developmental Medicine No. 61.* London: Spastics International Medical Publications.

Ounsted, M. K., V. A. Moar, and A. Scott. 1984. Children of Deviant Birthweight at the Age of Seven Years: Health, Handicap, Size and Developmental Status. *Early Human Development* 9:323-40.

Pandav, C. S. 1994. The Economic Benefits of the Elimination of IDD. In B. S. Hetzel and C. S. Pandav, eds., *S.O.S. for a Billion. The Conquest of Iodine Deficiency Disorders.* Delhi: Oxford University Press.

Parkinson, C. E., R. Scrivener, L. Graves, J. Bunton, and D. Harvey. 1986. Behavioural Differences of School-age Children Who Were Small-for-Dates Babies. *Developmental Medicine and Child Neurology* 28:498-505.

Parkinson, C. E., S. Wallis, and D. Harvey. 1981. School Achievement and Behaviour of Children Who Were Small-for-Dates at Birth. *Developmental Medicine and Child Neurology* 23:41-50.

Paz, I., R. Gale, A. Laor, Y. L. Danon, D. K. Stevenson, and D. S. Seidman. 1995. The Cognitive Outcome of Full-term Small for Gestational Age Infants at Late Adolescence. *Obstetrics and Gynecology* 85:452-56.

Pollitt, E. 1995. Functional Significance of the Covariance Between Protein Energy Malnutrition and Iron Deficiency Anemia. *Journal of Nutrition* 125:2272S-77S.

Pollitt, E., and K. Gorman. 1989. Long-term Developmental Implications of Motor Maturation and Physical Activity in Infancy in a Nutritionally At Risk Population. In B. Schürch and N. S. Scrimshaw, eds., *Activity, Energy Expenditure and Energy Requirements of Infants and Children.* IDECG (International Dietary Energy Consultative Group) Workshop, November 14-17, Cambridge, Mass.

Pollitt, E., K. S. Gorman, P. L. Engle, R. Martorell, and J. A. Rivera. 1993. Early Supplementary Feeding and Cognition. *Monographs of the Society for Research in Child Development.* Serial No. 235. 58(7):1-122.

Pollitt, E., K. S. Gorman, P. L. Engle, J. A. Rivera, and R. Martorell. 1995. Nutrition in Early Life and the Fulfillment of Intellectual Potential. *Journal of Nutrition* 125:1111S-18S.

Pollitt, E., K. S. Gorman, and E. Metallinos-Katsaras. 1991. Long Term Developmental Consequences of Intrauterine and Postnatal Growth Retardation in Rural Guatemala. In G. J. Suci and S. Robertson, eds., *Future Directions in Infant Development Research.* Cornell Symposium Series. New York: Springer-Verlag.

Pollitt, E., and E. Metallinos-Katsaras. 1990. Iron Deficiency and Behavior. Constructs, Methods, and Validity of the Findings. *Nutrition and the Brain* 8:101-46.

Pollitt, E., and S-Y Oh. 1994. Early Supplementary Feeding, Child Development, and Health Policy. *Food and Nutrition Bulletin* 15(3):208-14.

Pollitt, E., and C. Thomson. 1977. Protein-calorie Malnutrition and Behavior: A View from Psychology. In R. J. Wurtman and J. J. Wurtman, eds., *Nutrition and Brain.* Vol. 2. New York: Raven Press.

Pollitt, E., W. E. Watkins, and M. A. Husaini. n.d. Three-month Nutritional Supplementation among Indonesian Infants and Toddlers Benefits Memory Function Eight Years Later. Submitted to the *American Journal of Clinical Nutrition.* Forthcoming.

Pollock, J. I. 1994. Long-term Associations with Infant Feeding in a Clinically Advantaged Population of Babies. *Developmental Medicine and Child Neurology* 36:429-40.

Ramey, C. T., and S. L. Ramey. 1994. Which Children Benefit the Most from Early Intervention? *Pediatrics* 94:1064-66.

Ramsey, B. W., P. M. Farrell, P. Pencharz, and the Consensus Committee. 1992. Nutritional Assessment and Management in Cystic Fibrosis: A Consensus Report. *American Journal of Clinical Nutrition* 55:108-16.

Ricciuti, H. N. 1981. Adverse Environmental and Nutritional Influences on Mental Development: A Perspective. *Journal of the American Dietetic Association* 79:115-20.

Richardson, S.A., H. G. Birch, and C. Ragbeer. 1975. The Behaviour of Children at Home Who Were Severely Malnourished in the First 2 Years of Life. *Journal of Biosocial Science* 7:255-67.

Rivera, J. A., R. Martorell, M. T. Ruel, J-P Habicht, and J. D. Haas. 1995. Nutritional Supplementation during the Preschool Years Influences Body Size and Composition of Guatemalan Adolescents. *Journal of Nutrition* 125:1068S-77S.

Rogan, W. J., and B. C. Gladen. 1993. Breast-feeding and Cognitive Development. *Early Human Development* 13:181-93.

Rubin, R. A., C. Rosenblatt, and B. Balow. 1973. Psychological and Educational Sequelae of Prematurity. *Pediatrics* 52(3):352-63.

Saigal, S., P. Szatmari, P. Rosenbaum, D. Campbell, and S. King. 1991. Cognitive Abilities and School Performance of Extremely Low Birth Weight Children and Matched Term Control Children at Age 8 Years: A Regional Study. *Journal of Pediatrics* 118:751-60.

Salt, P., J. R. Galler, and F. C. Ramsey. 1988. The Influence of Early Malnutrition on Subsequent Behavioral Development. VII. The Effects of Maternal Depressive Symptoms. *Journal of Developmental and Behavioral Pediatrics* 9:1-5.

Schroeder, D. G., R. Martorell, J. A. Rivera, M. T. Ruel, and J-P Habicht. 1995. Age Differences in the Impact of Nutritional Supplementation on Growth. *Journal of Nutrition* 125:1051S-59S.

Sinisterra, L., H. McKay, A. McKay, H. Gómez, and J. Korgi. 1979. Response of Malnourished Preschool Children to Multidisciplinary Intervention. In J. Brozek, ed., *Behavioral Effects of Energy and Protein Deficits Proceedings*, International Nutrition Conference. NIH Publication No. 79-1906. Washington, D.C.: Government Printing Office.

Skuse, D., A. Pickles, D. Wolke, and S. Reilly. 1994. Postnatal Growth and Mental Development: Evidence for a "Sensitive Period." *Journal of Child Psychiatry* 35(3):521-45.

Smart, J. L. 1991. Critical Periods in Brain Development. In Gregory R. Bock and Julie Whelan, eds., *The Childhood Environment and Adult Disease.* Ciba Foundation Symposium 156. Chichester, England: John Wiley & Sons.

Smedler, A., G. Faxelius, K. Bremme, and M. Lagerström. 1992. Psychological Development in Children Born with Very Low Birth Weight after Severe Intrauterine Growth Retardation: A 10-year Follow-up Study. *Acta Paediatrica* 81:197-203.

Spurr, G. B. 1983. Nutritional Status and Physical Work Capacity. *Yearbook of Physical Anthropology* 26:1-35.

Stein, Z., M. Susser, G. Saenger, and F. Marolla. 1972. Nutrition and Mental Performance. Prenatal Exposure to the Dutch Famine of 1944-1945 Seems Not Related to Mental Performance at Age 19. *Science* 178:708-13.

Stjernqvist, K., and N. W. Svenningsen. 1995. Extremely Low-Birth-Weight Infants Less than 901 g: Development and Behaviour after 4 Years of Life. *Acta Paediatrica* 84:500-06.

Super, C. M., M. G. Herrera, and J. O. Mora. 1990. Long-term Effects of Food Supplementation and Psychosocial Intervention on the Physical Growth of Colombian Infants at Risk of Malnutrition. *Child Development* 61:29-49.

Teberg, A. J., F. J. Walther, and I. C. Peña. 1988. Mortality, Morbidity, and Outcome of the Small-for-Gestational Age Infant. *Seminars in Perinatology* 12(1):84-94.

Tenovuo, A., P. Kero, and H. Korvenranta. 1988. Developmental Outcome of 519 Small-for-Gestational Age Children at the Age of Two Years. *Neuropediatrics* 19:41-45.

The Infant Health and Development Program. 1990. Enhancing the Outcomes of Low-Birth-Weight, Premature Infants. *Journal of the American Medical Association* 263:3035-42.

Uauy, R., and I. de Andraca. 1995. Human Milk and Breast Feeding for Optimal Mental Development. *Journal of Nutrition* 125:2278S-80S.

United Nations Children's Fund. 1993. *The State of the World's Children 1993*. Oxford: Oxford University Press.

Villar, J., and J. M. Belizán. 1982. The Relative Contribution of Prematurity and Fetal Growth Retardation to Low Birth Weight in Developing and Developed Societies. *American Journal of Obstetrics and Gynecology* 143(7):793-98.

Villar, J., L. Altobelli, E. Kestler, and J. Belizán. 1986. A Health Priority for Developing Countries: The Prevention of Chronic Fetal Malnutrition. *Bulletin of the World Health Organization* 64(6):847-51.

Villar, J., U. Farnot, F. Barros, C. Victora, A. Langer, and J. Belizán. 1992. A Randomized Trial of Psychosocial Support during High-risk Pregnancies. *New England Journal of Medicine* 327:1266-71.

Villar, J., V. Smeriglio, R. Martorell, C. H. Brown, and E. Klein. 1984. Heterogeneous Growth and Mental Development of Intrauterine Growth-retarded Infants during the First 3 Years of Life. *Pediatrics* 74(5):783-91.

Waber, D. P., L. Vuori-Christiansen, N. Ortiz, J. R. Clement, N. E. Christiansen, J. O. Mora, R. B. Reed, and M. G. Herrera. 1981. Nutritional Supplementation, Maternal Education, and Cognitive Development of Infants at Risk of Malnutrition. *American Journal of Clinical Nutrition* 34:807-13.

Wachs, T. D. 1995. Relation of Mild-to-Moderate Malnutrition to Human Development: Correlational Studies. *Journal of Nutrition* 125:2245S-54S.

Walker, S. P., C. A. Powell, S. Grantham-McGregor, J. H. Himes, and S. M. Chang. 1991. Nutritional Supplementation, Psychosocial Stimulation, and Growth of Stunted Children: The Jamaican Study. *American Journal of Clinical Nutrition* 54:642-48.

Wallingford, J. C., and B. Underwood. 1986. Vitamin A Deficiency in Pregnancy, Lactation, and the Nursing Child. In J. C. Bauernfeind, ed., *Vitamin A Deficiency and Its Control*. Orlando: Academic Press, Inc.

Walther, F. J. 1988. Growth and Development of Term Disproportionate Small-for-Gestational Age Infants at the Age of 7 Years. *Early Human Development* 18:1-11.

Walther, F. J., and L. H. J. Ramaekers. 1982. Language Development at the Age of 3 Years of Infants Malnourished in Utero. *Neuropediatrics* 13:77-81.

Westwood, M., M. S. Kramer, D. Munz, J. M. Lovett, and G. V. Watters. 1983. Growth and Development of Full-term Nonasphyxiated Small-for-Gestational-Age Newborns: Follow-up through Adolescence. *Pediatrics* 71(3):376-82.

Winick, M., K. K. Meyer, and R. C. Harris. 1975. Malnutrition and Environmental Enrichment by Early Adoption. *Science* 190:1173-75.

World Health Organization. 1985. *Energy and Protein Requirements. Report of a Joint FAO/WHO/UNU Expert Consultation.* Technical Report Series 724. Geneva.

Zigler, E. 1994. Reshaping Early Childhood Intervention To Be a More Effective Weapon against Poverty. *American Journal of Community Psychology* 22(1):37-47.

———. 1995. Editorial: Can We "Cure" Mild Mental Retardation among Individuals in the Lower Socio Economic Stratus? *American Journal of Public Health* 85(3):302-04.

Zigler, E., C. S. Piotrkowski, and R. Collins. 1994. Health Services in Head Start. *Annual Review of Public Health* 15:511-34.

Early Child Development: Investing in our Children's Future
M.E. Young, editor.

Effects of Children's Ill Health on Cognitive Development

Robert J. Sternberg, Elena L. Grigorenko, and Catherine Nokes

Children's cognitive development does not occur independently of the development of their bodies. A complex reciprocal relation exists between children's physical health and their psychological development. The former influences the latter and the latter serves as a buffer between a variety of harmful biological agents and their effect on a child's health.

Many researchers have noted that a child's cognitive development does not take place in a sterile box and should be studied in the context of the developmental niche occupied by the child. Developmental niche refers to the (a) physical and social settings of a child's everyday life, (b) culturally determined patterns of childrearing, and (c) the psychology of caregivers (Harkness and Super 1994). Moreover, a child is born with a particular genetic endowment that predisposes him or her to certain patterns of development. This endowment might put the child at risk for the development of disorders characterized by specific symptoms of cognitive deficiency, such as phenylketonuria (PKU), fragile X syndrome, autism, and Tourette's syndrome. Alternatively, genetic endowment might make a child more susceptible to the adverse effect of biological agents. For example, the intensity of nematode infections seems to be mediated by the inherited characteristics of a child's immune system (Bundy 1994). And certain genetic characteristics have been shown to buffer the magnitude of cognitive impairment resulting from exposure to lead (Bellinger and others 1994).

The etiology of children's ill health is somewhat artificially separated into genetic and environmental causes. These two causes, however, are closely related to each other. For certain genetic conditions to be expressed, a child must be placed in an environment that allows phenotypic expression of the condition, and for certain environmental conditions to affect a child, he or she has to be genetically susceptible to their effect. Although the mechanisms of this genetic-environmental interplay are important, they are not well understood. Many researchers therefore continue to concentrate on understanding the main (noninteractive) effects of genes and environment.

Reflecting this tradition, this chapter reviews some of the effects of environmentally provoked conditions of ill health on children's cognitive development. The chapter complements the two preceding chapters, by Bundy and Martorell, which address related consequences of poor health and undernutrition. The present review is organized by the major manifestations of children's ill health that are caused by environmental agents: undernutrition, infections, and environmental toxins. The chapter highlights the buffering role of a child's microenvironment, that is, the home environment in which the child grows up. To best understand these effects, a model of children's cognitive development, and the effects of environment on this development, is presented first.

A Model of Cognitive Development

Models of cognitive development must address at least three questions. First, is development stagelike or continuous? Second, is development controlled primarily by maturation or by learning in the environment? Third, is development general or specific in particular domains?

In psychology, as in other sciences, researchers and theorists are tempted to take extreme positions on these questions and related issues. For example, the well-known developmental theory of Jean Piaget (1972) states that development is primarily stagelike, maturational, and domain-general. In contrast, most modern information-processing theories (Sternberg 1984; Sternberg and Powell 1983) state that development is primarily continuous, learning-based, and domain-specific.

Theories of cognitive development also differ in the importance ascribed to individual and developmental differences. For example, Piaget viewed the question of individual differences as the "American problem." He believed such differences are relatively minor in comparison with developmental ones. Anderson (1992) believes that individual and developmental differences are equally important, but that they result from distinct mechanisms. The author (Sternberg 1984, 1985) believes that both types of differences are equally important and result from the same mechanisms.

The Cognitive Activation Model

The cognitive activation model proposed in figure 1 is interactive, dealing with the effects of the environment on cognitive development. It proposes that (a) although all children have the capacity to develop cognitive expertise, enabling them to adapt to their environments, (b) a favorable environment activates cognitive mechanisms that are favorable to cognitive development, but (c) an unfavorable environment deactivates cognitive mechanisms, impeding development. In this view development is primarily continuous, although it can appear as stagelike changes when sets of new competencies unfold; maturation and learning can both contribute greatly to cognitive development; and development is domain-general in some aspects and domain-specific in others.

This cognitive activation model views cognitive development as the acquisition of expertise in many cognitive domains. Children start as novices in language, for example, and then acquire different levels of expertise in areas of language, such as reading, writing, speaking, and listening. The key assumption is that children will acquire the various kinds of expertise they need for adapting to the world if given a supportive social environment and if relatively free from noxious influences (both genetic and environmental). Because no environment is fully supportive or fully free from noxious influences, children develop only a portion of the expertise of which they are capable. But the children retain what Vygotsky (1978) refers to as a zone of potential (or proximal) development: If given more support, and if freed from noxious influences, they can acquire expertise in areas of development that might have been suppressed in the past, or they can compensate for previously impaired functions.

This model can be divided into the internal and external attributes shown in table 1, which interact with each other and are equally important. The five main kinds of interactive *internal attributes* include: (a) metacognitive skills, such as problem

Figure 1. The Cognitive Activation Model of Development

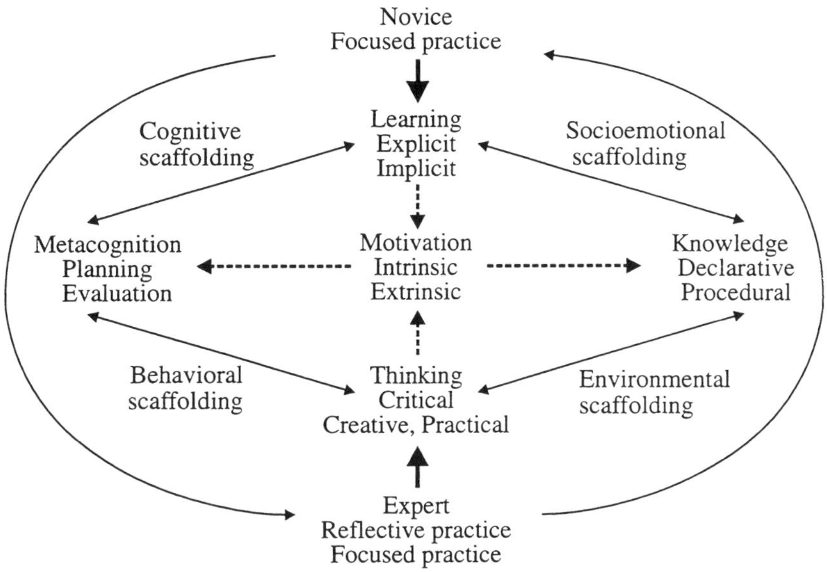

identification (what is the nature of the problem confronting me?), strategy formulation (how can I solve the problem?), and solution evaluation (is my solution to the problem correct?); (b) learning skills, such as selective combination (how do the things I am learning fit together?) and selective comparison (how does what I am learning relate to what I already know?); (c) thinking skills, such as critical thinking (how do I critique, judge, compare and contrast, evaluate, and analyze?), creative thinking (how do I discover, invent, imagine, suppose, hypothesize?), and practical thinking (how do I relate what I learn to my everyday life and to practical issues I face?); (d) motivational skills, such as achievement and motivation (is this a moderate risk or challenge?) and competence motivation (can I believe in my ability to meet this challenge?); and (e) knowledge-based skills, such as declarative knowledge (do I know what I need to know?) and procedural knowledge (do I know how to do what I need to do?).

The four main kinds of interactive *external attributes* include: (a) environmental scaffolding (support), such as adequate nutrition (is a child well nourished, both at a given time and in general?), freedom from infection (is a child in good health, both at a given time and in general?), and adequate quality of environment (is a child in danger of living in a toxic environment?); (b) cognitive scaffolding, such as cognitive stimulation and intervention and adequate education (is a child receiving cognitive support for thinking and learning in the home, school, and general environment?); (c) socioemotional scaffolding, such as formation of intrinsic motivation and emotional support and acceptance (is a child receiving socioemotional support for thinking and learning?); and (d) behavioral scaffolding, such as positive attitudes toward performance, adequate protection, and adequate levels of expectation (is a child receiving support for translating cognitive

Table 1. Interactive Attributes of the Cognitive Activation Model

Internal attributes	External attributes
Metacognitive skills	Environmental scaffolding
Problem identification	Adequate nutrition
Strategy formation	Freedom from infection
Solution evaluation	Adequate quality of environment (freedom from intoxication and danger)
Learning skills	
Selective combination	Cognitive scaffolding
Selective comparison	Cognitive stimulation and intervention
	Adequate education
Thinking skills	
Critical thinking	Socioemotional scaffolding
Creative thinking	Formation of intrinsic motivation
Practical thinking	Emotional support and acceptance
Motivational skills	Behavioral scaffolding
Achievement motivation	Positive attitudes toward performance
Competence motivation	Adequate protection
	Adequate levels of expectation
Knowledge-based skills	
Declarative knowledge	
Procedural knowledge	

development into behavior and for translating competencies into performance?). The concept of scaffolding as a supportive technique for intervention is described in greater detail in the accompanying chapter by Sternberg and Grigorenko (this volume).

A Comparable Model

Another model of cognitive development, proposed by Levinger (1994), was designed to address the effects of forces such as undernutrition, infection, and environmental toxins on children's cognitive development. In this model, Levinger refers to two kinds of characteristics that children bring to the classroom: primary variables and secondary variables. Primary variables include health and nutritional status, psychosocial support, and hunger level, all of which interact with each other. Secondary variables include prior learning experience, aptitude (such as intelligence quotient, IQ), and learning receptiveness. Primary and secondary variables interact with each other.

Levinger also suggests a different set of characteristics belonging to the classroom setting, called mitigating variables. These include intervention strategies, such as deworming and sensory impairment screening, and classroom characteristics, such as learning resources and teacher quality. Primary, secondary, and mitigating variables combine to produce active learning capacity.

The cognitive activation model differs from Levinger's model in three key respects. First, the cognitive activation model is one of developing expertise. It postulates that almost all children can reach levels of expertise enabling them to adapt to sociocultural demands. It rejects IQ and related measures as indicating limitations in the cognitive capacity of a child; such measures are narrow and bound by culture, and their scores frequently translate into self-fulfilling prophecies (Sternberg 1985, 1988, 1990). Although results of such measures can be reported, they must be interpreted with due caution.

Second, the cognitive activation model does not present external attributes (such as health and nutrition status) as primary variables and internal attributes (such as prior learning experience) as secondary variables. Both types of attributes are fully interactive, and assigning primary or secondary importance to them is not entirely meaningful. For example, children who do not develop learning or thinking skills will not exhibit these skills even if they are in perfect health, and children who have developed learning or thinking skills but have seriously compromised health are unlikely to be able to use or further develop these skills. Third, the cognitive activation model emphasizes maximizing actualized capacity, or accomplishment, instead of absolute capacity. Except in extreme cases, all children have the capacity to learn, and they need to be given the kinds of environments that allow them to fully use this capacity.

Summary

As illustrated in figure 1, the cognitive activation model postulates that various types of scaffolding, or external attributes, interact with internal attributes of a child and facilitate or impede cognitive development. The roles of socioemotional, cognitive, and behavioral supports (scaffolding) are addressed in other chapters of this volume. The effects of a child's ill health, caused by such environmental agents as undernutrition, childhood infection, and environmental toxins, on mental development are described below.

Undernutrition and Mental Development

Undernutrition remains a serious public health problem in today's world because of (a) an inability or unwillingness to control population growth in some countries, especially developing ones; (b) marginal food production worldwide; and (c) unbalanced food distribution, even within most industrialized countries (Freeman and others 1980). An estimated 3 percent of the world's children suffer one or more episodes of severe undernutrition before reaching 5 years of age (Behar 1968). About one-half of preschool children in developing countries and a small, yet significant proportion of children from low-income families in industrialized nations are undernourished (Freeman and others 1980).

Although some investigators believe in possible political and research bias in interpretation of existing evidence (Ricciuti 1991), the general consensus and several hypotheses link various types of undernutrition to cognitive impairment (Grantham-McGregor 1988). First, undernutrition may result in direct or indirect permanent anatomical or biochemical changes in the brain. Second, undernutrition may reduce activity, search for stimulation, and exploration, which all induce cognitive development in children. Third, altered cognitive and socioemotional behaviors of a child may cause a corresponding lack of reciprocal responsiveness, acceptance, and attachment in an adult, amplifying the magnitude of the problem.

Comprehensive reviews of the research literature on connections between undernutrition and cognitive development have been published (Lozoff 1988; Martorell, this volume; Pollitt and Metallinos-Katsaras 1990; Simeon and Grantham-McGregor 1990). Using the most recent research, this chapter presents the effects of various nutritional deficiencies on cognitive development in infants and school-aged children. Nutritional deficiencies include protein-energy malnutrition (PEM), short-term food deprivation, and inadequate levels of certain minerals and vitamins (micronutrients), such as zinc, iron, iodine, thiamine, and vitamin A.

PEM

PEM is a global term referring to various unfavorable conditions caused by nutrient deficiencies of varying type, severity, and duration. The deficiencies are inflicted at different stages of development and complicated by varying amounts of infection, resulting in children with inadequate ratios of weight for age, height for age, or weight for height (Grantham-McGregor 1988, 1990). PEM (undernutrition) is due mostly to inadequate nutrient intake; however, it might also result from infection, injury, chronic disease, or excessive nutrient loss (such as occurs with chronic diarrhea).

In childhood, undernutrition is the single most important cause of growth retardation. Severe PEM during critical phases of growth may significantly reduce the size and function of specific organs. In addition, undernutrition depresses the host's immune response and may increase susceptibility to infection. The severity of PEM often is determined by clinical signs and physical growth.

Severe undernutrition includes *kwashiorkor*, which is characterized by severe protein deficiency, growth retardation, changes in skin and hair pigment, edema, and pathological changes in the liver; *marasmic kwashiorkor*, which is characterized by a deficiency of calories and protein with severe wasting of the tissues, loss of subcutaneous fat, and usually dehydration; and *marasmus*, which is characterized by severe growth retardation, weight loss, and wasting of muscle and subcutaneous fat. Moderate PEM refers to weights and heights below 75 or 80 percent of age- and sex-specific standards (Simeon and Grantham-McGregor 1990). Severe PEM usually is restricted to infants (except during famine), and mild or moderate PEM is found more commonly in infants and school-age children.

The most frequent measures of body growth used to define PEM are: weight for age, which indicates acute and current nutritional status; height for age, which indicates chronic and past nutritional status; and weight for height, which indicates wasting. Ratios of height for age, weight for age, and weight for height are determined from sex- and age-specific reference tables and usually are expressed as Z scores.

A vast amount of evidence indicates that all serious, chronic nutritional deficiencies detrimentally affect cognitive functioning in children. Experimental research in this field is difficult to conduct for a number of ethical and organizational reasons. For example, severe PEM resulting from seasonal changes in food availability is difficult to study because the availability of food cannot be anticipated and the collection and distribution of food, not cognitive assessment, is given priority when food is scarce. For these reasons only one observational study has been conducted of a severe drought and temporary food shortage (McDonald and others 1994). Several studies have investigated the effects of long-term undernutrition (see Martorell, this volume). For example, severely chronically undernourished children, who were examined at the time of hospitalization, demonstrated cognitive and socioemotional deficits in comparison to a control group comprised of adequately nourished children treated for other diseases (Grantham-McGregor, Schofield, and Powell 1987).

To examine the long-term effects of chronic undernutrition, researchers have used four different types of studies: with matched controls, with sibling controls, in industrialized countries, and adoption studies. The results of these studies are equivocal; some of them show an association between poor nutrition and cognitive impairment, and others fail to establish this connection. However, similarities among the studies, despite their inevitable methodological and ethical complications, suggest a strong link between severe undernutrition and poor cognitive and socioemotional development. Table 2 summarizes the findings from studies of short- and long-term undernutrition in children of varying ages.

Table 2. Effects of Short- and Long-term Undernutrition

Severe undernutrition	Acute stage	Developmental outcomes
Short term Seasonal hunger	Impaired attention in school-age children, but no alteration of cognitive abilities in toddlers	Moderate or rapid improvements in cognitive functioning when adequately nourished
Long term Mixed severe PEM Kwashiorkor Marasmic kwashiorkor Marasmus	Cognitive and socioemotional impairment with little improvement at recovery	Tends to be associated with long-term deficits in global cognitive functioning unless the child is well nourished and placed in an enriched environment

Although mild and moderate PEM are much more prevalent than severe undernutrition, data regarding the effects of mild and moderate undernutrition are more controversial than data from studies of severe undernutrition (see Martorell, this volume). Two main design methodologies have been used to examine the effects of mild and moderate PEM on cognitive development. The first design methodology involves observational studies. Most of these have shown the association between nutritional status and cognitive development; height for age is more frequently related to cognitive impairment than weight for height (Simeon and Grantham-McGregor 1990).

The second design methodology involves supplementation studies. In industrialized countries supplementation of low-income pregnant women shows no conclusive results; in 75 percent of the studies, a high-protein supplementation did not benefit these women's offspring. In four preventive studies from developing countries, supplementation of pregnant women benefited their offspring; in three studies of undernourished children in these countries, supplementation alone had small or insignificant effects, but when combined with social stimulation it benefited children significantly. Mild and moderate undernutrition seem to result in a concurrent cognitive deficit (primarily motor-explorational skills) that appears to be reversible with proper supplementation and social stimulation.

Although these different studies of PEM have many complications and research design flaws, the flaws are different, lending credence to the combined results of the studies. The combined results show deficits in the mental functioning of severely undernourished children as well as significant effects from nutritional and stimulative rehabilitation and preventive supplementation. In particular, the findings consistently show that undernutrition in infancy primarily affects development of motor skills, whereas long-term effects are related to scholastic achievement and composite measures of cognitive performance, such as IQ.

Attempts to describe a "cognitive signature" of undernutrition by studying specific cognitive functions have not yet shown conclusive results. The effect of undernutrition is complex, and the extent to which PEM affects children's cognition varies according to the nature and severity of the undernutrition. However, little understanding exists of the differential effects of various types of PEM or of the differential significance of length of exposure or severity for specific cognitive functions.

Regarding the mechanism of PEM, the general consensus is that transient cognitive and socioemotional changes accompanying severe undernutrition have a metabolic basis (Simeon and Grantham-McGregor 1990). Understanding the mechanism that links PEM to long-term developmental impairments is more challenging. Two main hypotheses, which are not mutually exclusive, have been suggested regarding this mechanism. According to the first hypothesis, if transient behavior changes (such as reduced attention, activity, and exploration) occur repeatedly or continue for a long time, they result in developmental delays.

According to the second hypothesis, severe PEM results in irreversible effects on the brain that are manifested in cognitive and behavioral changes. For example, undernutrition may affect neurotransmitter synthesis; activation or inhibition of specific cell types in the brain; or precursors of cellular membrane receptors involved in intercellular recognition processes. Neither of the two hypotheses has been proven.

Short-term Food Deprivation

To understand the effects of short-term food deprivation on cognitive development, researchers have investigated the effects of a child missing breakfast. This event occurs in both industrialized and developing countries with only one difference: frequency. For this reason, comparing results across the two types of countries is more appropriate for these studies than for long-term food deprivation studies. Crossover designs also may be applied to missing-breakfast studies; the subjects' cognitive performance is compared using two treatment conditions: with and without breakfast.

Results of the missing-breakfast studies have been inconsistent (Craig 1986). Two studies showed a deterioration in cognitive performance after subjects missed breakfast (Conners and Blouin 1983; Tuttle and others 1954), but three other studies found no effects of missing breakfast (Dickie and Bender 1982; Upadhyay and others 1988). Results of two other studies, in which researchers controlled for the level of children's IQ, showed adverse effects of fasting on the children's problem solving performance, and children with low IQ were more disadvantaged than those with higher IQ (Pollitt, Leibel, and Greenfield 1981; Pollitt and others 1983). However in both studies controlling for IQ levels, fasting had a beneficial effect on immediate recall, irrespective of IQ.

The most consistent and comprehensive results of missing breakfast have been obtained in a carefully controlled study conducted in Jamaica (Simeon and Grantham-McGregor 1989). Effects of omitting breakfast were compared in matched groups of children with stunted growth (low height for age), without stunted growth, and severely undernourished. Cognitive performance in both undernourished groups deteriorated, while controls improved in arithmetic and in efficiency of problem solving. Wasted children (with low weight for height) from any group showed impairment in memory. Undernourished children in general are more at risk for deficient cognitive performance when missing breakfast.

No clear understanding exists of the mechanism connecting omitting breakfast to cognitive decline. Among the hypotheses are that: metabolic changes resulting from missing meals increase arousal levels which, in turn, influence the quality of cognitive performance; and metabolic changes related to missing meals may produce changes in neurotransmitter precursors that control behavior (Simeon and Grantham-McGregor 1990).

Mineral and Vitamin (Micronutrient) Deficiencies

Throughout research on the general impact of malnutrition on cognitive development, scientists have tried to understand the effect of element-specific deficiencies. Such deficiencies usually result from lack of a particular element in the overall diet of a population, whether through particular food consumption characteristics, characteristics of the soil where products are grown, or inefficient absorption of micronutrients from food.

All types of micronutrient deficiencies exist on a continuum ranging from element-deficient to element-replete. Extreme forms of element-specific deficiencies resulting in qualitatively distinct and usually irreversible states (such as endemic cretinism resulting from extreme iodine deficiency) have been described and fairly well studied. However, a large body of evidence, accumulated during the last few years, suggests that mild deficiencies of specific elements also are associated with impaired cognitive development, constituting an important public health problem.

Supplementation Effects. Significant interest in studying the effects of mineral and vitamin deficiency on cognitive functioning in otherwise adequately nourished children is grounded in a desire (a) to find alternatives for social ways of stimulating cognitive development among children of lower socioeconomic status (SES) in industrialized countries (Eysenck and Schoenthaler 1996) and (b) to understand the effect of nutrition on cognitive development.

The first objective is based on claims made by some researchers that vitamin and mineral supplementation (VMS) may raise IQ (Dean and Morgenthaler 1990; Dean, Morgenthaler, and Fowkes 1993) and that the recent worldwide increases in IQ (1 standard deviation during the past half-century) (Flynn 1987) are largely attributable to improved nutrition in industrialized nations (Lynn 1990). The second objective is based on the fact that a minority of individuals in industrialized countries have deficient or marginal vitamin and mineral intake (Benton 1992b). Some researchers (Yudkin 1991) argue that nutrient intake, classified as recommended dietary allowance and used as a criterion of normal nutrition in Western countries, is below the level corresponding to optimal cognitive functioning. Finding groups in a population of school-age children that are responsive to VMS may lead to a better understanding of the overall effects of nutrition on cognitive development.

During the past decade most of a number of well-designed, double-blind, placebo-controlled studies have shown an association between VMS and cognitive improvements (Eysenck and Schoenthaler 1996). However, much criticism and many unresolved questions surround these findings. Major criticisms of studies showing the positive effect of VMS are related to: the nutritional characteristics of the responding population; lack of dietary information in the population studied, which leads to unclear observed effects (presumably, respondents react to the component of the complex supplement that they lack); failure to account for practice effects in taking the test; and lack of specificity of related cognitive effects. For example, Benton (1992b) suggests that apparent improvement in nonverbal IQ could result from improved attention. However, the results of his attempt to test this hypothesis were inconclusive (Benton and Cook 1991).

In general, researchers (Benton 1992; Eysenck and Schoenthaler 1996; Nelson 1992) agree that:

- Inadequate levels of vitamins and minerals in the bloodstream reduce intellectual performance below a child's optimal level.

- VMS, in addition to a child's standard diet, seems to be associated with a rise in nonverbal (fluid) IQ, but not in verbal (crystallized) IQ. The improvement is not distributed equally; the worse the pretreatment academic performance, the larger the gain (Eysenck and Schoenthaler 1996).

- No effect of VMS has been shown for children already ingesting adequate levels of vitamins and minerals.

- Effects are significant for younger children, but little difference is made by VMS beyond adolescence.

- The observed gender effect may be attributable to the fact that adolescent girls benefit most because of a higher prevalence of iron deficiency that is related to menstrual cycles.

Because adequate levels of minerals and vitamins are important to a child's cognitive development and even mild deficiencies can impair that development, an understanding of specific, key elements is necessary. Effects from deficiencies in the minerals zinc, iron, and iodine and vitamins thiamine and A are described below.

Zinc Deficiency

Because zinc is essential to the mitotic division of cells, it is thought to be a critical element for neuronal growth and nucleic acid metabolism (Pfeiffer and Braverman 1982; Sandstead 1985). Zinc deprivation in prenatal, perinatal, and infant stages of development can result in nonspecific biochemical and morphological brain abnormalities and severe growth retardation (Bergmann and Bergmann 1985; Hambridge 1977; Hambridge and others 1972; Pollitt and Metallinos-Katsaras 1990; Walravens and Hambridge 1976). Although low levels of dietary zinc seem related to a range of children's cognitive and socioemotional problems, specific attempts to find a direct correspondence between dietary zinc intake and particular childhood deficits have not yet been rewarding; almost all of the accumulated data are primarily correlational.

Zinc deficiency has been linked to a number of poor health conditions and impairments. For example, *acrodermatitis enteropathica*, a human hereditary dysfunction of zinc absorption, is associated with apathy, lethargy, depression, amnesia, and mental retardation (Walravens and others 1981). Also, starvation increases the urinary excretion of zinc and worsens the effect of low dietary zinc intake. In addition, an experimentally induced deficiency of zinc has been associated with anorexia and impairment of taste and smell (Henkin and others 1973), suggesting that a vicious circle can become established; starvation leads to loss of zinc, which in turn, leads to suppression of taste and smell and a lack of desire for food. Grant and colleagues (1988) studied the concentration of zinc in the sweat and hair of dyslexics and found reduced amounts of zinc in the sweat. Even though zinc is, after iron, the most prevalent trace element in the brain, few attempts have been made to study psychological functioning while manipulating zinc levels. In one study of psychological functioning and zinc, Tucker and Sandstead (1984) followed five volunteers for 4 months who had been put on a diet deficient in zinc, but they did not find any effect of zinc deficiency on cognitive functioning.

Iron Deficiency

Iron deficiency is a highly prevalent problem globally (Scrimshaw 1991) and is considered to be the most frequent cause of anemia, which is manifest in an estimated 46 to 51 percent of children from less developed regions and in 7 to 12 percent of children from more developed regions throughout the world (DeMaeyer and Adiels-Tegman 1985). A number of studies have associated iron deficiency with impairment of cognitive functioning. However, many of the studies were confounded by poor nutrition and health and by social circumstance. Nutritional confounders of the effect of iron deficiency, especially in developing countries, are zinc deficiency and PEM. Iron also is important in the absorption of lead and cadmium, which in turn, are potentially detrimental to cognitive development, especially in metropolitan areas. The etiology of iron-deficiency anemia in populations where iron deficiency is highly prevalent could be heterogeneous, caused by factors such as low presence of iron in the diet, chronic blood loss from various parasitic infections, malaria, and the presence of some genetic blood diseases, such as sickle cell anemia and thalassemia (Pollitt and Metallinos-Katsaras 1990).

A large body of evidence also indicates that children with similar types of early nutritional trauma vary in developmental outcomes depending on their social and family environments, which could buffer or even neutralize adverse effects on cognitive functioning associated with biological assaults (Farran and McKinney 1986). These buffers, or naturally occurring confounders of iron deficiency, make accurate testing of causality between iron deficiency and impairment of cognitive development difficult.

Despite difficulties related to the study of iron deficiency, it is a public health problem, constituting a developmental risk factor that increases the probability of deviation from the expected path of development (Pollitt 1993). During the past decade an increasing number of experimental studies have been done with children deficient in iron, investigating the effects of iron treatment and controlling for confounding effects whenever possible.

Results of this research, although somewhat controversial, are highly consistent. Many observational studies demonstrate a statistical association between various types of iron deficiency and cognitive underachievement in infants and school-age children. Most experimental clinical trials show that iron treatment benefits some cognitive and psychomotor functions and academic achievements of infants and children. On average, iron deficiency "is associated with poor performance in infant developmental scales, IQ and learning tasks in preschool children, and educational achievement among school-age children" (Pollitt 1993: 524), even though about 30 percent of the studies listed show no or very little effect from iron treatment, and making definitive causal inferences on the basis of these findings is often impossible because of other adverse environmental and nutritional conditions occurring with iron deficiency.

Evidence of respectable magnitude shows that infants, toddlers, and school-age children with iron-deficiency anemia perform worse on cognitive tests than children of corresponding ages with sufficient levels of iron. Moreover, iron-anemic children consistently benefit from short- and long-term iron treatment. The majority of studies have demonstrated that iron therapy for these children improves their performance on selective learning and school achievement tests (Pollitt and Metallinos-Katsaras 1990). These studies are unique because consistent evidence links such specific cognitive processes as memory and attention of school-age children to a cognitive signature of iron anemia. Although findings in infancy and early childhood are more diffuse, they point repeatedly to deficient motor development.

Inconsistencies of findings on iron deficiency and its effects on cognitive development are related primarily to the presence of mild and moderate iron deficiency. Inconsistency also may be attributed to methodological imperfection of relevant studies as well as to a lack of understanding about the specific nature of psychological effects associated with iron deficiency.

Precise mechanisms for the effect of iron-deficiency anemia on cognition and behavior are unknown. Because iron is involved in synthesis and degradation of the neurotransmitters catecholamines and serotonin, iron deficiency is associated with reduced activity of monoamine oxidases (MAO) involved in the catabolism of catecholamines (reduced activity of MAO is related to an increased amount of noradrenaline). Iron deficiency also is associated with a decreased amount of aldehyde oxidase involved in the degradation of serotonin. Presumably, the biochemical activity of these iron-dependent enzymes can lead researchers to an understanding of the link between iron deficiency and cognitive functioning (Wharton 1995).

Iodine Deficiency

Iodine deficiency is the most common cause of mental retardation in the world, and endemic goiter is the most frequently observed iodine deficiency, having an estimated global prevalence of 190 million. Also, about 3.5 million people are thought to suffer from cretinism resulting from iodine deficiency. An estimated 800 million people are at risk from iodine deficiency disorders because of iodine poor environments (Hetzel 1987). These at-risk populations include more than 300 million people in China, 200 million in India, 150 million in Africa, and smaller but significant numbers in Latin America and other parts of Asia. The reason for persistent iodine deficiency among these populations is that most depend on local agriculture; they are locked into a cycle of iodine deficiency as long as they consume the local food (Hetzel 1989).

Iodine-deficiency disorders cover a broad spectrum of detrimental impairments resulting from deficiency of iron and occurring at all stages of development (intrauterine, neonatal, childhood, adulthood). Such disorders include goiter, endemic cretinism, hypothyroidism, neuromotor delays, and deaf-mutism, as well as increased pre- and postnatal mortality (Stanbury 1987; Stanbury and Hetzel 1980).

Endemic cretinism (neurological and myxedematous) results from severe iodine deficiency during pregnancy, causing deficits in fetal brain maturation (Ma and others 1993). The components of neurological cretinism are mental retardation, spastic-rigid motor disorder, and deaf-mutism. Symptoms of myxedematous cretinism include mental retardation and dwarfism. Halpern and colleagues (1991) studied both types of endemic cretinism in China and concluded that the same neurological disorder, reflecting a nonspecific insult to the developing fetal nervous system, is present in both types. Researchers believe that the effects of cretinism on mental function result from structural and functional damage to the brain and are irreversible, susceptible to remediation only to a very small degree. Whether endemic cretinism can be prevented in the neonatal period is unknown, but iodine treatment at birth does not prevent it (Pharoah, Buttfield, and Hetzel 1972).

Children who do not suffer from severe cretinism may experience subclinical deficits of motor and cognitive function from mild and moderate iodine deficiency (Connolly, Pharoah, and Hetzel 1979). Such deficits are manifested by low IQ scores, hyperactivity and short attention spans, impaired spatial orientation, specific mathematics disability, and difficulties with fine motor coordination (New England Congenital Hypothyroidism Collaborative 1981). Cognitive impairments milder than mental retardation occur approximately 5 times as frequently as cretinism in iodine-deficient populations (Boyages and others 1989; Ma and others 1989). The IQ curve in these populations shifts as much as ten points to the left (Bleichrodt and others 1989).

Researchers conducted a number of studies using iodine supplementation in geographic areas with a natural deficiency of iodine in the soil (Bautista and others 1982; Bleichrodt and others 1987; Connolly, Pharoah, and Hetzel 1979; Fierro-Benitez and others 1986; Xue-Yi and others 1994). In general, iodine deficiency is associated with mental and motor development impairments. These studies showed that when pregnant mothers received iodine supplements, their children performed better than children of mothers not receiving the supplements during pregnancy (Bleichrodt and others 1989; Connolly, Pharoah, and Hetzel 1979; Fierro-Benitez and others 1986; Xue-Yi and others 1994). Supplementation should be provided either before or during early stages of pregnancy.

Not much evidence exists about the effects of iodine supplementation in school-age children. Although in one study iodine supplementation significantly decreased thyroid function, no IQ differences were found for children in the treatment group compared with controls (Bautista and others 1982). However, a significant relationship between goiter reduction and IQ improvement was observed.

In general, iodine deficiency can be prevented, but early diagnosis of individuals who are at risk is crucial. Iodine supplementation must take place before conception or during early stages of pregnancy to prevent the neurological damage that develops from endemic cretinism at very early stages of fetal development (Hetzel and Mano 1989; New England Congenital Hypothyroidism Collaborative 1981). Whether cretinism can be prevented or ameliorated by treatment during late stages of pregnancy or after delivery is unknown (Xue-Yi and others 1994). Based on the results of rat studies, some researchers caution that supplementation be administered carefully because excess amounts of iodine may lead to acute inhibition of the thyroid (Kochupillai and others 1986). This concern, however, has not been supported (Pharoah and Connolly 1991).

Thiamine Deficiency

Thiamine is a vitamin necessary to release energy from carbohydrates. The amount of thiamine required by an organism is determined by the amount of carbohydrates in the diet. For example, much of the population in the Far East, where the main diet consists of rice, needs relatively more thiamine than other populations to release the energy of their high carbohydrate food. The precise effects of thiamine on cognitive development have not been well studied. A set of tests, conducted before and after supplementing a group of children with 2 milligrams of thiamine or a placebo every day for a year, showed significant improvements in the thiamine group. These children grew taller and had better eyesight, shorter reaction times, better memory, and higher scores on intelligence tests than children receiving the placebo (Benton 1992a).

Vitamin A Deficiency

Severe vitamin A deficiency could be a risk factor of childhood illness and mortality in developing countries. Some studies have indicated that intensive supplementation with vitamin A reduces mortality in populations deficient in the vitamin (Daulaire and others 1992; Muhilal and others 1988; Rahmathullah and others 1990; Sommer and others 1986; West and others 1991), although another study showed no beneficial effect (Vijayarghavan and others 1990).

Even mild and moderate vitamin A deficiencies can cause visual impairment (xerophthalmia) of various degrees of severity (Congdon and others 1995; WHO/UNICEF/International Vitamin A Consultative Group Task Force 1988). In general, the severity of the impairment parallels the severity of the deficiency, although no straightforward linear relation has been established and no implication exists that both eyes are involved. Xerophthalmia can be found in all age groups; however, preschool children (6 months to 6 years) are the group at highest risk. The mechanism of this effect is unknown. Xerophthalmia could result from lack of variety in younger children's diets as well as to the fact that school-age children have been studied less than preschool children. A preliminary estimate of the incidence of xerophthalmia blindness worldwide is 100,000, and the prevalence of noncorneal xerophthalmia is suggested to be much higher (8 million to 9 million). The prevalence of vitamin A deficiency among school-age children is estimated at about 85 million (Levinger 1994).

All formal studies investigating the cognitive or academic correlates of vitamin A deficiency have been done within the context of special education, partly because severe deficiency causes blindness, which often leads to placement in special education. However, blindness resulting from xerophthalmia certainly could affect school performance, especially in poorly lit classrooms. Because vitamin A helps maintain the mucosal epithelium, its deficiency can increase susceptibility to respiratory infections. Infections induced by vitamin A deficiency result in a higher mortality rate in infancy and could lead to a higher rate of absenteeism from school in school-age children.

Summary

Studying the effects of undernutrition, PEM, short-term food deprivation, and element-specific deficiencies on children's cognitive development shows that:

- Severe PEM or element-specific deficiencies adversely affect children's cognitive development, and some adverse effects are irreversible but may be prevented.

- Although the precise effect of moderate undernutrition is difficult to quantify, it is associated statistically with specific impairments in cognitive development, suggesting that undernutrition does not help children reach their optimal development.

- With the exception of outcomes from severe iodine deficiency, cognitive outcomes resulting from undernutrition can be reversed if a child is properly treated and socially rehabilitated in time.

- Remedial efforts for undernutrition should not stop at the moment of discharge from hospitals; without adequate nutrition and social stimulation in their developmental niche, children will most likely continue to suffer from dramatic long-term cognitive impairments throughout adolescence and adulthood.

Studies of the effects of undernutrition show truly interactive relationships, as illustrated by the cognitive activation model, among a child's nutritional status, various types of scaffolding provided by school systems and caregivers, and a child's motivation and ability to become an expert. Adequate nutrition is necessary, but without improving a child's support system it is not sufficient for a child's optimal cognitive development. The probability of children becoming experts in a particular activity depends on minimizing the probability of undernutrition and maximizing the probability of adequate scaffolding.

Several explanations are given for the uncertainty of conclusions and causal inferences from studies of less severe and moderate undernutrition. First, the main complication faced by researchers is the close link between undernutrition and other deficient socioeconomic conditions, which can significantly deter the cognitive development of children. Researchers readily admit that they do not have a satisfactory method of separating these social effects from the biological effects of undernutrition, and they are well aware of the methodological problems they face when conducting a study to yield causal inferences (Fairchild, Haas, and Habicht 1989).

Ricciuti (1993) suggests that many methodological flaws and inconsistencies result from the simplistic view of undernutrition as a direct, independent cause of significantly impaired learning and intellectual development. Leading to further inconsistencies is the false assumption that adequate nourishment alone can improve cognitive development. Under the influence of Ricciuti and other scientists, awareness has increased of the need to identify differential interactive (nutrition by social environment) effects. For example, the effects of additive coaction (Grantham-McGregor and others 1991; Super and others 1981, 1990) are demonstrated by greater levels of activity in infants who have received both food supplementation and psychosocial stimulation than in infants not receiving both. When children are exposed to both undernutrition and an inadequate psychosocial environment, the effects of synergetic interactions (Pollitt 1988) are detrimental and are associated with a higher probability of delay in cognitive development.

Buffering stimulation is an important part of interaction. It means establishing enriched psychosocial programs, providing better schooling, and educating parents to strengthen the scaffolding of a child's development. Buffering stimulation can protect children at risk for undernutrition from cognitive impairments and can ensure complete cognitive rehabilitation at recovery (Sigman and others 1988; Zeskind and Ramey 1981). The effects of buffering stimulation, however, are applicable only under conditions of long-term psychosocial stimulation and continuation of the intervention in supportive home environments (Cravioto and Arrieta 1979; Grantham-McGregor, Schofield, and Powell 1987; McKay and others 1978; McLaren and others 1973).

Other important interactions recognized by researchers include interaction among the constitution of an organism, the biological risk factor and its severity and chronicity, and the general environment in which an organism develops (Pollitt and Metallinos-Katsaras 1990). Another important interaction variable is related to duration of treatment or supplementation. Because the optimal length of treatment is unknown, a number of studies using short-term treatments may not have had enough time to show improvement. Researchers also tend to ignore individual differences in undernourished children while studying the effect of treatment and do not consider the individual specificity of children's developmental clocks.

Despite major methodological debates (concerning interaction, for example) and accomplishments, many recent studies of the effects of undernutrition are still limited by: inadequate characterization of subjects' overall nutritional status, lack of appropriate normal controls, omission of a group treated with placebo, or failure to demonstrate changes in behavior after nutrition therapy (Lozoff 1988; Pollitt and Metallinos-Katsaras 1990). However, even with methodological problems and other limitations, a few well-designed studies attempting to control for many confounding variables have distinctly shown adverse effects from undernutrition. The number of these studies is relatively small, but they provide robust and conclusive results: various forms of undernutrition have a detrimental effect on cognitive development.

A second explanation for the uncertainty of conclusions and causal inferences from studies of undernutrition is that measuring undernutrition status poses a serious problem. Diagnosis of undernutrition is not straightforward, and often researchers use indirect anthropometric or biochemical measures (such as hemoglobin value) as a substitute for nutritional status. These proxies can vary across different populations because they may be outcomes of evolutionary mechanisms specific to each population. For example, the anthropometric reference values of people in New Guinea can differ from those of Chinese. This population specificity makes comparing results obtained in various countries difficult (Pollitt 1990). The criterion of classifying children into deficient and replete groups also could be population-specific. Inconclusive results of studies conducted in different populations, therefore, may result from failing to adjust the categorizing threshold to population-specific reference values.

Other issues relevant to measuring undernutrition status are severity and duration of the insult. Even though a number of studies have tried to collect retrospective information on the severity and duration of undernutrition, only longitudinal studies that try to determine the severity of the insult for every child will be able to provide more conclusive information about specific cognitive profiles associated with different severity and duration of undernutrition.

Finally, one of the most obvious flaws in current studies of the effect of undernutrition on a child's cognitive and socioemotional development is failing to incorporate general developmental theory into the research. Few studies link psychological theory and undernutrition. Studies of undernutrition generally are characterized by mosaicism in psychological measures used, and most of these are aggregate measures. Aggregate measures of psychological development (for example, developmental and intellectual quotients), which often are culturally inappropriate, may add noise to research, suppressing the obvious effects of undernutrition.

Many researchers advocate testing a child's learning rather than a child's products (for example, Dietrich and Bellinger 1994). In line with the cognitive activation model, a measure of a child's expertise in a given activity may be used as an indicator of observed improvement or lack of improvement. This suggestion is costly because culturally specific dynamic tests must be developed to measure "live cognitive action" rather than measuring a repository of knowledge or skills already acquired, which intelligence tests usually measure. However, because conventional tests do not easily capture the process of acquiring expertise, culturally specific dynamic tests would be a wise investment.

Failure to account for the specificity of different developmental functions also can explain the controversy regarding evidence on the importance of time of the insult. Some researchers suggest that late onset of undernutrition is more detrimental than early onset, but others believe that the first weeks of life may be the most critical for nutrition (Lucas and others 1990). Both of these assumptions could be correct. Late onset of undernutrition could deter development of higher-order cognitive functions, which maturate at later stages of development. Early insult might result in deficiencies of more basic functions, such as attention and memory. If proper nutrition were provided, deficiencies of more basic functions could be compensated for by development of higher-order cognitive functions. Because study results are difficult to interpret, researchers should underscore the importance of developmental theory as a framework for future studies (Colletta and others 1993; Horowitz 1989).

These three considerations (the interaction of other elements with undernutrition, difficulties in measuring undernutrition, and the importance of developmental theory) may explain the inconsistency of current findings and suggest a new perspective for further studies. This new perspective is called the study of the ecology of undernutrition (Pollitt 1988; Ricciuti 1991).

Childhood Infections and Cognitive Development

From the moment of birth to mid-adolescence, children's contact with viruses, bacteria, and other microorganisms far exceeds their contact with other human beings. Various types of infection constitute the largest proportion of childhood diseases and can affect a child's cognitive development. Some major types of childhood infections, described below in their relation to cognitive development, include human immunodeficiency virus (HIV) infections, sensory infections (otitis media), respiratory illnesses, and helminth infections.

HIV Infections

As a result of the worldwide decline in transmission of HIV infection through blood products, mother-infant transmission has become the main route of HIV infection for young children. Infected mothers can transmit HIV to their offspring during pregnancy or birth (Andersen and others 1994). The reported rate of perinatal transmission ranges from 22 to 39 percent (Blanche and others 1989; Mok and others 1987; Ryder and others 1989). As the number of infected women increases, the number of cases of pediatric HIV infection also is anticipated to rise (Scott and others 1989). Some pediatric patients experience seroconversion after infancy (Loveland and Stehbens 1989).

At present, little is known about the early signs of HIV disease in school-age children and adolescents. Knowledge is limited by the relatively small size of this population and by the fact that pediatric patients infected later in infancy do not come to the attention of a medical professional until the disease is advanced. Available data suggest that the manifestations of HIV infection in school-age and adolescent patients is similar in some respects to the manifestations of HIV infection in adults.

HIV can affect a child's nervous system in any of three general ways. First, nonspecific illnesses can occur as HIV causes the immunocompromised host to become vulnerable to opportunistic infections of the nervous system. These opportunistic infections tend to have a short history and are sometimes treatable. Second, HIV can result in nonspecific developmental delays, such as impaired brain growth, progressive motor dysfunction, and loss of developmental milestones (Mintz 1992). Finally, HIV may lead to some specific neuropsychological outcomes by penetrating the brain early in the course of infection and directly affecting its function. This penetration results in chronic impairment of cognitive performance.

Various combinations of the second and third neurological manifestations of HIV infection in childhood are diagnosed as HIV-associated progressive encephalopathy (marked by further deterioration) or HIV-associated static encephalopathy (marked by a plateau or relative improvement) (Belman 1989; Janssen and others 1992; Working Group of the American Academy of Neurology AIDS Task Force 1991). Some researchers have suggested that progressive encephalopathy results from direct or indirect HIV infection of the brain, and the outcome is usually fatal (Epstein and others 1986; Mintz 1992).

HIV encephalopathy is associated with a number of cognitive changes: poor attention and concentration, frequently manifested as an attention deficit disorder with hyperactivity (Mintz 1992); decline in academic skills, particularly mathematics (Loveland and Stehbens 1989); decline in visual-spatial skills; impairment in verbal and nonverbal memory, learning and speech and language; and decline in abstract thinking and reasoning (Egan 1992; Tross and others 1988).

Formal developmental testing of infants infected with HIV prenatally and of young children has yielded conflicting results; some patients show developmental delays, and others show normal development (Belman 1989; Hittelman 1989). These results may be biased because most of the testing was conducted on a clinical population that could be characterized by many confounding variables. Confounding variables contributing to the poor outcomes of children infected by HIV include exposure to drugs in utero, prematurity, failure to thrive, prolonged hospitalization, psychosocial disruption, and environmental disadvantage (Coulter and Chase 1989).

Neuropsychological testing of pediatric patients infected later than infancy shows that manifestations of HIV brain disease in this age group are similar to manifestations of adult HIV encephalopathy (Loveland and Stehbens 1989). This analogy suggests that even significant cognitive impairment of these pediatric patients does not imply inevitable progression to severe dementia (Egan and Goodwin 1992). Prospective studies are in progress, although the high mortality rate of HIV brain disease makes them quite difficult to conduct.

Although neuropsychological research results do not converge on a specific developmental marker that can predict the onset of HIV encephalopathy, a majority of investigators have agreed that cognitive slowing, or decreased speed of information processing, predominates over other characteristics of the disease, including memory and attention loss, aphasia, agnosia, and apraxia (Cumming and Benson 1988; Egan and others 1990; Egan and others 1993; Goodin and others 1990; Navia and others 1986; Price and others 1988; Tross and others 1988). Furthermore, using cognitive tasks that differentiate various components of mental processing speed, researchers have suggested that such cognitive slowing is related to attention processes and possibly involves automatic and controlled components (Martin and others 1992a, 1992b), but the slowing is unrelated to speed of memory scanning (Martin and others 1993). More studies that include control groups of normal and other neuropsychiatric patients are needed to investigate the specificity of these findings in relation to acquired immunodeficiency syndrome (AIDS).

These findings seem appealing and theoretically plausible because they correspond to the current view that speed of basic information processing is an important correlate of cognitive functioning (Deary and Caryl 1993; Vernon 1987) and to the hypothesis that a major focus of HIV pathology is in subcortical structures (Everall, Luthert, and Lantos 1991; Navia and others 1986). Measures of mental speed might be useful in determining developmental disabilities, identifying school-age children who are at risk, and making appropriate placement and intervention. However, because the importance of mental speed in intelligence continues to be debated (Sternberg 1985), these results cannot be established definitely at this time.

Sensory Infections (Otitis Media)

Infections of the eyes, ears, and mouth are directly linked to children's cognitive development because these infections affect the visual, auditory, and taste channels for information to a child's cognitive system. Of the sensory infections in childhood, otitis media (OM) is the best studied in regard to its connection to children's cognitive development.

OM is inflammation of the middle-ear cavity caused by bacteria, resulting in the filling of the middle-ear space with fluid. Among several types of OM (Scheidt and Kavanagh 1986) are acute and chronic OM. Acute OM is an infection of recent onset with fluid that contains bacteria and pus. Chronic OM is an infection that persists beyond the period of time regularly observed for acute OM (3 months), and its clinical manifestations are characterized by less pain.

Otitis media is one of the most common childhood illnesses (Andersen and others 1994). It occurs most often in children 6-36 months of age, it is highly prevalent throughout the preschool years, and its incidence declines only after age 10. In industrialized countries, an estimated 50 percent of all children have at least one episode of OM before their first birthday; 10 percent have three or more such episodes. OM is more prevalent among boys, lower-SES groups, and malnourished children than among other groups.

The most common complication of OM is hearing loss, which occurs in an estimated 26 to 55 percent of cases (Bluestone and others 1983). Long-standing hearing losses in children and chronic OM alone have been linked to impaired cognitive skills and lowered school attainment (Leviton and Bellinger 1986; Zinkus 1986). Rates of OM tend to be higher among children with learning disabilities and attention disorders than among children without these conditions (Bennett, Ruuska, and Sherman 1980; Hagerman and Falkenstein 1987; Hartsough and Lambert 1985; Masters and Marsh 1978). Some recent studies suggest that even mild and fluctuating hearing losses relate to OM, when sustained in infancy and early childhood, are associated with later impairments in language and cognitive development (Chalmers and others 1989; Jenkins 1986; Matkin 1986; Teele, Klein, and Rosner 1984). However, it is unknown if OM-related linguistic difficulties are permanent or reversible.

Some researchers have found no significant relationship between OM in early childhood and motor performance (Von and others 1988) or school success (Black and Sonnenschein 1993; Roberts and others 1989; Stickler 1984). Although some researchers hypothesize that children with OM simply are less attentive and need more help from teachers when asked to work independently (Roberts and others 1989; Silva, Chalmers, and Stewart 1986), these findings have not been replicated (Arcia and Roberts 1993).

Another hypothesis explaining the controversial nature of findings related to OM suggests that positive and negative results cluster into two groups, depending on the SES of children with recurrent OM. OM seems to predict possible language delays in middle-class families, but not in lower-class families (Black and Sonnenschein 1993). This hypothesis suggests that OM acts differently based on the SES of a population; it is a risk factor in the middle-class population, but not in a population of lower SES where children's language development sometimes is compromised already.

Some researchers also believe that parent-child interaction is an important factor, buffering the effect of OM on language development. Parents' fostering of their children's cognitive growth may operate as a compensatory mechanism, counteracting the potentially negative effect of OM on language development (Black and Sonnenschein 1993; Hall and Hill 1986; Hemmer and Ratner 1994).

Dozens of studies have been conducted on associations between early recurrent OM and delays in language and cognitive development as well as learning problems (Bluestone and others 1983). This area of research, however, is no different from other studies of ill health and child development; despite repeatedly observed statistical associations between OM and children's cognitive characteristics, causal links have not been established conclusively. This inconclusiveness results primarily from lack of methodological sophistication or poor research methodology (Bluestone and others 1983; Paradise and Rogers 1986).

Studies in the field of OM differ from studies of other ill health and child development because the threat that chronic OM poses to developmental delay frequently results in surgery, which involves placing plastic or metal ventilating tubes in the middle ear after removing the fluid buildup. This surgery, however, may have some complications and side effects, and the question must be asked whether any cognitive impairments associated with OM are worth performing preventive surgery. If no cognitive effects are associated with ventilation, why subject a child to the possible complications of the operation? Despite the practical significance of research needed in this area, a definitive answer has not yet been obtained.

The leading hypotheses of the mechanism linking OM to possible later language and cognitive impairment relate to prelanguage development when children master the ability to distinguish phonemes. Some researchers hypothesize that the inconsistent auditory signal, which results from fluctuating hearing loss, may create difficulties for a child in partitioning the stream of speech. This inability to segment may impede a child's mastery of language (Bluestone and others 1983). According to another hypothesis, some common etiological factors predispose individuals both to OM and developmental impairments (Bluestone and others 1983).

In summary, current evidence regarding the adverse developmental consequences of OM is inconsistent. However, no persuasive contrary evidence exists either. If OM is hazardous to children's cognitive development, the mediating variable of this link is hearing loss. This hearing loss, especially if it takes place early in development, may result in a developmental lag, which could have ramifications for later development. More research is needed to understand the possible developmental sequelae of OM.

Respiratory Illnesses

Respiratory illness describes a wide spectrum of problems, covering the common cold to life-threatening illness. Respiratory illnesses no doubt represent the most common diseases of childhood. Among respiratory illnesses associated with some impairment of children's cognitive development are colds and influenza (flu) and infectious mononucleosis (IMN).

Colds and Flu

Colds and flu affect most children, and every child has an estimated one to three colds a year. More than 200 viruses, most commonly influenza A and B, produce respiratory tract infections, causing the flu. Influenza viruses are unstable, and new mutants appear

Inconclusive results may result from variability of the association between lead and outcome at different levels of these third variables and from differences in the distribution of these variables among samples.

No accepted hypothesis of the neurobiological mechanisms for lead poisoning exists, although several hypotheses have been formulated (Silbergeld 1992). These hypotheses are classified as neurodevelopmental (influencing cell and cell-connection development) and neuropharmacological (affecting cell interactions). Goldstein (1990, 1992) proposes that early neurodevelopmental lead poisoning may disturb establishment and elaboration of synapses in the cerebral cortex, in particular the hippocampal structures that are involved in memory and learning (Campbell and others 1982; Petit, Alfano, and LeBoutillier 1983). These alterations may lead to the development of a nervous system that appears structurally normal, but is functionally impaired. Lead's activity as a neuropharmacological toxicant might involve neurotransmission and signal transduction that depend on calcium (Pounds and Rosen 1988).

Pharmacological treatment of severe lead poisoning uses chelating agents such as edetate calcium disodium, succimer, or pencillamine to reduce the amount of lead sequestered in bone and soft tissues. In industrialized countries, special attention is given to educational programs in at-risk communities, pre- and perinatal protection of pregnant women against lead exposure, periodic screening of high-risk children, and remediation for poisoned children.

Despite their methodological and interpretational differences, studies of lead poisoning show a high degree of consistency in relating lead levels to overall deficits in children's cognitive functioning. The consensus is that lead has a real, albeit small, effect overall. However, the magnitude of this effect appears to vary across different populations. The data on lead poisoning have provided a solid foundation for public health policy. In the United States, the Centers for Disease Control and Prevention has redefined the threshold of lead exposure for clinical and social intervention from 25 milligrams/deciliter to 10 milligrams/deciliter. Much still remains to be discovered about the adverse effects of lead on a developing child.

Ionization

Ionization results from a number of natural causes (for example, radioactive substances in the soil, cosmic radiation, and the rapid movement of air over land) and from a number of man-made sources (for example, strong electrical fields and radiation exposure) (Farmer 1992). Research on ionization suggests that improved cognitive performance may be attributed to negative ions, which result from the addition of an electron to a molecule or from the separation of a single electron from a molecule, and impaired cognitive performance may be attributed to positive ions, which result from the loss of an electron by a molecule.

Using an auditory task and selective attention tasks, Morton and Kershner (1984, 1987, 1990) investigated the performance of children with and without learning disabilities in control situations and conditions enriched with negative ions. They found that negative ionization increased the performance of both normal and disabled learners. Other researchers have found no effects of ionization on a card-sorting task (Barron and Dreher 1964; Hedge and Collis 1987), verbal reasoning or inspection tasks (Albrechtsen and others

1978), memory tasks (Baron, Russell, and Arms 1985; Farmer and Bendix 1982), learning in a classroom environment (Britton 1984), or digit-symbol coding (Buckalew and Rizzuto 1984). These inconsistent data do not allow for reliable conclusions regarding the effects of ionization on cognitive processes.

Experimental studies of positive ions have not been conducted because of their potentially harmful effects to humans. However, since 1895 when X rays were discovered, many people have been voluntarily and involuntarily exposed to artificially created sources of radiation. Under these conditions, separating the effects of positive and negative ions is impossible, and the term *irradiation* is used.

Relatively little is known about the effects of irradiation on cognitive development. Similar to other teratogenic agents, ionizing radiation at different developmental stages causes organisms to react differently (Fritz-Niggli 1995). If irradiation occurs in the early stages of fetal development (during the preimplantation period), even very low dosages lead to cell death and, consequently, to fetus death. Later irradiation (at the stage of organogenesis) tends to result in various abnormalities, depending on which organ formation peaks in sensitivity at a given time; disturbances of the nervous system are the most prominent abnormalities. Even low dosages of irradiation at this stage of development result in approximately a twofold increase in mental retardation (Otake and Schull 1984) and intellectual impairment (UNSCEAR 1993). Postnatal irradiation of pediatric patients results primarily in the development of thyroid carcinomas (Nikiforov and Gnepp 1994), and cognitive impairments follow this debilitating, long-term condition.

Summary

The field of environmental toxins and their effects on children's cognitive development is a very new one, marking only its twentieth anniversary. In comparison with research on undernutrition and childhood infections, this field (with the possible exception of studies on lead poisoning) has accumulated significantly less consistent information. These environmental insults no doubt will attract the attention of more researchers in the near future because they are the inevitable side effects of civilization. Severe and acute teratogenic intoxication is most threatening for a child's cognitive activation because they affect not only the child's cognitive development, but also the whole system of scaffolding. For example, when acute irradiation results in the relocation of an entire community, not only is the cognitive functioning of children jeopardized, but also their whole system of social support—their environmental niche—is disturbed.

Conclusion

The results of the diverse studies cited in this chapter indicate that ill health during childhood, caused by undernutrition, infection, or environmental toxins, can adversely affect cognitive development. At severe levels of insult, these consequences are potentially serious. Sufficient evidence also demonstrates that, at least in some cases, remediation of the physical condition can have a positive effect on cognitive development. Delay in suitable interventions only can result in millions of children with cognitive skills that function at levels well below the children's potential.

The results of the studies described are inconsistent and sometimes controversial. But how realistic is expecting results to totally converge? Total convergence is possible only with an implicit expectation that a true link between environmental insult and cognition exists which all valid studies can find. Because researchers have attempted to overcome inconsistencies by concentrating on better assessment and statistical control of confounding, discrepancies often are interpreted in terms of how valid or well designed a particular study is. Such interpretations notwithstanding, nature may be slightly more complicated than even the better-designed studies.

Unfortunately, in many cases, methodological debates have focused on issues of internal and external validity, such as the blindness of experimenters, sampling procedures, subject recruitment, and methodology for statistical analyses (Pollitt and Metallinos-Katsaras 1990). These issues are doubtless important; however, they frequently overshadow questions of adequacy regarding the characterization of exposure and measurement of an insult (that is, questions of the duration and severity of the insult), the theoretical framework for selecting outcome variables, and characterization of the evaluation of exposure and outcome.

Issues of double-blind studies of placebo and treatment must be dealt with, but better theories underlying research on children's ill health and mental development also are needed. "Our models are not yet sophisticated [enough] to characterize the interactions governing this process" (Bellinger 1995: 202). Should the main question asked in these studies be changed from "Does insult X result in Y units of cognitive impairment?" to "Under what environmental conditions do different patterns of lead exposure produce measurable impairments at what ages in which behavioral endpoints in which types of populations?" (Bellinger 1995: 210).

Nutritional and medical interventions that provide environmental scaffolding are jointly necessary, but they are not sufficient for improving cognitive functioning. They place children in the position to profit from cognitive, socioemotional, and behavioral scaffolding, but they do not actually provide this scaffolding. They are prerequisites rather than substitutes for educational interventions. Without nutritional and medical interventions, children may not benefit from educational interventions, but without educational interventions, healthy children will be without the stimulation needed to show the benefit. Ideally, educational interventions will include information about health, teaching children to take care of themselves and not to rely on others to care for them.

Health intervention followed by educational intervention actualizes children's potential and accomplishments. Both interventions are necessary to ameliorate the effects of children's ill health on cognitive development. Without both, children are deprived of opportunities to become productive and happy contributors to their societies and to the world.

Note

Preparation of this chapter was supported by the Partnership for Child Development, University of Oxford, England, and by the Javits Act Program (Grant #R206R50001) as administered by the U.S. Department of Education, Office of Educational Research and Improvement.

References

Abel, E. L. 1980. The Fetal Alcohol Syndrome: Behavioral Teratology. *Psychological Bulletin* 87:29-50.

Ader, R. 1983. Developmental Psychoneuroimmunology. *Developmental Psychobiology* 16:251-67.

Adetunji, J. A. 1991. Response of Parents to Five Killer Diseases among Children in a Yoruba Community, Nigeria. *Social Science and Medicine* 32:1379-87.

Ahmed, F., M. Mohiduzzaman, and A. A. Jackson. 1993. Vitamin A Absorption in Children with Ascariasis. *British Journal of Nutrition* 69:817-25.

Ahmed, N., M. F. Zeitlin, A. S. Beiser, C. M. Super, and S. N. Gershoff. 1993. A Longitudinal Study of the Impact of Behavioral Change Intervention on Cleanliness, Diarrhoeal Morbidity and Growth of Children in Rural Bangladesh. *Social Science and Medicine* 37:159-71.

Albrechtsen, O., V. Clausen, F. G. Christense, J. G. Jensen, and T. Møller. 1978. The Influence of Small Atmospheric Ions on Human Well-being and Mental Performance. *International Journal of Biometeorology* 22:249-62.

Anderson, M. 1992. *Intelligence and Development: A Cognitive Theory*. Oxford: Blackwell.

Andersen, R. D., J. F. Bale, Jr., J. A. Blackman, and J. P. Murph. 1994. *Infections in Children*. Gaithersburg, Md.: Aspen Publishers, Inc.

Arcia, E., and J. E. Roberts. 1993. Otitis Media in Early Childhood and its Association with Sustained Attention in Structured Situations. *Developmental and Behavioral Pediatrics* 14:181-83.

Baghurst, P., A. McMichael, N. Wigg, G. Vimpani, E. Robertson, R. Roberts, and S.-L. Tong. 1992. Environmental Exposure to Lead and Children's Intelligence at the Age of Seven Years. *New England Journal of Medicine* 327:1279-84.

Baron, R. A., G. W. Russell, and R. L. Arms. 1985. Negative Ions and Behavior: Impact on Mood, Memory, and Aggression among Type A and Type B Persons. *Journal of Personality and Social Psychology* 48:746-54.

Barron, C. I., and J. J. Dreher. 1964. Effects of Electric Fields and Negative Ion Concentrations on Test Pilots. *Aerospace Medicine* 35:716-30.

Bautista, A., P. A. Barker, J. T. Dunn, M. Sanchez, and D. L. Kaiser. 1982. The Effects of Oral Iodized Oil on Intelligence, Thyroid Status, and Somatic Growth in School-age Children from an Area of Endemic Goiter. *American Journal of Clinical Nutrition* 35:127-34.

Behar, M. 1968. Prevalence of Malnutrition among Preschool Children in Developing Countries. In N. S. Scrimshaw and J. E. Gordon, eds., *Malnutrition, Learning and Behavior*. Cambridge, Mass.: MIT Press.

Bellinger, D. C. 1995. Interpreting the Literature on Lead and Child Development: The Neglected Role of the "Experimental System." *Neurotoxicology and Teratology* 17:201-12.

Bellinger, D., H. Hu, L. Titlebaum, and H. Needleman. 1994. Attentional Correlates of Dentin and Bone Lead Levels in Adolescents. *Archives of Environmental Health* 49:98-105.

Bellinger, D., K. Stiles, and H. Needleman. 1992. Low-level Lead Exposure, Intelligence, and Academic Achievement: A Long-term Follow-up Study. *Pediatrics* 90:855-61.

Belman, A. L. 1989. Neurologic Syndromes Associated with Symptomatic Human Immunodeficiency Virus Infection in Infants and Children. In P. B. Kozlowski, D. A. Snider, P. M. Vietze, and H. M. Wisniewski, eds., *Brain in Pediatric AIDS*. Basel, Switzerland: Karger.

Belopol'skaia, N. L., and N. V. Grebennikova. 1996. Neuropsychology and Psychological Diagnosis of Abnormal Development. In E. L. Grigorenko, P. Ruzgis, and R. J. Sternberg., eds., *Russian Psychology: Past, Present, and Future*. Commack, N.Y.: Nova Science.

Bennett, F. C., S. H. Ruuska, and R. Sherman. 1980. Middle Ear Function in Learning-disabled Children. *Pediatrics* 66:254-60.

Benton, D. 1992a. Vitamin and Mineral Intake and Human Behaviour. In A. P. Smith and D. M. Jones, eds., *Handbook of Human Performance*. New York: Harcourt Brace Jovanovich.

———. 1992b. Vitamin-Mineral Supplements and Intelligence. *Proceeding of the Nutrition Society* 51:295-302.

Benton D., and R. Cook. 1991. The Impact of Selenium Supplementation on Mood. *Biological Psychiatry* 29(11):1092-98.

Bergmann, K. E., and R. L. Bergmann. 1985. Gestational Zinc Deficiency. *The American Journal of Clinical Nutrition* 42:342-46.

Bithoney, W. G., A. M. Vandeven, and A. Ryan. 1993. Elevated Lead Levels in Reportedly Abused Children. *Journal of Pediatrics* 122:719-20.

Black, M. M., and S. Sonnenschein. 1993. Early Exposure to Otitis Media: A Preliminary Investigation of Behavioral Outcome. *Developmental and Behavioral Pediatrics* 14:150-55.

Blanche, S., C. Rouzioux, M-LC. Moscato, F. Veber, M-J. Mayaux, C. Jacomet, J. Tricore, A. Deville, M. Vial, G. Firton, A. de Cerpy, D. Douard, M. Robin, C. Courpotin, N. Ciraru-Vigneron, F. le Deist, C. Griscelle, and the HIV Infection in Newborns French Collaboration Study Group. 1989. A Prospective Study of Infants Born to Women Seropositive for Human Immunodeficiency Virus Type 1. *New England Journal of Medicine* 320:1643-48.

Bleichrodt, N., F. Ecobar del Rey, G. Morreale de Escobar, I. Garcia, and C. G. Rubio. 1989. Iodine Deficiency, Implications for Mental and Psychomotor Development in Children. In G. R. DeLong, J. Robbins, and P. G. Condliffe, eds., *Iodine and the Brain*. New York: Plenum Press.

Bleichrodt, N., I. Garcia, C. Rubio, G. Morreale de Escobar, and F. Ecobar del Rey. 1987. Developmental Disorders Associated with Severe Iodine Deficiency. In B. Hetzel, J. Dunn, and J. Stanbury, eds., *The Prevention and Control of Iodine Deficiency Disorders*. Amsterdam: Elsevier.

Bluestone, C. D., J. O. Klein, J. L. Paradise, H. Eichenwals, F. H. Bess, M. P. Downs, M. Green, J. Berko-Gleason, I. M. Ventry, S. W. Gray, B. J. McWilliams, and G. A. Gates. 1983. Workshop on Effects of Otitis Media on the Child. *Pediatrics* 71:639-49.

Boivin M., and B. Giordani. 1993. Improvements in Cognitive Performance for School Children in Zaire, Africa Following an Iron Supplement and Treatment for Intestinal Parasites. *Journal of Pediatric Psychology* 8:249-64.

Boyages, S. C., J. K. Collins, G. F. Maberly, J. J. Jupp, J. Morris, and C. J. Eastman. 1989. Iodine Deficiency Impairs Intellectual and Neuromotor Development in Apparently-normal Persons: A Study of Rural Inhabitants of North-central China. *Medical Journal* 150:676-82.

Britton, J. E. 1984. The Effects of Negative Air Ions on Learning in an Educational Environment. *Dissertation Abstract International* 45:1245A.

Bruce-Jones, W. D. A., P. D. White, J. M. Thomas, and A. W. Clare. 1994. The Effects of Social Adversity on the Fatigue Syndrome, Psychiatric Disorders and Physical Recovery, Following Glandular Fever. *Psychological Medicine* 24:651-59.

Buckalew, L. W., and A. P. Rizzuto. 1984. Negative Air Ion Effects on Human Performance and Physiological Condition. *Aviation, Space, and Environmental Medicine* 55:731-34.

Bundy, D. A. P. 1994. Immunoepidemiology of intestinal helminthic infections. 1. The Global Burden of Intestinal Nematode Disease. *Transactions of the Royal Society of Tropical Medicine and Hygiene* 88:259-61.

Campbell, N., D. Wooley, V. Vijayan, and S. Overmann. 1982. Morphometric Effects of Postnatal Lead Exposure on Hippocampal Development of the 15 Day Old Rat. *Developmental Brain Research* 3:595-612.

Carek, D. J., and A. B. Santos. 1984. Atypical Somatoform Disorder Following Infection in Children—A Depressive Equivalent? *Journal of Clinical Psychiatry* 45:108-11.

Cerf, B. J., J. E. Rohde, and T. Soesanto. 1981. Ascaris and Malnutrition in a Balinese Village: A Conditional Relationship. *Tropical and Geographical Medicine* 33:367-73.

Chakraverty, P., P. Cunningham, G. Z. Shen, and M. S. Pereira. 1986. Influenza in the United Kingdom 1982-1985. *Journal of Hygiene* 97:347-58.

Chalmers, D., I. Stewart, P. Silva, and A. Mulvena. 1989. *Otitis Media with Effusion in Children—The Deunedin Study*. London: MacKeith Press.

Chan, M. S., G. F. Medley, D. Jamison, and D. A. P. Bundy. 1994. The Evaluation of Potential Global Morbidity Attributable to Intestinal Nematode Infections. *Parasitology* 109:373-87.

Chasnoff, I. J., M. E. Bussey, R. Savich, and C. Stack. 1986. Perinatal Cerebral Infarction and Maternal Cocaine Use. *Journal of Pediatrics* 108:456-59.

Chiriboga, C. A. 1993. Fetal Effects. *Neurologic Clinics* 11:707-28.

Cohen, S., D. A. J. Tyrrell, and A. P. Smith. 1991. Psychological Stress and Susceptibility to the Common Cold. *New England Journal of Medicine* 325:606-12.

Cohen, S., and G. M. Williamson. 1991. Stress and Infectious Disease in Humans. *Psychological Bulletin* 109:5-24.

Colletta, N. D., S. Sockalingham, and M. Zeitlan. 1993. The Child Development Milestone Chart—An Approach to Low Cost Programming in Indonesia. *Early Child Development and Care* 96:161-71.

Congdon, N., A. Sommer, M. Severns, J. Humphrey, D. Friedman, L. Clement, L.-S.-F. Wu, and G. Natadisastra. 1995. Pupillary and Visual Threshold in Young Children as an Index of Population Vitamin A Status. *American Journal of Clinical Nutrition* 61:1076-82.

Conners, C. K., and A. G. Blouin. 1983. Nutritional Effects on Behavior of Children. *Journal of Psychiatric Research* 17:193-201.

Connolly, K. J., and J. D. Kvalsvig. 1993. Infection, Nutrition and Cognitive Performance in Children. *Parasitology* 107:S187-S200.

Connolly, K. J., P. O. D. Pharoah, and B. S Hetzel. 1979. Fetal Iodine Deficiency and Motor Performance during Childhood. *Lancet* ii:1149-51.

Cooney, G. H. 1995. Lead Research: Where Do We Go from Here? *Neurotoxicology and Teratology* 17:215-18.

Cooney, G., A. Bell, W. McBride, and C. Carter. 1989. Low-level Exposure to Lead: The Sydney Lead Study. *Developmental Medicine and Child Neurology* 31:640-49.

Cooper, E. S., C. A. M. Whyte-Alleng, J. S. Finzi-Smith, and T. T. MacDonald. 1992. Intestinal Nematode Infections in Children: The Pathophysiological Price Paid. *Parasitology* 104:S91-S103.

Coulter, D. L., and C. Chase. 1989. Neurological Assessment of Infants and Young Children with HIV Infection. In P. B. Kozlowski, D. A. Snider, P. M. Vietze, and H. M. Wisniewski, eds., *Brain in Pediatric AIDS*. Basel, Switzerland: Karger.

Craig, A. 1986. Acute Effects of Meals on Perceptual and Cognitive Efficiency. *Nutrition Reviews* 44(suppl.):163-71.

Cravioto, J., and R. Arrieta. 1979. Stimulation and Mental Development of Malnourished Infants. *Lancet* 2:899.

Cumming, J. L., and D. F. Benson. 1988. Psychological Dysfunction Accompanying Subcortical Dementia. *Annual Review of Medicine* 39:53-61.

Daugherty, S. A., B. E. Henry, D. L. Peterson, R. L. Swarts, S. Bastein, and R. S. Thomas. 1991. Chronic Fatigue Syndrome in Northern Nevada. *Reviews of Infectious Diseases* 13:39-44.

Daulaire, N. M. P., E. S. Starbuck, R. M. Houston, M. S. Church, T. A. Stukel, and M. R. Pandy. 1992. Childhood Mortality after a High Dose of Vitamin A in a High Risk Population. *BJM* 304:207-10.

Dean, W., and J. Morgenthaler. 1990. *Smart Drugs and Nutrients*. Santa Cruz, Calif.: B. & J. Publications.

Dean, W., J. Morgenthaler, and S. Fowkes. 1993. *Smart Drugs II: The Next Generation*. Menlo Park, Calif.: Health Freedom Publications.

Deary, I. J., and P. G. Caryl. 1993. Intelligence, EEG and Evoked Potentials. In P. A. Vernon, ed., *Biological Approaches to the Study of Human Intelligence*. Norwood, N.J.: Ablex.

DeMaeyer, E., and M. Adiels-Tegman. 1985. The Prevalence of Anemia in the World. *World Health Statistics Quarterly* 38:302-16.

Dickie, N., and A. Bender. 1982. Breakfast and Performance. *Human Nutrition: Applied Nutrition* 36A:46-56.

Dietrich, K., and R. Bellinger. 1994. The Assessment of Neurobehavioral Development in Studies of the Effects of Prenatal Exposure to Toxicans. In H. Needleman and D. Bellinger, eds., *Prenatal Exposure to Environmental Toxicans: Developmental Consequences*. Baltimore: The Johns Hopkins University Press.

Dietrich, K., O. Berger, P. Succop, and P. Hammond. 1993. The Developmental Consequences of Low to Moderate Prenatal and Postnatal Lead Exposure: Intellectual Attainment in the Cincinnati Lead Study Cohort Following School Entry. *Neurotoxicology and Teratology* 15:37-44.

Egan, V. 1992. Neuropsychological Aspects of HIV Infection. *AIDS Care* 4:3-10.

Egan, V., A. Chiswich, R. Brette, and G. Goodwin. 1993. The Edinburgh Cohort of HIV-positive Drug Users: The Relationship Between Auditory P3 Latency, Cognitive Function and Self-rated Mood. *Psychological Medicine* 23:613-22.

Egan, B. G., J. R. Crawford, R. P. Brettle, and G. M. Goodwin. 1990. The Edinbourgh Cohort of HIV-positive Drug Users: Current Intellectual Function Is Impaired, but Not Due to Early AIDS Dementia Complex. *AIDS* 4:651-56.

Egan, V., and G. Goodwin. 1992. HIV and AIDS. In A. P. Smith and D. M. Jones, eds., *Handbook of Human Performance*. Vol. 2. New York: Harcourt Brace Jovanovich.

Epstein, L. G., L. R. Sharer, J. M. Oleske, E. M. Connor, J. Goudsmith, L. Bagdon, M. R. Guroff, and M. R. Koenigsberger. 1986. Neurological Manifestations of Human Immunodeficiency Virus Infection in Children. *Pediatrics* 78:678-87.

Ernhart, C., M. Morrow-Tlucak, A. Wolf, D. Super, and D. Drotar. 1987. Low Level Lead Exposure in the Prenatal and Early Postnatal Periods: Intelligence Prior to School Entry. *Neurotoxicology and Teratology* 11:161-70.

Everall, I. P., P. J. Luthert, and P. L. Lantos. 1991. Neuronal Loss in the Frontal Cortex in HIV Infection. *Lancet* 337:1119-21.

Eysenck, H. J., and S. L. Schoenthaler. 1996. Raising IQ Level by Vitamin and Mineral Supplementation. In R. J. Sternberg and E. L. Grigorenko, eds., *Intelligence, Heredity, and Environment*. New York: Cambridge University Press.

Fairchild, M. W., J. D. Haas, and J.-P. Habicht. 1989. Iron Deficiency and Behavior: Criteria for Testing Causality. *American Journal of Clinical Nutrition* 50:566-74.

Farmer, E. W. 1992. Ionization. In A. P. Smith and D. M. Jones, eds., *Handbook of Human Performance*. Vol. 1. New York: Harcourt Brace Jovanovich.

Farmer, E. W., and A. Bendix. 1982. Geophysical Variables and Behavior: V. Human Performance in Ionized Air. *Perceptual and Motor Skills* 54:403-12.

Farran, D. C., and J. D. McKinney, eds. 1986. *Risk in Intellectual and Psychosocial Development*. New York: Academic Press.

Feldman, R. G., and R. G. White. 1992. Lead Neurotoxicity and Disorders of Learning. *Journal of Child Neurology* 7:354-59.

Fierro-Benitez, R., R. Casar, J. Stanbury, P. Rodriguez, F. Garces, F. Fierro-Renoy, and E. Estrella. 1986. Long-term Effects of Correction of Iodine Deficiency on Psychomotor Development and Intellectual Development. In J. Dunn, E. Pretell, C. Daza, and F. Viteri, eds., *Towards the Eradication of Endemic Goiter, Cretinism and Iodine Deficiency*. Washington, D.C.: Pan American Health Organization.

Finnigan, F., and R. Hammersley. 1992. The Effects of Alcohol on Performance. In A. P. Smith and D. M. Jones, eds., *Handbook of Human Performance*. Vol. 2. New York: Harcourt Brace Jovanovich.

Flynn, J. R. 1987. Massive IQ Gains in 14 Nations: What IQ Tests Really Measure. *Psychological Bulletin* 101:171-91.

Freeman, H. E., R. E. Klein, J. W. Townsend, and A. Lechtig. 1980. Nutrition and Cognitive Development among Rural Guatemalan Children. *American Journal of Public Health* 70(12):1277-85.

Fritz-Niggli, H. 1995. 100 Years of Radiobiology: Implications for Biomedicine and Future Perspectives. *Experimentia* 51:652-64.

Gadie, M., F. J. Nye, and P. Storey. 1976. Anxiety and Depression after Infectious Mononucleosis. *British Journal of Psychiatry* 128:559-64.

Gillett, J. D. 1985. The Behavior of *Homo Sapiens*, the Forgotten Factor in the Transmission of Tropical Diseases. *Transactions of the Royal Society of Tropical Medicine and Hygiene* 79:12-20.

Golding, J. F. 1992. Cannabis. In A. P. Smith and D. M. Jones, eds., *Handbook of Human Performance*. Vol. 2. New York: Harcourt Brace Jovanovich.

Goldstein, G. 1990. Lead Poisoning and Brain Cell Function. *Environmental Health Perspective* 89:91-94.

———. 1992. Developmental Neurobiology of Lead Toxicity. In H. Needleman, ed., *Human Lead Exposure*. Boca Raton, Fla.: CRC Press.

Goodin, D. S., M. J. Aminoff, D. N. Chernoff, and H. Hollander. 1990. Long-latency Event-related Potentials in Patients Infected with Human Immunodeficiency Virus. *Annals of Neurology* 27:414-19.

Grant, E. C. G., J. M. Howard, S. Davies, H. Chasty, B. Hornsby, and J. Galbraith. 1988. Zinc Deficiency in Children with Dyslexia: Concentrations of Zinc and Other Minerals in Sweat and Hair. *British Medical Journal* 296:607-09.

Grantham-McGregor, S. 1988. Studies in Behaviour and Malnutrition in Jamaica. *Transactions of the Royal Society of Tropical Medicine and Hygiene* 82:7-9.

———. 1990. Malnutrition, Mental Function, and Development. In R. M. Suskind and L. Lewinter-Suskind, eds., *The Malnourished Child.* New York: Raven Press.

Grantham-McGregor, S., C. A. Powell, S. P. Walker, and J. H. Himes. 1991. Nutritional Supplementation, Psychosocial Stimulation, and Mental Development of Stunted Children: The Jamaican Study. *Lancet* 338:1-5.

Grantham-McGregor, S., W. Schofield, and C. Powell. 1987. Development of Severely Malnourished Children Who Received Psychosocial Stimulation: Six-year Follow-up. *Pediatrics* 79:247-54.

Gunderson, E. K., and R. H. Rahe, eds. 1974. *Life Stress and Illness*. Springfield, Il.: Thomas.

Guyatt, H. L., D. A. P. Bundy, G. F. Medley, and B. T. Grenfell. 1990. The Relationship Between the Frequency Distribution of *Ascaris lumbricoides* and the Prevalence and Intensity of Infection in Human Communities. *Parasitology* 101:139-43.

Hagerman, R. J., and A. R. Falkenstein. 1987. An Association Between Recurrent Otitis Media in Infancy and Later Hyperactivity. *Clinical Pediatrics* 26:253-57.

Hall, A. 1993. Intestinal Parasitic Worms and the Growth of Children. *Transactions of the Royal Society of Tropical Medicine and Hygiene* 87:241-42.

Hall, D. M. B., and P. Hill. 1986. When Does Secretory Otitis Media Affect Language Development? *Archives of Disease in Childhood* 61:42-47.

Halpern, J.-P., S. C. Boyages, G. F. Maberly, J. K. Collins, C. Eastman, and J. G. L. Morrie. 1991. The Neurology of Endemic Cretinism. *Brain* 114:825-41.

Hambridge, K. M. 1977. The Role of Zinc and Other Trace Metals in Pediatric Nutrition and Health. *Pediatric Clinics of North America* 24:95-106.

Hambridge, K. M., C. Hambridge, M. Jacobs, and J. D. Baum. 1972. Low Levels of Zinc in Hair, Anorexia, Poor Growth, and Hypogeusia in Children. *Pediatric Research* 6:868-74.

Hansen, O., J. Nerup, and B. Holbek. 1986. A Common Specific Origin of Specific Dyslexia and Insulin-dependent Diabetes Mellitus? *Heteridas* 105:165-67.

Hanson, J. W., A. P. Streissguth, and D. W. Smith. 1978. The Effect of Moderate Alcohol Consumption during Pregnancy on Fetal Growth and Morphogenesis. *Journal of Pediatrics* 92:457-60.

Harkness, S., and C. M. Super. 1994. The Developmental Niche: A Theoretical Framework for Analyzing the Household Production of Health. *Social Science and Medicine* 38:217-26.

Hartsough, C. S., and N. M. Lambert. 1985. Medical Factors in Hyperactive and Normal Children: Prenatal Developmental and Health History Findings. *American Journal of Orthopsychiatry* 55:190-201.

Heazlett, M., and R. F. Whaley. 1976. The Common Cold: Its Effect on Perceptual Ability and Reading Comprehension among Pupils of a Seventh Grade Class. *Journal of School Health* 46:145-47.

Hedge, A., and M. D. Collis. 1987. Do Negative Ions Affect Human Mood and Performance? *Annals of Occupational Hygiene* 31:285-90.

Hemmer, V. H., and N. B. Ratner. 1994. Communicative Development in Twins with Discordant Histories of Recurrent Otitis Media. *Journal of Communicative Disorders* 27:91-106.

Hendler, N., and W. Leahy. 1978. Psychiatric and Neurologic Sequelae of Infectious Mononucleosis. *American Journal of Psychiatry* 135:842-44.

Henkin, R. I., B. M. Patten, P. K. Re, and D. A. Bronzert. 1973. A Syndrome of Acute Zinc Loss: Cerebellar Dysfunction, Mental Changes, Anorexia, and Taste and Smell Dysfunction. *Archives of Neurology* 32:745-51.

Hertzman, C. n.d. *Environment and Health in Central and Eastern Europe*. Washington, D.C.: World Bank. Forthcoming.

Hetzel, B. 1987. An Overview of the Prevention and Control of Iodine Deficiency Disorders. In B. Hetzel, J. Dunn, and J. Stanbury, eds., *The Prevention and Control of Iodine Deficiency Disorders*. Amsterdam: Elsevier.

Hetzel, B. S. 1989. Iodine and the Brain. In G. R. DeLong, J. Robbins, and P. G. Condliffe, eds., *Iodine and the Brain*. New York: Plenum Press.

Hetzel, B. S., and M. T. Mano. 1989. A Review of Experimental Studies of Iodine Deficiency during Fetal Development. *Journal of Nutrition* 119:145-51.

Hittelman, J. 1989. Neurodevelopmental Aspects of HIV Infections. In P. B. Kozlowski, D. A. Snider, P. M. Vietze, and H. M. Wisniewski, eds., *Brain in Pediatric AIDS*. Basel, Switzerland: Karger.

Horowitz, F. D. 1989. Using Developmental Theory to Guide the Search for the Effects of Biological Risk Factors on the Development of Children. *American Journal of Clinical Nutrition* 50:589-97.

Janssen, R. S., O. C. Nwanyanwe, R. M. Selik, and J. K. Stehr-Green. 1992. Epidemiology of Human Immunodeficiency Virus Encephalopathy in the United States. *Neurology* 42:1472-76.

Jenkins, J. J. 1986. Cognitive Development in Children with Recurrent Otitis Media: Where Do We Stand? In J. F. Kavanagh, ed., *Otitis Media and Child Development*. Parkton, Md.: York Press.

Kasl, S. V., A. S. Evans, and J. C. Neiderman. 1979. Psychosocial Risk Factors in the Development of Infectious Mononucleosis. *Psychosomatic Medicine* 41:445-66.

Kemeny, M. E., F. Cohen, L. A. Zegans, and M. A. Conant. 1989. Psychological and Immunological Predictors of Genital Herpes Recurrence. *Psychosomatic Medicine* 51:195-208.

Kochupillai, N., M. M. Godbole, C. S. Pandav, A. Mithal, and M. M. S. Ahuya. 1986. Environmental Iodine Deficiency, Neonatal Chemical Hypothyroidism (NCH) and Iodised Oil Prophylaxis. In N. Kochupillai, M. G. Karmarkar, and V. Ramalingaswmi, eds., *Iodine Nutrition, Thyrozine and Brain Development*. New Delhi: Tata McGraw-Hill.

Koller, L. D. 1979. Effects of Environmental Contaminants on the Immune System. *Advances in Veterinary Science and Comparative Medicine* 23:267-95.

Lahita, R. G. 1988. Systemic Lupus Erythematosus: Learning Disability in the Male Offspring of Female Patients and Relations to Laterality. *Psychoneuroendocrinology* 13:385-96.

Levav, M., M. E. Cruz, and A. F. Mirsky. 1995. EEG Abnormalities, Malnutrition, Parasitism and Goiter: A Study of Schoolchildren in Ecuador. *Acta Pediatrica* 84:197-202.

Levinger, B. 1994. *Nutrition, Health and Education for All*. New York: United Nations Development Programme.

Leviton, A., and D. Bellinger. 1986. Is There a Relationship between Otitis Media and Learning Disorders? In J. F. Kavanagh, ed., *Otitis Media and Child Development*. Parkton, Md.: York Press.

Loveland, K. A., and J. A. Stehbens. 1989. Early Neurodevelopmental Signs of HIV Infection in Children and Adolescents. In P. B. Kozlowski, D. A. Snider, P. M. Vietze, and H. M. Wisniewski, eds., *Brain in Pediatric AIDS*. Basel, Switzerland: Karger.

Lozoff, B. 1988. Behavioral Alterations in Iron Deficiency. *Advances in Pediatrics* 35:331-60.

Lucas, A., R. Morley, T. J. Cole, S. M. Gore, P. J. Lucas, P. Crowle, R. Pearse, A. J. Boon, and R. Powell. 1990. Early Diet in Preterm Babies and Developmental Status at 19 Months. *Lancet* 335:1477-81.

Lynn, R. 1990. The Role of Nutrition in Secular Increases in Intelligence. *Personality and Individual Differences* 11:273-85.

Ma, T., Z. C. Lian, S. P. Qi, E. R. Heinz, and G. R. DeLong. 1993. Magnetic Resonance Imaging of Brain and the Neuromotor Disorder in Endemic Cretinism. *Annals of Neurology* 34:91-94.

Ma, T., Y. Y. Wang, D. Wang, Z. P. Chen, and S. P. Chi. Neurological Studies in Iodine Deficiency Areas in China. 1989. In G. R. DeLong, J. Robbins, and P. G. Condliffe, eds., *Iodine and the Brain*. New York: Plenum Press.

Martin, E. M., L. C. Robertson, H. E. Edelstein, W. J. Jagust, D. J. Sorensen, D. San Giovanni, and V. A. Chirurgi. 1992a. Performance of Patients with Early HIV-I Infection on the Stroop Task. *Journal of Clinical and Experimental Neuropsychology* 14:840-51.

Martin, E. M., L. C. Robertson, D. J. Sorensen, W. J. Jagust, K. F. Malon, and V. A. Chirurgi. 1993. Speed Memory Scanning Is Not Affected in Early HIV-1 Infection. *Journal of Clinical and Experimental Neuropsychology* 15:311-20.

Martin, E. M., D. J. Sorensen, L. C. Robertson, H. E. Edelstein, and V. A. Chirurgi. 1992b. Spatial Attention in HIV-1 Infection: A Preliminary Report. *Journal of Neuropsychiatry and Clinical Neurosciences* 4:288-93.

Masters, L., and G. E. Marsh. 1978. Middle Ear Pathology as a Factor in Learning Disabilities. *Journal of Learning Disabilities* 11:54-57.

Matkin, N. D. 1986. The Role of Hearing in Language Development. In J. F. Kavanagh, ed., *Otitis Media and Child Development*. Parkton, Md.: York Press.

McDonald, M. A., M. Sigman, M. P. Espinosa, and C. G. Neumann. 1994. Impact of a Temporary Food Shortage on Children and Their Mothers. *Child Development* 65:404-15.

McKay, H., L. Sinesterra, A. McKay, H. Gomez, and P. Lloredo. 1978. Improving Cognitive Ability in Chronically Deprived Children. *Science* 200:270.

McLaren, D. S., U. S. Yatkin, A. A. Kanawati, S. Sabbagh, and Z. Kadi. 1973. The Subsequent Mental and Physical Development of Rehabilitated Marasmic Infants. *Journal of Mental Deficiency Research* 17:273-81.

Minder, B., E. A. Das-Smaal, E. F. J. M. Brand, and J. F. Orlebeke. 1994. Exposure to Lead and Specific Attention Problems in Schoolchildren. *Journal of Learning Disabilities* 27:393-99.

Mintz, M. 1992. Neurologic Abnormalities. In R. Yogev and E. Connor, eds., *Management of HIV Infection in Infants and Children*. St. Louis, Mo.: Mosby-Year Book, Inc.

Mody, C.K., B. I. Miller, H. B. McIntyre, S. K. Cobb, and M. A. Goldberg. 1988. Neurologic Complications of Cocaine Abuse. *Neurology* 38:1189-93.

Mok, J. Q., C. Giaquinto, A. De Rossi, I. Grosch-Wörner, A. E. Ades, and C. S. Peckham. 1987. Infants Born to Mothers Seropositive for Human Immunodeficiency Virus: Preliminary Findings from a Multi-center European Study. *Lancet* 1:1164-68.

Morton, L. L., and J. R. Kershner. 1984. Negative Air Ionization Improves Memory and Attention in Learning-disabled and Mentally Retarded Children. *Journal of Abnormal Child Psychology* 12:353-65.

———. 1987. Negative Ion Effects on Hemispheric Processing and Selective Attention in the Mentally Retarded. *Journal of Mental Deficiency Research* 31:169-80.

Morton, L. L., and J. R. Kershner. 1990. Differential Negative Air Ion Effects on Learning Disabled and Normal-achieving Children. *International Journal of Biometeorology* 34:35-41.

Mott, S. H., R. J. Packer, and S. J. Soldin. 1994. Neurologic Manifestations of Cocaine Exposure in Childhood. *Pediatrics* 93:557-60.

Muhilal, P. D., Y. R. Idjradinata, Muherdiyantiningsih, and D. Karyadi. 1988. Vitamin A Fortified Monosodium Glutamate and Health, Growth, and Survival of Children: A Controlled Field Trial. *American Journal of Clinical Nutrition* 48:1271-76.

National Research Council. 1992. *Environmental Neurotoxicology*. Washington, D.C.: National Academy Press.

Navia, B. A., E. S. Cho, C. K. Petito, and R. W. Price. 1986. The AIDS Dementia Complex II: Neuropathology. *Annals of Neurology* 19:525-35.

Needleman, H. L., C. Gunnoe, A. Leviton, R. Reed, H. Peresie, C. Maher, and P. Barrett. 1979. Deficits in Psychologic and Classroom Performance in Children with Elevated Dentine Lead Levels. *New England Journal of Medicine* 300:689-95.

Nelson, M. 1992. Vitamin and Mineral Supplementation and Academic Performance in Schoolchildren. *Proceedings of the Nutrition Society* 51:303-13.

New England Congenital Hypothyroidism Collaborative. 1981. Effects of Neonatal Screening for Hypothyroidism: Prevention of Mental Retardation by Treatment before Clinical Manifestations. *Lancet* 2(8255):1095-98.

Nikiforov, Yu., and D. R. Gnepp. 1994. Pediatric Thyroid Cancer after the Chernobyl Disaster. *Cancer* 74:748-66.

Nokes, C., and D. A. P. Bundy. 1994. Does Helminth Infection Affect Mental Processing and Educational Achievement? *Parasitology Today* 10:14-18.

Nokes, C., S. M. Grantham-McGregor, A. W. Sawyer, E. S. Cooper, and D. A. Bundy. 1992. Parasitic Helminth Infection and Cognitive Function in School Children. *Proceedings of the Royal Society of London - Series B: Biological Sciences* 247(1319):77-81.

Nordin, J. D., S. J. Rolnick, and J. M. Griffin. 1994. Prevalence of Excess Lead Absorption and Associated Risk Factors in Children Enrolled in a Midwestern Health Maintenance Organization. *Pediatrics* 93:172-77.

Otake, M., and W. J. Schull. 1984. In Utero Exposure to A Bomb Radiation and Mental Retardation: A Reassessment. *British Journal of Radiology* 57:409-14.

Paradise, J. L., and K. D. Rogers. 1986. On Otitis Media, Child Development, and Tympanostomy Tubes: New Answers or Old Questions? *Pediatrics* 77:88-92.

Penman, H. G. 1970. Fatal Infectious Mononucleosis: A Critical Review. *Journal of Clinical Pathology* 23:765-69.

Petit, T. L., D. P. Alfano, and J. C. LeBoutillier. 1983. Early Lead Exposure and the Hippocampus. A Review of Recent Advances. *Neurotoxicology* 4:79-94.

Pfeiffer, C. C., and E. R. Braverman. 1982. Zinc: The Brain and Behavior. *Biological Psychiatry* 17:513-32.

Pharoah, P. O. D., I. H. Buttfield, and B. S. Hetzel. 1972. The Effects of Iodine Prophylaxis on the Incidence of Endemic Cretinism. *Advanced Experimental Medical Biology* 30:201-21.

Pharoah, P. O. D., and K. J. Connolly. 1991. Effects of Maternal Iodine Supplementation during Pregnancy. *Archives of Disease in Childhood* 66:145-47.

Piaget, J. 1972. *The Psychology of Intelligence*. Totowa, N.J.: Littlefield Adams.

Plaut, S. M., and S. B. Friedman. 1981. Psychosocial Factors, Stress, and Disease Processes. In R. Ader, ed., *Psychoneuroimmunology*. New York: Academic Press.

Pocock, S. J., M. Smith, and P. Baghurst. 1994. Environmental Lead and Children's Intelligence: A Systematic Review of the Epidemiological Evidence. *BMJ* 309:189-97.

Pollitt, E. 1988. A Critical View of Three Decades of Research on the Effects of Chronic Energy Malnutrition on Behavioral Development. In B. Schurch and N. Scrimshaw, eds., *Chronic Energy Deficiency: Consequences and Related Issues*. Lausanne: IDECG (International Dietary Energy Consultative Group).

———. 1990. *Malnutrition and Infection in the Classroom*. Paris: United Nations Educational, Scientific, and Cultural Organization.

———. 1993. Iron Deficiency and Cognitive Function. *Reviews in Nutrition* 13:521-37.

Pollitt, E., R. L. Leibel, and Greenfield, D. 1981. Brief Fasting, Stress, and Cognition in Children. *American Journal of Clinical Nutrition* 34:1526-33.

Pollitt, E., C. Lewis, C. Garza, and R. J. Shulman. 1983. Fasting and Cognitive Function. *Journal of Psychiatric Research* 17:169-74.

Pollitt, E., and E. Metallinos-Katsaras. 1990. Iron Deficiency and Behavior: Constructs, Methods, and Validity of the Findings. In R. J. Wurtman and J. J. Wurtman, eds., *Nutrition and the Brain*. Vol. 8. New York: Raven Press.

Pounds, J., and J. Rosen. 1988. Cellular Ca^{2+} Homeostasis and Ca^{2+}-Mediated Cell Processes as Critical Targets for Toxicant Action: Conceptual and Methodological Pitfalls. *Toxicology and Applied Pharmacology* 94:331-41.

Price, R. W., B. Brew, J. J. Sidtis, M. Rosenblum, A. C. Scheck, and P. Cleary. 1988. The Brain in AIDS: Central Nervous System HIV-1 Infection and AIDS Dementia Complex. *Science* 239:586-92.

Rahmathullah, L., B. A. Underwood, R. D. Thulasiraj, R. C. Milton, K. Ramaswamy, R. Rahmathullah, and G. Babu. 1990. Reduced Mortality among Children in Southern India Receiving a Small Weekly Dose of Vitamin A. *New England Journal of Medicine* 323:929-35.

Randall, C. L., and E. P. Riley. 1981. Prenatal Alcohol Exposure: Current Issues and the Status of Animal Research. *Neurobehavioral Toxicological Teratology* 3:111-15.

Ricciuti, H. N. 1991. Malnutrition and Cognitive Development: Research-Policy Linkages and Current Research Directions. In R. J. Sternberg and L. Okagaki, eds., *Directors of Development*. Hillsdale, N.J.: Lawrence Erlbaum and Associates.

———. 1993. Nutrition and Mental Development. *Current Directions in Psychological Science* 2(2):43-46.

Roberts, J. E., M. R. Burchinai, A. M. Collier, C. T. Ramey, M. A. Koch, and F. W. Henderson. 1989. Otitis Media in Early Childhood and Cognitive, Academic, and Classroom Performance of the School-aged Children. *Pediatrics* 83:477-85.

Rodier, P. 1986. Time of Exposure and Time of Testing in Developmental Neurotoxicology. *Neurotoxicology* 7:69-76.

Ryder, R. W., W. Nsa, S. E. Hassig, F. Behets, M. Rayfield, B. Ekungola, A. M. Nelson, U. Mulenda, H. Frances, K. Mwandagalirwa, F. Davach, M. Rogers, N. Nzilambi, A. Greenberg, J. Mann, T. C. Quinn, P. Pilot, and J. W. Curran. 1989. Perinatal Transmission of the Human Immunodeficiency Virus Type 1 to Infants of Seropositive Women in Zaire. *New England Journal of Medicine* 320:1637-42.

Sachs, H., and D. I. Moel. 1993. Lead Poisoning: Twenty Years After. *Pediatrics* 92:505.

Sandstead, H. H. 1985. W. O. Atwater Memorial Lecture. Zinc: Essentiality for Brain Development and Function. Review. *Nutrition Reviews* 43(5):129-37.

Scheidt, P. C., and J. F. Kavanagh. 1986. Common Terminology for Conditions of the Middle Ear. In J. F. Kavanagh, ed., *Otitis Media and Child Development*. Parkton, Md.: York Press.

Schwartz, J. 1994. Low Level Lead Exposure and Children's IQ: A Meta Analysis and Search for a Threshold. *Environmental Research* 65:42-55.

Scott, G. D., C. Hutto, R. W. Makuch, M. T. Mastrucci, T. O'Connor, C. D. Mitchell, E. J. Tradiro, and W. P. Parks. 1989. Survival in Children with Perinatally Acquired Human Immunodeficiency Virus Type 1 Infection. *New England Journal of Medicine* 321:1791-96.

Scrimshaw, N. S. 1991. Iron Deficiency. *Scientific American* 11:46-52.

Shaheen, S. 1984. Neuromaturation and Behavior Development: The Case of Childhood Lead Poisoning. *Developmental Psychology* 20:542-50.

Sigman, M., C. Neumann, E. Carter, and D. J. Cattle. 1988. Home Interactions and the Development of Embu Toddlers in Kenya. *Child Development* 59:1251-61.

Silbergeld, E. 1992. Neurological Perspective on Lead Toxicity. In H. Needleman, ed., *Human Lead Exposure*. Boca Raton, Fla.: CRC Press.

Silva, P. A., D. Chalmers, and I. Stewart. 1986. Some Audiological, Psychological, Educational and Behavioral Characteristics of Children with Bilateral Otitis Media with Effusion: A Longitudinal Study. *Journal of Learning Disabilities* 19:165-69.

Simeon, D. T., and S. M. Grantham-McGregor. 1989. Effects of Missing Breakfast on the Cognitive Functions of School Children of Differing Nutritional Status. *American Journal of Clinical Nutrition* 49:646-53.

———. 1990. Nutrition and Mental Development in Children. *Nutrition Research Reviews* 3:1-24.

Simeon, D. T., S. M. Grantham-McGregor, J. E. Callender, and M. S. Wong. 1995. Treatment of Trichuris Trichiura Infections Improves Growth, Spelling Scores and School Attendance in Some Children. *Journal of Nutrition* 125(7):1875-83.

Smith, A. 1990. Viral Infections, Immune Responses and Cognitive Performance. *International Journal of Neuroscience* 51:355-56.

Smith, A. P. 1992a. Chronic Fatigue Syndrome and Performance. In A. P. Smith and D. M. Jones, eds., *Handbook of Human Performance*. Vol. 2. New York: Harcourt Brace Jovanovich.

———. 1992b. Colds, Influenza and Performance. In A. P. Smith and D. M. Jones, eds., *Handbook of Human Performance*. Vol. 2. New York: Harcourt Brace Jovanovich.

Smith, A. P., D. A. J. Tyrrell, W. Al-Nakib, G. I. Barrow, P. G. Higgins, S. Leekam, and S. Trickett. 1989. Effects and After-effects of the Common Cold and Influenza on Human Performance. *Neuropsychobiology* 21:90-93.

Smith, A. P., D. A. J. Tyrrell, W. Al-Nakib, K. B. Coyle, C. B. Donovan, P. G. Higgins, and J. S. Willman. 1988. The Effects of Experimentally-induced Respiratory Virus Infections on Performance. *Psychological Medicine* 18:65-71.

Smith, A. P., D. A. J. Tyrrell, K. B. Coyle, and J. S. Willman. 1987. Selective Effects of Minor Illnesses on Human Performance. *British Journal of Psychology* 78:183-88.

Snodgrass, S. R. 1994. Cocaine Babies: A Result of Multiple Teratogenic Influences. *Journal of Child Neurology* 9:227-33.

Sommer, A., I. Tarwotjo, E. Djunaedi, K. P. West, Jr., A. A. Loeden, and R. Tilden, and L. Mele. 1986. Impact of Vitamin A Supplementation on Childhood Mortality. *Lancet* 1:169-73.

Stanbury, J. B. 1987. Iodine Deficiency Disorders: Introduction and General Aspects. In B. Hetzel, J. Dunn, and J. Stanbury, eds., *The Prevention and Control of Iodine Deficiency Disorders*. Amsterdam: Elsevier.

Stanbury, J. B., and B. S. Hetzel, eds. 1980. *Endemic Goiter and Endemic Cretinism. Iodine Nutrition in Health and Disease*. New York: Wiley and Sons.

Stephenson, L. 1987. *Impact of Helminth Infections on Human Nutrition*. London: Taylor & Francis.

Stephenson, L., M. C. Latham, E. J. Adams, S. N. Kinoti, and A. Pertet. 1993. Physical Fitness, Growth and Appetite of Kenyan School Boys with Hookworm, *Trichuris trichiura* and *Ascaris lumbricoide* Infections Are Improved Four Months after a Single Dose of Albendazole. *Journal of Nutrition* 123:1036-46.

Stephenson, L., M. C. Latham, S. N. Kinoti, K. M. Kurz, and H. Brigham. 1990. Improvements in Physical Fitness in Kenyan Schoolboys Infected with Hookworm, *Trichuris trichiura* and *Ascaris lumbricoides* Following a Single Dose of Albendazole. *Transactions of the Royal Society of Tropical Medicine and Hygiene* 84:277-82.

Sternberg, R. J., ed. 1984. *Mechanisms of Cognitive Development*. New York: Freeman.

———. 1985. *Beyond IQ: A Triarchic Theory of Human Intelligence*. New York: Cambridge University Press.

———. 1988. *The Triarchic Mind*. New York: Viking-Penguin.

———. 1990. *Metaphors of Mind*. New York: Cambridge University Press.

Sternberg, R. J., and Powell, J. S. 1983. The Development of Intelligence. In J. H. Flavell and E. M. Markman, eds., *Handbook of Child Psychology*. Vol. III. *Cognitive Development*. 4th ed. New York: Wiley.

Stickler, G. B. 1984. The Attack on the Tympanic Membrane. *Pediatrics* 74:291-92.

Super, C., J. Clement, L. Vuoir, N. Christianse, J. Mora, and M. Herrera. 1981. Infant and Caretaker Behavior as Mediator of Nutritional and Social Intervention in the Varrios of Bogota. In T. Field, ed., *Culture and Early Interaction*. Hillsdale, N.J.: Lawrence Erlbaum and Associates.

Super, C. M., and S. Harkness. 1986. The Developmental Niche: A Conceptualization at the Interface of Child and Culture. *International Journal of Behavioral Development* 9:545-69.

Super, C., M. Herrera, and J. Mora. 1990. Long-term Effects of Food Supplementation and Psychosocial Intervention on the Physical Growth of Colombian Infants at Risk for Malnutrition. *Child Development* 61:29-49.

Teele, D. W., J. O. Klein, and B. A. Rosner. 1984. Otitis Media with Effusion during the First Three Years of Life and Development of Speech and Language. *Pediatrics* 74:283-87.

Tross, S., R. W. Price, B. Navia, H. T. Thaler, J. Gold, D. A. Hirsh, and J. J. Sidtis. 1988. Neurological Characterisation of the AIDS Dementia Complex: A Preliminary Report. *AIDS* 2:81-88.

Tucker, D. M., and H. M. Sandstead. 1984. Neuropsychological Function in Experimental Zinc Deficiency in Humans. In C. J. Frederickson, G. A. Howell, and E. J. Kasarkis, eds., *The Neurology of Zinc*. New York: Alan Liss.

Tuttle, W. W., K. Daum, R. Larsen, J. Salzano, and L. Roloff. 1954. Effect on School Boys of Omitting Breakfast. Physiologic Responses, Attitudes, and Scholastic Attainments. *Journal of the American Dietetic Association* 30:674-77.

UNSCEAR (United Nations Scientific Committee on the Effects of Atomic Radiation). 1993. *Report to the General Assembly with Scientific Annexes. Annex H: Radiation Effects on the Developing Human Brain.* New York: United Nations.

Upadhyay, S., D. Agarwal, K. Agarwal, K. Srivastava, and G. Adhikari. 1988. Brief Fasting and Cognitive Functions in Rural School Children. *Indian Pediatrics* 25:288-89.

Vernon, R. E., ed. 1987. *Intelligence and Speed of Information Processing*. Norwood, N.J.: Ablex.

Vijayaraghavan, K., G. Radhaiah, B. S. Prakasam, K. V. R. Sarma, and V. Reddy. 1990. Effect of Massive Dose Vitamin A on Morbidity and Mortality in Indian Children. *Lancet* 336:1342-45.

Volpe, J. 1992. Effect of Cocaine Use on the Fetus. *New England Journal of Medicine* 6:399-407.

Von, T., J. C. Deitz, J. McLaughlin, S. DeButts, and M. Richardson. 1988. The Effects of Chronic Otitis Media on Motor Performance in 5- and 6-year-old Children. *American Journal of Occupational Therapy* 42:421-26.

Vygotsky, L. S. 1978. *Mind in Society: The Development of Higher Psychological Processes.* Cambridge: Harvard University Press.

Wachsmuth, J. R., and H. L. MacMillan. 1991. Effective Treatment for an Adolescent with Chronic Fatigue Syndrome. *Clinical Pediatrics* 30:488-90.

Walravens, P. A., and K. M. Hambridge. 1976. Growth of Infants Fed a Zinc Supplementated Formula. *American Journal of Clinical Nutrition* 29:1114-21.

Walravens, P. A., W. J. Van Doornick, and K. M. Hambridge. 1981. Metals and Mental Function. *Journal of Pediatrics* 93:535.

Warm, J. S., and E. A. Allusi. 1967. Behavioral Reactions to Infection: Review of the Psychological Literature. *Perceptual Skills* 24:755-61.

Wasserman, G., J. Graziano, P. Factor-Litvak, D. Popovac, N. Morina, A. Musabegovic, N. Vrenezi, S. Capuni-Paracka, V. Lekis, E. Preteni-Redjepi, S. Hasdzialjevic, V. Slavkovich, J. Kline, P. Shrout, and Z. Stein. 1992. Independent Effects of Lead Exposure and Iron Deficiency Anemia on Developmental Outcome at Age 2 Years. *Journal of Pediatrics* 121:695-703.

Watkins, W. E., and E. Pollitt. n.d. "Stupidity of Worms": Do Intestinal Worms Impair Mental Performance? *Psychological Bulletin*. Forthcoming.

Weiner, H. 1977. *Psychobiology and Human Disease*. New York: Elsevier.

West, K. P., R.-N. P. Pokhrel, J. Katz, S. C. LeClerq, S. K. Khatry, S. R. Shrestha, E. K. Pradhan, J. M. Tielsch, M. R. Pandey, and A. Sommer. 1991. Efficacy of Vitamin A in Reducing Preschool Child Mortality in Nepal. *Lancet* 338:67-71.

Wharton, B. 1995. Iron Deficiency and the Brain: Mathematics and Mechanisms (abstr.). *A Healthy Body and a Healthy Mind*. Oxford: Dormy Meeting.

WHO (World Health Organization)/UNICEF (United Nations Children's Fund)/International Vitamin A Consultative Group Task Force 1988. *Vitamin A Supplements. A guide to their Use in the Treatment and Prevention of Vitamin A Deficiency and Xerophthalmia*. Geneva.

Working Group of the American Academy of Neurology AIDS Task Force. 1991. Nomenclature and Research Case Definitions for Neurological Manifestations of Human Immunodeficiency Virus-type 1 (HIV-1) Infection. *Neurology* 41:778-85.

Xue-Yi, C., J. Xin-Min, D. Zhi-Hong, M. A. Rakeman, Z. Ming-Li, K. O'Donnell, M. Tai, K. Amette, N. DeLong, and G. R. DeLong. 1994. Timing of Vulnerability of the Brain to Iodine Deficiency in Endemic Cretinism. *New England Journal of Medicine* 331:1739-44.

Yudkin, J. 1991. Intelligence of Children and Vitamin-Mineral Supplements: The DRF Study. Discussion, Conclusion and Consequences. *Personality and Individual Differences* 12:363-65.

Zeskind, P., and C. Ramey. 1981. Preventing Intellectual and Interactional Sequelae of Fetal Malnutrition. *Child Development* 52:213-18.

Zinkus, P. W. 1986. Perceptual and Academic Deficits Related to Early Chronic Otitis Media. In J. F. Kavanagh, ed., *Otitis Media and Child Development*. Parkton, Md.: York Press.

Interventions for Cognitive Development in Children 0-3 Years Old

Robert J. Sternberg and Elena L. Grigorenko

Intelligence is one of the most important attributes of an individual because it is a principal means by which individuals adapt to the environment. Indeed, major theorists of intelligence have defined it as the ability to adapt to the environment (Intelligence and Its Measurement 1921; Sternberg and Detterman 1986). Given the importance of intelligence, it is no wonder that ever since ancient Greek times, and probably well before, philosophers such as Plato and many others have speculated on how one might develop it.

The preceding chapters explore the synergistic effects of health and nutrition in relation to children's cognitive development. Studies show that ill health and malnutrition adversely affect cognitive development. These effects are complex, vary according to the nature and severity of poor health or nutrition, and may be long term. Ill health and malnutrition can be particularly devastating for newborns, infants, and toddlers, who are just beginning to develop the cognitive abilities and pathways that will direct and sustain their later development. Yet, as suggested in the preceding chapter, appropriate, timely, and coordinated interventions can remediate these effects and help stimulate cognitive development.

Three messages are paramount: Cognitive abilities, which represent a major part of intelligence, can be developed; cognitive development efforts should begin at the earliest possible ages and ideally in the first 3 years of life; and appropriate techniques are available to stimulate positive cognitive development.

This chapter presents evidence to show that cognitive ability can be promoted by environmental interventions and that these interventions can and should be started at an early age. By starting early, one can maximize the number of years for optimal cognitive development, prevent the likelihood of inadequate development, reduce or eliminate the need for later remediation or catch-up, and give children the means to develop their abilities autonomously from the earliest possible age.

The chapter begins with a definition of terms. The next three sections convey the state of knowledge on cognitive abilities, as revealed by alternative models of intelligence; the heritability of cognitive abilities and its informativeness regarding the modifiability of these abilities; and the effects of environment on cognitive development. The next two sections focus on interventions: examples and their efficacy, and programmatic considerations and intervention models. A final section summarizes conclusions. The main themes are that cognitive abilities are heritable and molded by environment and that intervention is worthwhile and can be effective even with the youngest children.

Definitions

Highlighted in this chapter is one technique for stimulating cognitive development. Known as *scaffolding* (Wood 1980; Wood, Bruner, and Ross 1976), this technique derives theoretically from modern notions that children's cognitive abilities emanate from their desire and ability to cope with appropriate levels of relative novelty. Scaffolding is an interactive intervention that supports a child's optimal development by adjusting environmental input to the child's internal readiness and by equipping the child with resources to enhance development and maturation. Critical to the notion of scaffolding are the ideas that the unit of intervention is the dyad of caregiver and child and that the support of the caregiver is key to fostering development.

Scaffolding contrasts with the conventional notion of *stimulation*, which derives theoretically from more traditional views that infants' cognitive abilities emanate from their sensorimotor capabilities. Stimulation is a unidirectional intervention of external input from caregiver to child and is significantly less sensitive to a child's internal readiness to accept and process the input. The main unit of intervention in stimulation is the infant.

Reference is made to both scaffolding and stimulation in the following sections on the state of knowledge, and they are addressed in more detail in the section on programmatic considerations and models. It is important to note that scaffolding and stimulation are not mutually exclusive and are complementary concepts. They can be used together to develop cognitive abilities. Evidence shows, however, that scaffolding is a particularly effective intervention.

Models of Intelligence

Psychologists have sought to understand cognitive abilities by using a number of theoretical models. Four of the major theoretical models are described below: the psychometric, Piagetian, cognitive information-processing, and systems models (Sternberg 1990; Sternberg and Berg 1990).

The Psychometric Model

The psychometric model is based on the idea that the structure of cognitive abilities can be identified through a statistical method called factor analysis, which is applied to tables of correlations or covariances between psychometric tests of ability. Factors represent underlying or covert sources of individual differences, in contrast to psychometric tests, which represent overt sources of such differences. A number of psychometric tests measure the intelligence of infants. Perhaps the most well-known are the revised Bayley Scales of Mental and Motor Development (the Bayley) (Bayley 1993) and the Wechsler Preschool and Primary Scale of Intelligence (WPPSI) (Wechsler 1989). The Bayley is a downward extension of the Stanford-Binet, which is the modern version of scales originally proposed by Alfred Binet in turn-of-the-century France.

The psychometric model may not be the best basis for developing cognitive abilities of infants for various reasons. First, because the psychometric model emphasizes mental structure more than cognitive processes, it may not suggest optimally what cognitive processes should be developed (Sternberg 1977). Second, and perhaps more crucial, the sensorimotor tasks that underlie scores on psychometric tests of intelligence for infants show a zero correlation, on average, with scores on psychometric intelligence tests, which become relevant in middle childhood and remain relevant through adulthood (Bornstein and Sigman 1986). For these two reasons, the kinds of abilities defined by the psychometric model and developed in an intervention based on it [using, for example, the Bayley to indicate the effects of the intervention (Andrews and others 1982; Ramey, Yeates, and Short 1984)] may not have clear relevance to intelligence, as conventionally defined, in the years after infancy.

The Piagetian Model

The Piagetian model is based on Jean Piaget's (1972) theory of intellectual development. According to this theory, intelligence develops as an equilibration between two cognitive operations: assimilation, by which new information is incorporated into already existing schema; and accommodation, by which new information is incorporated into new schemas. Also according to this theory, intelligence develops in four stages: sensorimotor, preoperational, concrete-operational, and formal-operational.

Tasks that derive from this theory are used to measure intelligence. For example, intelligence in the concrete-operational stage might be measured by a test of liquid conservation that shows whether a child understands that pouring liquid from a tall, thin beaker into a short, stout one does not change the amount of liquid available. In the infancy period, sensorimotor tests are used to measure intelligence, much as in the psychometric model, because of the nature of the abilities that Piaget (1952, 1972) believed to develop during infancy. Tests for later periods have moderate to strong correlations with conventional psychometric tests of intelligence for corresponding age levels (Tuddenham 1962, 1970), but sensorimotor tests for infants do not correlate with scores on intelligence tests administered postinfancy, as noted earlier.

The Cognitive Information-Processing Model

According to this model (Sternberg and Powell 1983), intelligence develops through acquisition, organization, and efficient use of cognitive operations. A number of information-processing theories have been proposed (Sternberg 1984), but they share the view that intelligence can be measured through children's performance on age-appropriate cognitive tasks.

During infancy, tasks measure infants' habituation to relatively familiar stimuli and dishabituation to relatively new stimuli. The idea is that more intelligent infants will become bored more quickly by looking at relatively familiar stimuli and become interested more easily in relatively new stimuli than less intelligent infants. Infants' scores on these tests moderately correlate, even in the 0.40s, with scores on intelligence tests during middle and later childhood. Interestingly, the correlations seem to increase with the age of the children at retest, called a "sleeper effect" (Bornstein and Sigman 1986; Fagan 1984, 1985; Lewis and Brooks-Gunn 1981; McCall 1989).

This theoretical model seems quite promising as a basis for programs that foster infants' intellectual development. Because what is relatively new for one infant may not be so for another, the Piagetian model gives rise to programs based on scaffolding. Such programs use adult mediation to provide appropriate levels of novelty, in contrast to familiarity, for individual children.

Systems Models

Although an offshoot of cognitive information-processing models, systems models are broader in scope. Two main systems models are those of Gardner (1983, 1993) and Sternberg (1985, 1988, 1996).

According to Gardner (1983), intelligence comprises seven relatively autonomous, multiple intelligences: linguistic, logical-mathematical, spatial, musical, bodily-kinesthetic, interpersonal, and intrapersonal. Gardner has not conducted direct empirical tests of his theory, but supports it with a number of converging sources of evidence, such as developmental progressions, prodigies, evidence from brain damage, and psychometric evidence.

According to Sternberg (1985), intelligence has three main aspects that are largely, but not totally, distinct: analytical, creative, and practical. Sternberg (1996; Sternberg and others 1995, 1996) has found that the three aspects of intelligence are quite distinct psychometrically; other research supports this contention (Carraher, Carraher, and Schliemann 1985; Ceci and Liker 1988; Scribner 1984).

These systems models add to cognitive information-processing a broader scope of what constitutes intelligence. For example, Sternberg's theory basically agrees with cognitive theory but includes a broader range of abilities than are studied in conventional cognitive paradigms. Sternberg uses tasks measuring creative and practical, everyday competencies that would not appear on a conventional intelligence test or a narrowly conceived cognitive test. A broader scope of intelligence also enlarges the frame for possible intervention. Instead of targeting the unknown structure of an entity known as psychometric intelligence quotient (IQ), system models allow the design of specific interventions targeted to enhance particular components of intelligence.

In summary, available data suggest that the cognitive information-processing model, perhaps as extended through systems theories, is particularly suitable for and susceptible to intervention. With an understanding of how intelligence develops, its modifiability can be examined. Two factors, what is given (stable) and what is acquired (changeable), are considered determinants of the modifiability of intelligence. Researchers believe that genes control the stable component of intelligence and the environment controls its changeable component. How much intelligence is heritable and how much is environmental is not understood. A key question is: Can intelligence be heritable and still modifiable?

Heritability of Cognitive Abilities

The preponderance of evidence suggests that cognitive abilities, including those centrally involved in intelligence, can be inherited to some degree (Sternberg and Grigorenko 1996). Heritability is quantified by the coefficient h^2. This coefficient is an estimate of the proportion of variations among individual differences presumably resulting from genetic effects. Current estimates of heritability for various cognitive abilities vary between 0.15

to 0.90, depending on the ability, the age when it is measured, and the sample size used to estimate the coefficient. Thirteen factors about this statistic are important to remember:

- It applies to populations, not individuals.

- Its value varies across populations: For yet unknown reasons, significant discrepancies in h^2 estimates exist across different populations.

- Its value is affected by the range of environments in the assessed population: Global environmental changes may cause h^2 to fluctuate even within a given population.

- It encompasses some nonenvironmental effects: It does not necessarily take into account effects of genotype-environment interactions and correlations.

- It reflects some genetic effects, namely, those that result in measured individual differences, not group differences.

- It can be estimated in different ways based on the type of relatives involved in the analyses, and different methods of estimation typically result in different values that must be subjected to multirelative group analysis to correct for sample specificity.

- Its estimate depends on strong assumptions that are constantly debated and questioned by researchers, such as the assumption that identical and fraternal twins will grow up in similar environments or that separate identical twins are normally assigned randomly to nonmatching environments.

- Its value varies across ages (generally increasing with age), nonspecifically reflecting changes in the age-specific breakdown of genetic and environmental influences on traits as well as changes in age-to-age genetic effects.

- When calculated within groups, it does not generalize across groups.

- It involves error, like all descriptive statistics.

- It contains no necessary implications for social, economic, or educational policy.

- It does not translate into an understanding of the biological mechanisms underlying the development of intelligence.

- Most importantly, its value does not convey anything about the modifiability of a trait.

Two of the factors noted above are important limitations of the h^2 statistic of heritability in relation to intelligence. First, because the value of the statistic does not address a trait's modifiability, intelligence could have zero, moderate, or even total heritability and, in any of these conditions, be not at all, partially, or fully modifiable. The h^2 statistic deals with correlations, but modifiability deals with mean effects. Correlations, however, are independent of score levels. For example, adding a constant to a set of scores will not affect the correlation of that set with another set of scores.

Consider height as an example of the limitation of h^2 in addressing modifiability. Height is highly hereditary with an h^2 value of more than 0.90. Yet height also is highly modifiable, as shown by the fact that average heights have risen dramatically throughout the past several generations. As an even more extreme example, consider phenylketonuria (PKU). PKU is a genetically determined, autosomal recessive condition (with an h^2 of 1), and yet its effects are highly modifiable. Feeding an infant with PKU a diet free of phenylalanine prevents the development of mental retardation that otherwise would become manifest.

The second important limitation of heritability noted above is that the h^2 statistic does not indicate the actual biological mechanisms involved in development of intelligence. A global estimate of the genotypic effect reflected by h^2 does not bring researchers any closer to understanding the biological mechanisms behind intellectual development or to defining the limits of its modifiability.

In summary, whether intelligence is hereditary has nothing to do with its modifiability. Researchers can believe in high heritability, as do Herrnstein and Murray (1994) or Jensen (1969), while believing in modifiability. The two issues are separate and should not be confused.

Environmental Effects on Cognitive Abilities

Environment has a powerful effect on levels of cognitive ability. Perhaps the simplest and most potential demonstration of this is called the "Flynn effect" (Flynn 1987, 1994). The basic phenomenon of the Flynn effect is an increase in IQ throughout successive generations around the world during the past 30 years.

The effect is powerful, showing an increase in IQ of about 20 points per generation for tests of fluid intelligence (Cattell 1971; Horn and Cattell 1966) such as the Raven Progress Matrices, which measure a person's ability to cope effectively with relatively new stimuli. The mean effect has been inexplicably greater for tests of fluid ability than for tests of crystallized knowledge-based abilities. But if linearly extrapolated, the difference would suggest that a person at the 90th percentile on the Raven test in 1892 would score at the 5th percentile in 1992.

This effect must be environmental because a successive stream of genetic mutations could not have occurred and exerted such influence in such a short period of time. Psychometric tests of intelligence indicate that environment must be exerting a powerful effect on intelligence; intelligence can be, and is being, modified.

Several explanations for the Flynn effect are given below. Although they may seem contradictory, they share the element of scaffolding, as described earlier. The explanations show that scaffolding successfully promotes cognitive development even when provided incidentally through changes in a child's environment.

The first explanation of the Flynn effect is *increased schooling*. Education has been repeatedly associated with a wide variety of developmental outcomes, and time in school is related to improvements in cognitive performance (Ceci 1991). Bronfenbrenner and colleagues (1996; Ceci 1996) point out that in the 1930s, for example, mean educational attainment was 8 to 9 years; today it is 14 years.

Cahan and Cohen (1980) studied more than 11,000 fourth, fifth, and sixth graders in Israel, comparing children separated in age by only a couple of weeks but in different grades because of the birthday cutoff for entering school in a given year. The study compared, for example, 10-year-olds with 4 or 5 years of schooling. Effects of schooling, seen in tests measuring fluid and crystallized abilities, were twice the effect of age. The effect of just 1 year of schooling was larger in nine of the twelve tests than the effect of 1 year of age.

A second explanation of the Flynn effect is *greater educational attainment of parents*, especially minority parents, which enables them to be more effective mediators for their children. For example, in developing countries, a large body of research has established strong links between maternal education and improved cognitive performance in children (LeVine and others 1991; McGowan and Johnson 1984). The importance of parent education for children's development is addressed in detail in two later chapters (see Kagitcibasi and Lombard, this volume).

Some programs educate mothers about health care, helping them provide optimal nutrition and engage in adequate health practices for their children. For example, Lansdown (1995) reports that when mothers understand how to promote health and nutrition, children are more likely to attend school for more total years, to perform better on various tests, and to succeed better in the school environment. The mother-child relationship can increase children's IQ scores if mothers have more knowledge of health and nutrition and if they behave in accordance with this knowledge, training children in good health and nutrition practices.

Along these lines, Feuerstein (1980) argues that most intellectual development in children does not occur as a result of direct instruction in school or other environments, but occurs through learning experiences mediated by parents, usually the mother. A mother's interpretation of the environment for her child in an experientially and age-appropriate way, rather than a child's experience of the environment, fosters intellectual development. Providing appropriate mediated learning experiences may be considered a form of scaffolding. In more recent generations, families tend to have fewer total children and greater financial resources per child, both of which may result in greater intellectual development (Zajonc 1976).

A third explanation of the Flynn effect may be related somehow to the effect of *increased scaffolding by parents* toward their infants. Bronfenbrenner and Ceci (1994) studied changes over time in the nature and type of parental attention given to young children. They found that mothers' perceptions and ideas about how to mother have changed from the 1940s to the present, especially for middle-class mothers. Old perceptions emphasized feeding on a strict schedule and using ample discipline. Since the 1940s, however, mothers have moved toward feeding on demand and responding to their children. Parenting norms have changed toward responsiveness, or scaffolding.

Even though the study by Bronfenbrenner and Ceci is retrospective, comparing parental attitudes toward their infants across 50 years, other research suggests the importance of early home environment for cognitive development. For example, Hess and colleagues (1984) found that maternal measures taken during the preschool years predicted school readiness at age 5 and predicted achievement test performance at grade 6. The prediction was stronger for age 5 than age 12, indicating that a mother's influence on school achievement is stronger during the preschool years, precisely those years during which interventions should begin. Elardo, Bradley, and Caldwell (1977) found that language development at age 3 related to various scaffolding aspects of the early home environment. These aspects of scaffolding included emotional and verbal responsivity of the mother, provision of appropriate play materials, and mother-child interaction.

The effects visible at age 3 start early. In a study of parental responsiveness to infants, Riksen-Walraven (1978) examined the interactions of 100 Dutch mothers with their 9-month-olds. Mothers were assigned randomly to four groups. The length of interaction time was constant across the groups, but the interactions differed in quality and the behavior of the mothers differed in accordance with the instructions they received.

One group of mothers was instructed not to direct their children's activities too much, but to give the children an opportunity to find things out for themselves, to praise them for their efforts, and to respond to their initiation of interactions. Another group of mothers was told to speak to their infants a lot and to initiate interactions frequently; these mothers controlled the interactions instead of responding to the children. A third group was instructed to combine the approaches of the first two groups. A fourth (control) group was given no instruction.

After 3 months all infants were tested. Infants of mothers who had been encouraged to be responsive showed higher levels of exploratory behavior than infants in any other group, and they preferred new to familiar objects. These infants, randomly assigned to conditions of greater maternal responsiveness, showed enhanced cognitive functioning.

In summary, the Flynn effect convincingly illustrates environmental effects on IQ. Explanations for the effect support the modifiability of cognitive abilities. This evidence for the potency of the environment in molding cognitive abilities has been accepted as valid by even the most conservative critics (for example, Herrnstein and Murray 1994). Studies in which attempts have been made to modify cognitive abilities are reviewed below.

Cognitive Intervention: Examples and Efficacy

In the face of data such as those summarized above, behavioral scientists should be uniformly in favor of early cognitive intervention, but they are not. Some behavioral scientists still believe that cognitive abilities cannot be modified substantially, despite considerable evidence to the contrary. In their writings, they tend to select interventions that have been less successful or to interpret the results of cognitive interventions in a way that minimizes their effectiveness (for example, Herrnstein and Murray 1994). They often seem to set up a straw man, arguing that unless cognitive interventions show massive, durable, and transferable gains, they are not worthwhile. However, such standards are not applied elsewhere in the sciences. For example, a treatment for cancer may be considered extraordinarily effective even though it does not result in permanent and total remission for every patient. But today, many more behavioral scientists seem to favor than disfavor cognitive intervention.

Evidence in support of early intervention comes from two sources. The first is *natural experiments*, such as adoption studies. Two adoption studies were conducted in orphanages, one by Dennis (1973) in Iran and one by Rutter (1996) in Romania. Dennis found that children placed in Iranian orphanages had low IQs. Probably because they were reared in institutions of different quality, girls had a mean IQ of about 50 and boys of about 80. Children adopted out of an Iranian orphanage by the age of 2 had IQs that averaged 100 during later childhood; they were able to overcome the effects of early deprivation. Children adopted after the age of 2 showed normal intellectual development from that point, but never overcame the effects of early deprivation; they remained mentally retarded. These results suggest that interventions to foster cognitive development need to start as early as possible.

Rutter's Romanian project showed increases in mean IQ from 60 to 109 for orphans who came to the United Kingdom before 6 months of age. These children showed complete recovery from early mental retardation. Those who came to the United Kingdom after 6 months of age showed, on average, continuing deficits. This finding again argues for early interventions.

The second source of evidence in support of cognitive intervention is *intervention studies*. The general purpose of intervention programs is to ensure adequate cognitive development of children from low-income families by involving parents in educating their children (the family support model of intervention) or providing children with early education programs in preschool settings (the educational model of intervention). In the first model the target is the family, and the benefits to children are secondary to benefits for the family. Because the second model is child-centered, children are the primary beneficiaries of the intervention. Some studies have tried to target both parents and children.

Regardless of the form of intervention, the underlying logic of these models for intervention programs is the same: to enhance a child's cognitive development through cognitive and environmental scaffolding. The goal is to promote children's physical, cognitive, and socioemotional development, enabling children to negotiate successfully the transition to school (Schweinhart and Weikart 1988). In the long run, the goal is to prevent such maladaptations as school failure and delinquent behaviors.

Intervention Models and Examples

Data supporting the effectiveness of intervention studies have been accumulating since the 1960s, when the U.S. Head Start program was first launched (Chafel 1992). A meta-analysis of 210 research reports on the effects of Head Start on children (McKey and others 1985) showed immediate gains on cognitive and socioemotional tests for children enrolled in the program. Although the gains of participants did not remain relative to the gains of nonparticipants over time, Head Start children were less likely to repeat grades or require special education help.

Since the 1960s a vast number of studies, including large-scale federal programs, university-based interventions, and small-scale research projects, have estimated the effects of early cognitive intervention on child development. Results from the three types of studies, which target parents, children, or both, support the importance of early intervention. In addition to having different primary targets, intervention programs differ in a number of other ways. For example, programs may have different delivery settings (home, school, center, clinic), timing of onset (prenatal, infant, toddler), duration (length of intervention), intensity (amount of intervention per unit of time), curriculum content, intervener-to-child ratios, and staff education.

Table 1 summarizes the targets, projects, duration, and outcomes for the two major types of intervention models: family support models, and educational models. Major findings that have emerged in 30 years of providing cognitive intervention to children are described briefly below for each of these models and for center-based childcare, which combines both family support and educational components.

Table 1. Two Types of Cognitive Intervention Models

Intervention model	Primary target	Projects	Duration	Outcomes
Family support model	Family	Improving mother-child interaction Teaching mothers to solve problems and meet their children's meets Improving mothers' socioemotional functioning and self-esteem Improving mother's socioeconomic status by ensuring their participation in the job market Enhancing maternal knowledge of child development	3 years (average)	Short-term effects include immediate developmental gains in participants in contrast to nonparticipants Long-term effects are inconsistent
Educational model	Child	Direct, child-centered educational intervention	Between 1 and 10 years	Short-term effects include better academic performance of participants in contrast to nonparticipants Long-term effects include fewer referrals to special education, lower grade retention rates, and higher percentage of school graduation for participants compared with matched nonparticipants.

Family Support Model of Intervention

The major goal of this approach, illustrated in table 1, is changing parenting practices to strengthen children's cognitive and socioemotional outcomes. These programs (Benasich, Brooks-Gunn, and Clewell 1992) use various strategies including (a) helping mothers improve their child interactions and teaching skills; (b) teaching mothers to solve problems and respond to their children's needs; (c) raising mothers' self-esteem and socioemotional functioning; (d) ensuring maternal enrollment in school or participation in the job market; and (e) enhancing maternal knowledge and understanding of child development.

For example, the Yale Child Welfare Research Project (Provence and Naylor 1983) enrolled seventeen impoverished women who were expecting their first child. Services, provided for 30 months, included pediatric care, regular home visits, day care, and regular developmental examination of the children. At the end of the intervention, significant results were limited to children's language development (Rescorla, Provence, and Naylor 1982), and the follow-up study revealed no differences in IQ scores or achievement test results, but showed better school attendance and school adjustment in participants (Seitz, Rosenbaum, and Apfel 1985).

The Florida Parent Education Program (Gordon, Guinagh, and Jester 1977) was a home-based, parent-mediated intervention program for children from infancy to age 3. The follow-up study showed no significant IQ or academic differences between participants and controls by grade 5, but the participants were significantly less likely to be placed in special education.

Another large-scale intervention effort was undertaken for infants of Black teenage mothers in Washington, D.C. This program provided pediatric care and parenting education for 3 years. The participants demonstrated IQ gains when compared to controls at age 3 (Gutelius and others 1972). Unfortunately, no longitudinal follow-up study was done.

The Parent Child Developmental Center (Johnson 1988) conducted a large-scale, parent-centered intervention study involving 458 Mexican-American families randomly assigned to treatment conditions. The results of the Texas follow-up study, which took place when children were 7-10 years of age, showed that participants performed significantly better than controls in reading and mathematics. However, no differences were shown in grade retention or placement in special education (Johnson and Walker 1991).

Since the 1970s Hebrew University has been using two unique, home-based preschool programs to train mothers from disadvantaged families to act as home teachers for their young children (Lombard 1994, this volume). The first program, the Home Instruction Program for Preschool Youngsters (HIPPY), teaches mothers of children ages 3-6 how to improve their children's learning profiles. HIPPY was so successful that researchers constructed a second program, the Home Activities for Toddlers and Their Families (HATAF), which was developed for children ages 10-36 months to complement HIPPY.

Lombard's HIPPY methodology has been implemented in Turkey as part of the Turkish Early Enrichment Project (TEEP) for low-income families of Istanbul and in the Netherlands for ethnic minorities. Although the implementation was successful in Turkey (see Kagitcibasi, this volume), the program's effects in Holland were negligible (Eldering and Vedder 1993).

Although the majority of intervention programs using the family support model resulted in significant short- or long-term differences between participants and nonparticipants, the effects of some programs were negligible. A number of factors may explain the inconsistency in findings. First, most of these programs had certain methodological difficulties, principally: limited duration of the intervention, unmeasured magnitude of the intervention, and absence of supporting scaffolding after the intervention. For example, the variability in project results could be explained by the different numbers of home visits and the different magnitude and quality of the interventions during visits.

A second factor that may explain some inconsistencies is that, in the overwhelming majority of parent-mediated studies, parents were viewed and treated as supplemental interveners. Turning parents into interveners is cost-efficient and developmentally beneficial. For example, in analyses of outcomes for fifty-two early intervention studies, White, Bush, and Casto (1985) found parental involvement highly beneficial to intervention. Of course, parental participation is not solely responsible for the outcomes of infant intervention programs (White, Taylor, and Moss 1992). Indeed, programs could serve infants and parents better by viewing both as the target of intervention.

Educational Model of Intervention

The major assumption underlying the educational model, also illustrated in table 1, is that intervention should be direct and child-centered. The Carolina Early Intervention Program (Ramey 1988) is one of the most successful developmental day-care projects of this kind. Also known as the Abecedarian Project, this program was designed for children from poor families and required their full-time participation, beginning at 3 months of age, in a high-quality early childhood curriculum for infants and toddlers that was theory-based. During 5 years, 112 families were admitted to the program, and approximately one-half were assigned randomly to the experimental group while the others became the control group.

Although the data from this program (Campbell and Ramey 1994; Ramey 1988) showed no difference in cognitive performance between intervention and control groups during the first year of study (Ramey, Yeates, and Short 1984), a significant difference emerged by age 4 and persisted through 7 years of school (Campbell and Ramey 1994). In other words, early cognitive scaffolding appears to prevent a possible decline in cognitive development during preschool and school years (Rauh and others 1988).

Results of the Abecedarian Project led researchers to develop an extension, Project CARE (Wasik and others 1990). This project, a component of the Abecedarian educational day-care curriculum, provided family support and home visiting. It included teaching parents how to solve problems effectively and how to acquire specific knowledge and skills related to positive child development. The design included a control group and two intervention groups: center-based educational day care plus family education, and family education only. The results showed no effects of cognitive intervention for the family education group (Roberts and others 1989; Wasik and others 1990).

Researchers of the Milwaukee Project (Garber 1988), also a child-centered approach, followed a sample of forty Black children born to low-income mothers with IQs below 75. The final group included seventeen experimental and eighteen control families. The purpose was to prevent retardation in the children by providing extensive educational enrichment during the preschool years. The reported preschool IQ scores for participants were dramatically higher (29.5 points) than those of the controls. However, after 7 years in school, no differences were found between participants and nonparticipants (Campbell and Ramey 1994).

The most widely publicized evidence concerning outcomes of early intervention was gathered by the Consortium for Longitudinal Studies, which was formed by leaders of eleven projects collectively serving economically disadvantaged children between 1962 and 1973. Even though the main profile of consortium projects was an educational intervention program, more than one-half of the studies also used frequent home visits to involve parents. And even though some consortium projects did not include home visits, they involved parents through parent-teacher conferences at school, through allowing parents to observe cognitive stimulation sessions, and so on (Seitz 1990). Educational outcomes were encouraging. Overall, participants in the projects had significantly fewer placements and referrals to special education programs; fewer grade retentions (Lazar and others 1982); and a 12.3 percent increase in high school graduation (Royce, Darlington, and Murray 1983). Evidence also showed that early intervention contributes to long-term outcomes, such as reduced dropout and delinquency and increased employment (Berrueta-Clement and others 1984; Schweinhart and others 1993; Young 1996). However, IQ gains of participants largely disappeared after 3 years of public school, and the significance of IQ differences between participants and controls generally did not continue past 5 or 6 years after the project (Lazar and others 1982; McKey and others 1985; White 1985).

In summary, three consistent types of outcomes have been reported for the educational model. First, participants usually show a short-term IQ gain, which is maintained for a number of years in some programs. Second, despite the higher IQs observed at school entry in participants compared with nonparticipants, participants do not show commensurably stronger school performance. Third, in a number of studies, the most notable differences between participants and nonparticipants relate to better school adjustment (higher graduation rates, lower dropout rates) and general life outcomes (better job placement, less delinquency).

Center-based Childcare

Traditional childcare should not be confused with intervention programs such as Head Start (Zigler and Lang 1991). Nevertheless, researchers (Cronbach 1982; McCartney and others 1985) argue for using quality indicators of day-care programs as substitutes for treatment intensity, in effect viewing childcare programs of different quality as intervention programs of different treatment magnitude.

Because center-based childcare is becoming a primary way to care for infants and young children around the world (Kisker and others 1991; Young 1996), issues of particular importance now relate to the quality of center-based infant associated with infant development and identification of child and family characteristics that serve as risk or protective factors. Addressing these issues in research settings and finding links between infant care and infant development should result in programs to regulate infant childcare and promote infant development.

Recent research has focused on identifying family and child factors that moderate the association between childcare and child developmental outcomes (Burchinal and others 1995). Of particular interest is whether high-quality childcare can buffer child outcomes from stressful and developmentally risky, poor home care (Scarr and Eisenberg 1993). The hope is that childcare can protect children who come from potentially risky family backgrounds, such as poverty or single-parent homes, that negatively affect development (Sameroff and others 1993). Despite the societal importance of the effect of early childcare on further development, this protective factor has not yet been well described or quantified, and it remains a central point of debate in developmental psychology.

A significant amount of evidence indicates the positive influence of high-quality day care on child development. For example, improved cognitive performance has been reported in low- and middle-income children participating in average Swedish day-care programs (Andersson 1989, 1992) and in U.S. community-based day care (Burchinal, Lee, and Ramey 1989; Clarke-Stewart 1991). In these studies, day-care participants had cognitive test scores between those of participants in specially designed intervention centers and those of children with minimal or no center-based experience.

Similarly, a long-term follow-up study in West Germany (Tietz 1987), conducted with a sample of representative cohorts, showed that children who attended high-quality childcare centers had significantly better academic performance and social skills at 8-13 years of age than children who attended lower-quality centers. Some evidence also indicates that, on average, factors relating to quality of day care better predict children's social development (for example, school adjustment) than their cognitive (IQ) development (Dunn 1993; Kontos 1991).

These findings, showing positive effects of high-quality day care on child development, have been challenged by data from the U.S. National Longitudinal Survey of Youth (NLSY), which was conducted on a national probability sample. The NLSY data reveal a range of findings. One study reported a negative association between participation in day care during the first year of life and cognitive indices, as measured by the Peabody Picture Vocabulary Tests at ages 3-4 (Baydar and Brooks-Gunn 1991). In another study, Desai, Chase-Landsdale, and Michel (1989) demonstrated finer interaction effects, showing that negative effects of nonmaternal childcare are specific only to high-income families. Another group of researchers (Caughy, DiPetro, and Strobino 1994) found a significant interaction effect between type of day care and quality of home environment. Specifically, participation in center-based care was associated with higher reading and mathematics scores for 5- and 6-year-old children from impoverished home environments but was associated with lower scores for children of comparable ages from more nearly optimal and stimulating home environments.

Significant evidence (Clark-Stewart 1989) indicates a connection between infant day care and maladaptive social development, such as increased aggression with peers and lowered compliance with adult demands. For example, researchers (Vandell and Corsaniti 1990) reported that academic and social skills in a sample of middle-class 8-year-olds in Texas who had received extensive infant day care of dubious or poor quality were poorer than among children who did not attend day-care centers.

Some of the short-term outcomes of center-based childcare also tend to be controversial. A series of reports on a study in Bermuda showed that children attending higher-quality day-care centers had higher scores than nonattenders on measures of language development, regardless of socioeconomic status (SES) (McCartney 1984; McCartney and others 1985; Phillips, McCartney, and Scarr 1987). Analogous results indicating that day care enhances child language development were obtained in a study of 20-month-old infants of low SES (O'Connell and Farran 1982). This study demonstrated that infants in high-quality centers tend to have higher indices of language development than infants reared at home in low-income families.

Similarly, results of a Canadian study (Schliecker, White, and Jacobs 1991) indicated that SES and day-care quality are related significantly to breadth and sophistication of vocabulary, with quality of care being especially important for children of single parents. In this study, fifty-seven socioeconomically disadvantaged children were assigned randomly to three different treatment conditions. However, other researchers (Melhuish and others 1990) found that infants in lower-quality center-based care tend to have poorer language development than infants receiving better-quality care at home. Investigators also reported that SES, family values, and maternal education significantly predict child development, but the quality of center-based care does not (Goelman and Pence 1987; Kontos and Fiene 1987).

A number of large-scale studies in industrialized countries have investigated the quality of center-based care for infants, based on structural and process measures. On average, these studies have revealed an adequate level of structural care (for example, group size, child-adult ratios, teacher education) but a poor level of process care (for example, dimensions of adult-child interactions) (Burchinal and others 1996).

Researchers (Dunn 1993; Scarr and others 1993) have reviewed current literature on children's developmental correlates and day-care quality. Their analysis of structural characteristics suggests that smaller groups in childcare centers lead to higher compliance, cooperation, and considerateness; engagement in more sophisticated play; better academic progress; and fewer antisocial responses. In contrast, larger groups are linked to more aimless wandering and poorer social adjustment. These analyses also show that lower ratios of children to caregivers relate to higher levels of social competence, more sophisticated social play, higher compliance and cooperation, and more advanced academic progress. Higher caregiver-child ratios correlate with more aimless wandering, more peer interaction, and less optimal social adjustment. Higher, more specialized education of caregivers also is associated with children's displaying higher levels of social competence, more compliance, more cooperation, and better academic progress, but also lower levels of independence and social competence.

Research on procedural aspects of center-based care indicates that positive, attentive caregiver interactions with children (especially when conducted through planned, goal-directed activities such as play) relate to positive outcomes for children on all developmental dimensions. The review by Burchinal and colleagues (1996) suggests that, although many centers are adequately staffed and hygienically appropriate, procedural aspects are inadequate. Infants do not receive responsive and stimulating interactions with adults that provide the emotional, motor, and linguistic scaffolding crucial for cognitive and language development (Bradley and others 1989; Snow 1983; Tomasello and Farrar 1986).

Building on the ideology of Head Start and other center-based programs of early cognitive intervention, large-scale studies have been conducted in Asia, the Middle East, and Latin America. Many of these studies are described by Myers (1995) and Young (1995, 1996). The studies demonstrate the link between early intervention, increased school readiness, lower dropout and grade repetition rates, and enhanced academic achievement.

The spectrum of international research has increased greatly since the 1990s, when the World Bank initiated several programs targeted to early development (Young 1995). These programs include: parental education in India, Mexico, and Nigeria addressing issues of children's well-being during the first 3 years of life; home day care or center-based day care in Bolivia and Colombia providing direct services to children 2-6 years old; and nonformal or formal preschool education programs in Chile, Ecuador, El Salvador, and Venezuela. These programs are ongoing endeavors that provide rich and extensive data on the effects of early childhood intervention on cognitive and socioemotional development.

In summary, two findings obtained from research on center-based childcare seem most important. First, a significant interaction effect appears to exist between childcare quality and family environment, which suggests the need to carefully evaluate the appropriateness of childcare in relation to the type and quality of upbringing at home. In other words, childcare that would be beneficial to a child from an impoverished family environment could be quite detrimental to a child from an enriched family environment. Second, ensuring the high quality of structural characteristics is not enough. Successful outcomes of center-based childcare depend on process aspects, that is, adequate scaffolding by childcare staff. For more discussion of the elements of quality in early childhood programs, see Schweinhart (this volume).

Effectiveness of Early Cognitive Intervention

Because of the many successful intervention programs in the past decade, the focus of research on early childhood intervention programs has shifted from proving that they work to showing how they work. The goal now is to investigate why and for how long the programs are effective. Researchers warn that premature and unqualified interpretations of the powerful outcome data from interventions might lead to overgeneralization and could perpetuate simplistic models of child development that exaggerate the role of early intervention (Haskins 1989; Woodhead 1988).

With this new focus and caution, researchers today devote attention to asking more sophisticated questions about how to ensure the short- and long-term effects of intervention and to understanding how these effects are embedded in a wider context of family, community, schooling, and employment, as well as what their psychological mechanisms are and how interventions can foster their long-term duration (Woodhead 1988). From their studies, researchers have suggested two major hypotheses to explain the long-term effectiveness of intervention (Reynolds and others 1996). The first is the cognitive-advantage hypothesis, and the second is the family-scaffolding hypothesis.

Long-term Effectiveness

According to the *cognitive-advantage hypothesis*, the positive effects of preschool result in cognitive readiness, which in turn, triggers a positive chain of academic achievements and commitments that continues throughout adolescence (Bloom 1976; Royce and others 1983; White 1985). This hypothesis has been used to explain the long-term effects of the High/Scope Perry Preschool Program. Early cognitive advantages gained from this program arguably lead to a series of positive developments throughout the school years (Berrueta-Clement and others 1984; Schweinhart and others 1993; Schweinhart and

Weikart 1980). These positive developments build up, supporting the "Matthew effect" (Merton 1968; Walberg and Tsai 1983), in which initial advantages multiply over time and ultimately lead to better outcomes.

The *family-scaffolding hypothesis* links longer-term effects of early childhood interventions with improvement in family functioning. The central assumption of this hypothesis is that an intervention must affect family processes to produce long-term effects because much of early development is based heavily on interactions between infants and parents. Family processes refer to parental attitudes toward, beliefs about, and understanding of child development (Scott-Jones 1984).

The relevant scientific literature covers a vast number of issues relating to child development and family processes: partnerships between families and schools (Epstein 1990; Kroth 1989); teaching effective parenting and childrearing skills (Gamson, Hornstein, and Borden 1989; Nye 1989); and appropriate parental roles in the normal developmental process (Vartuli and Winter 1989; White 1985). Researchers have conducted a number of studies with interventions that targeted parental attitudes, beliefs, and understandings. The results of these studies demonstrate the positive effects of family process interventions (Affholter, Connell, and Nauta 1983; Jester and Guinagh 1983; Johnson and Walker 1991; Seitz, Rosenbaum, and Apfel 1985).

In addition, much independent literature demonstrates the importance of family processes for infant development. For example, researchers (Benasich and Brooks-Gunn 1996; Fry 1985; Snyder, Eyres, and Barnard 1979; Stevens 1984a, b) have identified links between maternal knowledge of child development and concepts of childrearing as well as links between quality of the home environment and cognitive and behavioral outcomes for children. In a prospective longitudinal study of a low-birthweight, preterm cohort, Benasich and Brooks-Gunn (1996) found that measures of maternal knowledge at 12 months were significantly associated with quality of the home environment, number of child behavioral problems, and children's IQ at 36 months.

A number of studies (McGillicuddy-DeLisi 1985; Ninio 1979; Snyder, Eyres, and Barnard 1979; Stevens 1984b) have investigated relationships between parental understanding of developmental milestones and child outcomes. The literature on child outcomes, although sparse, suggests that parental knowledge of developmental norms and parental beliefs about the influence of these norms on infant learning are significantly related to parental and child competence. For example, Dichtelmiller and colleagues (1992), in a study of extremely-low-birthweight, preterm infants, found that parental knowledge about infant development (evaluated at a child's birth) was positively related to performance of the child on the Bayley at 8 months. Sameroff and colleagues (Sameroff and others 1987; Seifer and Sameroff 1987) report that the complexity and depth of maternal understanding of childrearing makes a significant contribution to a child's IQ at 4 years of age.

Reynolds and colleagues (1992) suggest that even though the two hypotheses explaining the long-term effectiveness of early childhood intervention (cognitive readiness and family scaffolding) have been investigated separately, they appear to be compatible and may bear implications crucial for the success of cognitive interventions. For example, in a large-scale longitudinal study, researchers found that preschool participation at ages 3 or 4 was significantly related to higher reading and math achievement and lower incidence of grade repetition at age 12 (Reynolds and others 1996). The researchers showed that cognitive readiness and parental involvement in school significantly mediated the effects of preschool intervention. Modifications in school and family contexts appear to significantly facilitate the effect of preschool programs.

Negative Influences on Outcome

In addition to understanding factors that may ensure long-term effects of early intervention, researchers are investigating influences that might destroy or mask positive outcomes. A review of the literature suggests that long-lasting effects of early intervention are less likely to be found if:

- Postprogram educational experiences do not support or reinforce the acquired gains (for example, if scaffolding is withdrawn at the end of intervention)
- Parental involvement does not persist (for example, if no family-based scaffolding exists)
- Teachers do not encourage and support scholastic development
- Children frequently change schools, school environments are unstable, or children discontinue school attendance (Gorman and Pollitt 1996)
- A child's family faces continuing economic hardship and its attendant stresses (Sampson and Laub 1994)
- Motivation to achieve is low (Zigler and others 1982)
- Physical health is jeopardized (Hale, Seitz, and Zigler 1990; Neumann and others 1991; Pollitt 1990)
- Nutrition is inadequate (Grantham-McGregor and others 1991; Wachs and others 1993)
- Adverse environmental effects, such as exposure to teratogenic agents, are present (Kopp and Krakow 1983).

Any one or a combination of these factors may eliminate or mask the effects of early intervention. A linear relationship also has been shown between the number of active adverse factors and negative outcomes of cognitive development (Sameroff and others 1993; Gorman and Pollitt 1996). For example, when these effects occur in clusters, intervention programs have difficulty succeeding.

Methodological Drawbacks

In addition to these complications of real life that might jeopardize the effectiveness of intervention programs, current intervention studies also have a number of methodological drawbacks. These drawbacks may have caused the efficacy of preschool interventions to be underestimated. First, restricted sampling is a special problem for many intervention studies. Random assignment, the preferred method for evaluating program effects, rarely can be used in large-scale, government-supported programs because denying services to those who are predetermined as eligible is not possible (McKey and others 1985). Lack of experimental control, as well as lack of purity in administering treatment, may mask effects of an intervention or result in the inability to detect them statistically.

A second serious complication is related to heterogeneity of populations, both nonparticipant (Schnur, Brooks-Gunn, and Shipman 1992) and participant (Duncan and Rogers 1988; Furstenberg, Brooks-Gunn, and Morgan 1987; Gordon and Shipman 1979). This issue is especially important for federal programs that traditionally enroll the poorest and least developmentally able children (Hebbeler 1985; Schnur, Brooks-Gunn, and Shipman 1992). Also, few intervention programs control for other variables (for example, family functioning and parental sensitivity) that have been shown to be important developmentally. Failing to control for additional variance introduced into analyses by other relevant factors may mask effects of the efficiency of early intervention. And last but not least, much more careful estimation of the magnitude and quality of interventions should be made.

Evaluation Issues

Special consideration has been given to determining the most beneficial age of onset for cognitive intervention. Should intervention begin between ages 0 and 3, 2 and 5, or 3 and 6? For example, Weikart (1996) argues that the optimal time for intervention is between 2½ to 6, and that infancy and toddler interventions have not yet demonstrated their effectiveness. This statement is simultaneously fair and unfair. It is fair in saying that the results of infant-toddler intervention studies are inconsistent. However, significantly fewer of these studies exist than do studies of preschool children. Randomly selecting a few preschool intervention studies to match the number of early intervention studies will most likely show some inconsistencies in results of the former; judging the overall potential of early intervention studies based on the few available studies is unfair.

Quality of the programs also should be considered when evaluating these studies. Designing a good intervention program for infants and toddlers is more difficult than creating a good program for preschoolers. If the history of preschool educational programs is centuries old, the field of early cognitive intervention is very young. In other words, the fact that no cure has been found yet does not mean that one does not exist.

Another important issue relating to the effectiveness of early intervention programs is cost-benefit ratio. Early intervention programs tend to be more expensive than preschool programs because they usually enroll children, parents, and professionals. Investing money in something, like early interventions, means taking it away from something else, like subsequent health and educational interventions. However, early intervention programs increase the value of human capital by providing an early chance for adequate development; investing early saves on later investments. Both van der Gaag and Barnett expand on this issue in this volume.

In summary, some conclusions can be drawn from these diverse examples and studies of the efficacy of cognitive intervention described above: cognitive intervention is indeed worthwhile; it needs to incorporate effective scaffolding; and it should begin as early as possible in a child's life. The most effective outcome can be reached when there is "a convergence of support structures in children's family and school environments that persists over time" (Reynolds and others 1996: 1135). Based on these conclusions, certain criteria must be adopted when designing an intervention.

Programmatic Considerations and Models

To be maximally effective, an intervention must meet certain criteria. These criteria, which should be considered when designing cognitive interventions for early childhood, are outlined below.

Design Criteria

- *Theory-based.* The intervention program should be based on a psychological developmental theory, which takes into account psychological and developmental characteristics of a targeted developmental stage and defines the roles of interveners, parents, and children within a large family and care-center context.

- *Appropriate goals.* The program should have well-pronounced, clear, and reachable goals that can be met using available resources.

- *Simplicity.* The program must be simple and easily implemented, even in the harshest of circumstances.

- *Low-tech.* The program must not require equipment or devices that will be unavailable to parents once investigative teams leave.

- *Parental education.* The program must teach parents to understand the developmental stage of a targeted child. It must not assume any particular level of parental education, whether through schooling or otherwise. Special attention should be given to hands-on techniques, which will ensure that parents provide the necessary, age-appropriate cognitive, behavioral, and socioemotional scaffolding.

- *Autonomy.* The program must be teachable and adaptable, able to be carried out in full by local educators and other childcare professionals after the investigative team leaves.

- *Cultural appropriateness and relevance.* The program must be appropriate and relevant for the culture in which it is being conducted, taking into consideration what the members of the culture are trying to accomplish in rearing their young. This consideration is particularly important because different cultural groups have different conceptions of socializing an intelligent child (Okagaki and Sternberg 1993).

- *Development of diverse intellectual skills.* The program should foster the development of diverse intellectual skills, such as analytical, creative, and practical skills, rather than foster the development of a narrow band of skills, such as those needed to succeed on conventional psychometric tests of intelligence.

- *Motivation.* The program should motivate parents and children alike to maximize the likelihood of continued use and effectiveness.

- *Emotional connections.* The program should take into account children's emotional, as well as cognitive, needs.

- *Testable.* The program's effects should be scientifically testable and, ideally, positively verifiable through a design that includes control as well as experimental groups. The program also should involve a set of instructions allowing adequate estimate of the effect of intervention.

- *Inexpensive.* The program should be inexpensive to implement to ensure the likelihood of continued use after investigators leave.

- *Adequate duration and optimal onset.* Early interventions should last longer to be more effective. A program with limited resources should take into account the most optimal time for intervention.

- *Outcomes in multiple domains.* The program should evaluate outcomes in multiple domains, including cognitive, socioemotional, and behavioral domains.

- *Contextual.* The program should involve various niches of child functioning to ensure that the necessary scaffolding is provided within the family and at school.

Three Approaches

Keeping these criteria in mind, previous models of intervention for developing cognitive skills can be classified into three categories. The first category might be termed negative-influence models. Models in this category depict one or more negative influences impeding cognitive development; when these influences are removed, cognitive development will be optimized or proceed in a highly satisfactory manner.

Two variants differ depending on whether the intervention removes one or more than one of the negative influences. For example, researchers who view the administration of anthelmintic pills or micronutrients as the single key to cognitive development subscribe to the first subcategory. Although anthelmintic pills (Watkins and Pollitt, forthcoming) and micronutrient supplementation (Ricciuti 1991) have some effect, no evidence exists to support the idea that any single medical or nutritional intervention unleashes powerful cognitive growth. They may be necessary but not sufficient conditions for optimal cognitive development.

The second variant, targeting multiple negative influences, also may be a necessary but not sufficient approach. Eliminating these influences does not ensure that cognitive development will proceed, because other influences may arise.

The second major category might be termed positive-influence models. Models in this category emphasize positive factors that stimulate cognitive development (such as reading to children or responding to their cues) rather than remove negative factors (such as ill health or undernutrition). Two variants differ, again depending on whether the intervention focuses on a single factor to unleash accelerated cognitive development or multiple factors. In the first instance, a single positive factor is viewed as sufficient for cognitive development. The single positive factor might be cognitive stimulation, sensorimotor stimulation, or any intervention administered in isolation from other kinds of interventions. In the second instance, multiple positive factors are viewed as necessary for cognitive development (for example, a home-based program that includes socioemotional, cognitive, and behavioral stimulation).

The third major category of models combines the second variants of each of the first two categories. Interveners first eliminate multiple impediments to cognitive development, such as poor nutrition or ill health, and then seek positive cognitive interventions. Such a model might seem obvious, yet many respected medical professionals choose other models, preferring to believe that a pill, injection, or other medical intervention, for example, will somehow provide accelerated cognitive development without any cognitive-behavioral program of intervention.

This third type of model can be implemented successfully when medical professionals collaborate with psychological professionals as teams that first focus on health problems (both disease and poor nutrition) and then focus on cognitive-behavioral interventions. Although medical needs must be met first, the medical intervention will not necessarily be complete before beginning a cognitive-behavioral intervention.

Scaffolding: The Key to Intervention

Scaffolding is an excellent technique for accomplishing combined interventions. Indeed, scaffolding is key to stimulating cognitive development. The main element of a scaffolding intervention is teaching parents, especially mothers, to respond to their infants and young children (Anderson and Sawin 1983; Barrera, Rosenbaum, and Cunningham 1986). Such an intervention guides adults to respond to children in ways that fit the children. Although this emphasis differs from earlier emphases on stimulation (Scarr-Salapatek and Williams 1973), the two types of interventions are potentially compatible.

Scaffolding contrasts with stimulation by originating in cognitive theory instead of psychometric or Piagetian theory, by seeking balance instead of maximization, and by targeting the dyad instead of the infant. Like stimulation, however, scaffolding can respond to children's developed and developing socioemotional needs, behavioral repertoire, and cognitive abilities.

Three converging lines of evidence demonstrate the importance of scaffolding for early development. First, socioemotional, behavioral, and cognitive scaffolding adequate for a child's development are significantly associated with subsequent outcomes of cognitive development (see Sternberg, Grigorenko, and Nokes, this volume).

Second, scaffolding is a crucial part of any intervention program. Its importance is twofold. Scaffolding is important, either instead of or in addition to stimulation, for intervention programs targeting families. Parents need to respond to their children's needs. Scaffolding requires that parents provide carefully designed guidance. This guidance is based on a child's actualized capacity, targeted to a child's absolute capacity, and unique and sensitive to a given child's needs. Many expensive intervention studies where parents were additional interventionists did not show any positive effects of intervention because parents were taught what to do but were not taught how to respond to their child's needs, how to read behavioral and socioemotional clues, or how to deliver adequate interventions without overstimulating a child.

Scaffolding also is important for interventions targeting education, where the intervention is delivered in a centralized manner by professionals. Because scaffolding, especially that supporting the socioemotional needs of a child, is crucial within the family, the most effective intervention programs intertwine active educational intervention at preschools with adequate scaffolding at home.

Third, studies of the long-term effects of intervention indicate that without adequate duration of a program and without adequate scaffolding after the program, cognitive gains tend to disappear. Inadequate or lack of scaffolding minimizes treatment effects and shrinks the window of educational opportunity for children in need of services. To foster and ensure long-term effects of early intervention, scaffolding should be present within families and schools.

Conclusion

This review leads to five main conclusions. First, scaffolding (socioemotional, behavioral, cognitive) combined with appropriate health interventions is key to fostering cognitive development in early childhood. Second, a scaffolding model of intervention derives from extended cognitive information-processing models of cognitive abilities, in which infants who respond well to and process new information better than other infants show higher levels of intelligence later. Third, although cognitive abilities are partially hereditary, such heritability has no implications for the efficacy of cognitive interventions and does not jeopardize efforts to modify cognitive abilities. Fourth, the power of the environment in affecting cognitive abilities can be seen at birth (and even in the intrauterine environment) and continues throughout the life span. Thus, earlier intervention ensures more opportunity for greater cognitive developments later. Finally, an effective intervention involves eliminating negative influences *and* adding positive supports.

Note

We are grateful to Wendy M. Williams for her valuable contributions to the section of this chapter about the Flynn effect.

References

Affholter, D. P., D. Connell, and M. J. Nauta. 1983. Evaluation of the Child and Family Resource Program. *Education Review* 7:65-79.

Anderson, C. J., and D. Sawin. 1983. Enhancing Responsiveness in Mother-Infant Interaction. *Infant Behavior and Development* 6:361-68.

Andersson, B. E. 1989. Effects of Public Daycare: A Longitudinal Study. *Child Development* 60:857-66.

———. 1992. Effects of Day-care on Cognitive and Socioemotional Competence of Thirteen-year-old Swedish School Children. *Child Development* 63:20-36.

Andrews, S. R., J. B. Blumenthal, D. L. Johnson, A. J. Kahn, C. J. Ferguson, T. M. Lasater, P. W. Malone, and D. B. Wallace. 1982. The Skills of Mothering: A Study of Parent-Child Development Centers. *Monographs of the Society for Research in Child Development* 46(6). Serial No. 198.

Barrera, M. E., P. L. Rosenbaum, and C. E. Cunningham. 1986. Early Home Intervention with Low-birthweight Infants and Their Parents. *Child Development* 57:20-33.

Baydar, N., and J. Brooks-Gunn. 1991. Effects of Maternal Employment and Child-care Arrangements on Preschoolers' Cognitive and Behavioral Outcomes: Evidence from the Children of the National Longitudinal Survey of Youth. *Developmental Psychology* 27:932-45.

Bayley, N. 1993. *The Bayley's Scales of Mental and Motor Development*. Rev. New York: Psychological Corporation.

Benasich, A. A., and J. Brooks-Gunn. 1996. Maternal Attitudes and Knowledge of Child-rearing: Associations with Family and Child Outcomes. *Child Development* 67:1186-1205.

Benasich, A. A., J. Brooks-Gunn, and B. C. Clewell. 1992. How Do Mothers Benefit from Early Intervention Programs? *Journal of Applied Developmental Psychology* 13:311-62.

Berrueta-Clement, J. R., L. J. Schweinhart, W. S. Barnett, A. S. Epstein, and D. P. Weikart. 1984. *Changed Lives: The Effects of the Perry Preschool Program on Youths through Age 19*. Ypsilanti, Mich.: High/Scope Press.

Bloom, B. S. 1976. *Human Characteristics and School Learning*. New York: McGraw-Hill.

Bornstein, M. H., and M. D. Sigman. 1986. Continuity in Mental Development from Infancy. *Child Development* 57:251-74.

Bradley, R. H., B. M. Caldwell, S. L. Rock, C. T. Ramey, K. E. Barnard, C. Gray, M. A. Hammond, S. Mitchell, A. W. Gottfried, L. Seigel, and D. L. Johnson. 1989. Home Environment and Cognitive Development in the First Three Years of Life: A Collaborative Study Involving Six Sites and Three Ethnic Groups in North America. *Developmental Psychology* 25:217-35.

Bronfenbrenner, U., and S. J. Ceci. 1994. Nature-Nurture Reconceptualized in Developmental Perspective: A Bioecological Model. *Psychological Review* 101:568-86.

Bronfenbrenner, U., P. McClelland, E. Wethington, P. Moen, and S. J. Ceci. 1996. *State of Americans: This Generation and the Next*. New York: Free Press.

Burchinal, M., M. W. Lee, and C. T. Ramey. 1989. Type of Day-care and Preschool Intellectual Development in Disadvantaged Children. *Child Development* 60:128-37.

Burchinal, M. R., S. L. Ramey, M. K. Reid, and J. Jaccard. 1995. Early Child Care Experiences and their Association with Family and Child Characteristics during Middle Childhood. *Early Childhood Research Quarterly* 10:33-61.

Burchinal, M. R., J. E. Roberts, L. A. Nabors, and D. M. Bryant. 1996. Quality of Center Child Care and Infant Cognitive and Language Development. *Child Development* 67:606-20.

Cahan, S., and N. Cohen. 1980. Age Versus Schooling Effects on Intelligence Development. *Child Development* 60:1239-49.

Campbell, F. A., and C. T. Ramey. 1994. Effects of Early Intervention on Intellectual and Academic Achievement: A Follow-up Study of Children from Low-income Families. *Child Development* 65:684-98.

Carraher, T. N., D. Carraher, and A. D. Schliemann. 1985. Mathematics in the Streets and in Schools. *British Journal of Developmental Psychology* 3:21-29.

Cattell, R. B. 1971. *Abilities: Their Structure, Growth and Action*. Boston: Houghton Mifflin.

Caughy, M., J. A. DiPietro, and D. Strobino. 1994. Day-care Participation as a Protective Factor in the Cognitive Development of Low-income Children. *Child Development* 65:457-71.

Ceci, S. J. 1991. How Much Does Schooling Influence General Intelligence and Its Cognitive Components: A Reassessment of the Evidence. *Developmental Psychology* 27:703-22.

———. 1996. *On Intelligence*. Cambridge, Mass.: Harvard University Press.

Ceci, S. J., and J. Liker. 1988. Stalking the IQ-expertise relationship: When the critics go fishing. *Journal of Experimental Psychology: General* 117:96-100.

Chafel, J. A. 1992. Funding Head Start: What Are the Issues? *American Journal of Orthopsychiatry* 62:9-21.

Clarke-Stewart, K. A. 1989. Infant Day Care: Maligned or Malignant? *American Psychologist* 44:266-73.

———. 1991. A Home Is Not a School: The Effects of Child Care on Children's Development. *Journal of Social Issues* 47:105-23.

Cronbach, L. J. 1982. *Designing Evaluations of Educational and Social Programs.* San Francisco: Jossey-Bass.

Dennis, W. 1973. *Children of the Creche.* New York: Appleton-Century-Crofts.

Desai, S., P. L. Chase-Lansdale, and R. T. Michael. 1989. Mother or Market? Effects of Maternal Employment on the Intellectual Ability of 4-Year-old Children. *Demography* 26:545-61.

Dichtelmiller, M., S. J. Meisels, J. W. Plunkett, M. E. A. Bozynski, C. Claflin, and S. C. Mangelsdorf. 1992. The Relationship of Parental Knowledge to the Development of Extremely Low Birth Weight Infants. *Journal of Early Intervention* 13:210-20.

Duncan, G. J., and W. L. Rogers. 1988. Longitudinal Aspects of Childhood Poverty. *Journal of Marriage and the Family* 50:1007-21.

Dunn, L. 1993. Proximal and distal features of day care quality and children's development. *Early Childhood Research Quarterly* 8:167-92.

Elardo, R., R. Bradley, and B. M. Caldwell. 1977. A Longitudinal Study of the Relation of Infants' Home Environments to Language Development at Age Three. *Child Development* 48:595-603.

Eldering, L., and P. Vedder. 1993. Culture-sensitive Home Intervention: The Dutch Hippy Experiment. In L. Eldering and P. Leseman, ed., *Early Intervention and Culture.* Paris: United Nations Educational, Scientific, and Cultural Organization.

Epstein, J. L. 1990. School and Family Connections: Theory, Research, and Implications for Integrating Sociologies of Education and Family. In D. G. Unger and M. B. Sussman, eds., *Families in Community Settings: Interdisciplinary Perspectives.* New York: Haworth.

Fagan, J. F. 1984. The Intelligent Infant: Theoretical Implications. *Intelligence* 8:1-9.

———. 1985. A New Look at Infant Intelligence. In D. K. Detterman, ed., *Current Topics in Human Intelligence.* Vol 1. *Research Methodology.* Norwood, N.J.: Ablex.

Feuerstein, R. 1980. *Instrumental Enrichment: An Intervention Program for Cognitive Modifiability.* Baltimore: University Park Press.

Flynn, J. R. 1987. Massive IQ Gains in 14 Nations: What IQ Tests Really Measure. *Psychological Bulletin* 101:171-91.

———. 1994. IQ Gains Over Time. In R. J. Sternberg, ed., *The Encyclopedia of Human Intelligence.* New York: Macmillan.

Fry, P. S. 1985. Relations Between Teenagers' Age, Knowledge, Expectations, and Maternal Behavior. *British Journal of Developmental Psychology* 3:47-55.

Furstenberg, F. F., Jr., J. Brooks-Gunn, and P. Morgan. 1987. *Adolescent Mothers in Later Life.* New York: Cambridge University Press.

Gamson, B., H. Hornstein, and B. Borden. 1989. Adler-Dreikurs Parent Study Group Leadership Training. In M. J. Fine, ed., *The Second Handbook on Parent Education.* San Diego: Academic.

Garber, H. L. 1988. *The Milwaukee Project: Prevention of Mental Retardation in Children at Risk.* Washington, D.C.: American Association of Mental Retardation.

Gardner, H. 1983. *Frames of Mind.* New York: Basic Books.

———. 1993. *Multiple Intelligences: The Theory in Practice.* New York: Basic Books.

Goelman, H., and A. Pence. 1987. Effects of Child Care, Family, and Individual Characteristics on Children's Language Development: The Victoria Day Care Research Project. In D. A. Phillips, ed., *Quality in Child Care: What Does Research Tell Us?* Washington, D.C.: National Association for the Education of Young Children.

Gordon, E. W., and S. Shipman. 1979. Human Diversity, Pedagogy, and Educational Equality. *American Psychologist* 34:1030-36.

Gordon, I. J., B. Guinagh, and R. E. Jester. 1977. The Florida Parent Education Infant and Toddler Programs. In M. C. Day and R. K. Parker, eds., *The Preschool in Action: Exploring Early Childhood Programs.* Boston: Allyn & Bacon.

Gorman, K. S., and E. Pollitt. 1996. Does Schooling Buffer the Effects of Early Risk? *Child Development* 67:314-26.

Grantham-McGregor, S. M., C. M. Powell, S. P. Walker, and J. H. Himes. 1991. Nutritional Supplementation, Psychosocial Stimulation, and Mental Development of Stunted Children: The Jamaican Study. *Lancet* 338:1-5.

Gutelius, M. R., A. D. Kirsch, S. MacDonald, M. E. Brooks, T. McErlean, and C. Newcomb. 1972. Promising Results from a Cognitive Stimulation Program in Infancy: A Preliminary Report. *Clinical Pediatrics* 11:585-93.

Hale, B. A., V. Seitz, and E. Zigler. 1990. Health Services and Head Start: A Forgotten Formula. *Journal of Applied Developmental Psychology* 11:447-58.

Haskins, R. 1989. Beyond Metaphor: The Efficacy of Early Childhood Education. *American Psychologist* 44:274-82.

Hebbeler, K. 1985. An Old and a New Question on the Effects of Early Education for Children from Low Income Families. *Educational Evaluation and Policy Analysis* 7:207-16.

Herrnstein, R. J., and C. Murray. 1994. *The Bell Curve*. New York: The Free Press.

Hess, R. D., S. D. Holloway, W. P. Dickson, and G. G. Price. 1984. Maternal Variables as Predictors of Children's School Readiness and Later Achievement in Vocabulary and Mathematics in Sixth Grade. *Child Development* 55:1902-12.

Horn, J. L., and R. B. Cattell. 1966. Refinement and Test of the Theory of Fluid and Crystallized Intelligence. *Journal of Educational Psychology* 57:253-70.

Intelligence and Its Measurement: A Symposium. 1921. *Journal of Educational Psychology* 12:123-47, 195-216, 271-75.

Jensen, A. R. 1969. How Much Can We Boost IQ and Scholastic Achievement? *Harvard Educational Review* 39(1):1-123.

Jester, R. E., and B. J. Guinagh. 1983. The Gordon Parent Education and Infant and Toddler Program. In The Consortium for Longitudinal Studies, ed., *As the Twig Is Bent: Lasting Effects of Preschool Programs*. Hillsdale, N.J.: Lawrence Erlbaum and Associates.

Johnson, D. L. 1988. Primary Prevention of Behavior Problems in Young Children: The Houston Parent-Child Development Center. In R. H. Price, E. L. Cowen, R. P. Lorion, and J. Ramos-McKay, eds., *14 Ounces of Prevention: A Casebook for Practitioners*. Washington, D.C.: American Psychological Association.

Johnson, D. L., and T. Walker. 1991. A Follow-up Evaluation of the Houston Parent-Child Development Center: School Performance. *Journal of Early Intervention* 15:226-36.

Kisker, E. E., S. L. Hoffereth, D. A. Phillips, and E. Farquhar. 1991. *A Profile of Child Care Settings: Early Education and Care in 1990*. Vol. 1. Princeton, N.J.: Mathematical Policy Research.

Kontos, S. 1991. Child Care Quality, Family Background, and Children's Development. *Early Childhood Research Quarterly* 6:249-62.

Kontos, S., and R. Fiene. 1987. Predictors of Quality and Children's Development in Day Care. In D. Phillips, ed., *NAEYC Research Monograph*. Washington, D.C.: National Association for the Education of Young Children.

Kopp, C. B., and J. B. Krakow. 1983. The Developmentalist and the Study of Biological Risk: A View of the Past with an Eye Toward the Future. *Child Development* 54:1086-1108.

Kroth, R. 1989. School-based Parent Involvement Programs. In M. J. Fine, ed., *The Second Handbook on Parent Education*. San Diego: Academic.

Lansdown, R. June 1995. Context and Assessment. Presentation and comments at Wellcome Trust conference, A Healthy Body and a Healthy Mind? Worcestershire, England.

Lazar, I., R. Darlington, H. Murray, J. Royce, and A. Snipper. 1982. Lasting Effects of Early Education: A Report from The Consortium for Longitudinal Studies. *Monographs of the Society for Research in Child Development* 47(2-3). Serial No. 195.

LeVine, R. A., S. E. LeVine, A. Richman, F. M. Tapia Uribe, C. Sunderland Correa, and P. M. Miller. 1991. Women's Schooling and Child Care in Demographic Transition: A Mexican Case Study. *Population and Development Review* 17:459-96.

Lewis, M., and J. Brooks-Gunn. 1981. Visual Attention at Three Months as a Predictor of Cognitive Functioning at Two Years of Age. *Intelligence* 5:131-40.

Lombard, A. D. 1994. *Success Begins at Home: The Past, Present, and Future of the Home Instruction Program for Preschool Youngsters.* 2nd ed. Guilford, Conn.: Dushkin Publishing Group.

McCall, R. B. 1989. The Development of Intellectual Functioning in Infancy and the Prediction of Later IQ. In S. D. Osofsky, ed., *The Handbook of Infant Development.* New York: Wiley.

McCartney, K. 1984. Effect of Quality of Day Care Environment on Children's Language Development. *Developmental Psychology* 20:244-60.

McCartney, K., S. Scarr, D. Phillips, and S. Grajek. 1985. Day care as intervention: Comparisons of Varying Quality Programs. *Journal of Applied Developmental Psychology* 6:247-60.

McGillicuddy-DeLisi, A. V. 1985. The Relationship Between Parental Beliefs and Children's Cognitive Level. In I. E. Sigel, ed., *Parental Belief Systems.* Hillsdale, N.J.: Lawrence Erlbaum and Associates.

McGowan, R. J., and D. L. Johnson. 1984. The Mother-Child Relationship and Other Antecedents of Childhood Intelligence: A Causal Analysis. *Child Development* 55:810-20.

McKey, R. H., K. Condelli, H. Granson, B. Barrett, C. McConkey, and M. Plants. 1985. *The Impact of Head Start on Children, Families, and Communities.* Washington, D.C.: CSR.

Melhuish, E. C., E. Lloyd, S. Martin, and A. Mooney. 1990. Type of Child Care at 18 Months: II. Relations with Cognitive and Language Development. *Journal of Child Psychology and Psychiatry and Allied Disciplines* 31:861-70.

Merton, R. K. 1968. The Matthew Effect in Science. *Science* 175:56-63.

Myers, Robert. 1995. *The Twelve Who Survive: Strengthening Programs of Early Childhood Development in the Third World.* 2nd ed. Ypsilanti, Mich.: High/Scope Press.

Ninio, A. 1979. The Naive Theory of the Infant and Other Maternal Attitudes in Two Subgroups in Israel. *Child Development* 50:976-80.

Neumann, C., M. A. McDonald, M. Sigman, N. Bwibo, and M. Marquardt. 1991. Relationships Between Morbidity and Development in Mild-to-moderately Malnourished Kenyan Toddlers. *Pediatrics* 88:934-42.

Nye, B. A. 1989. Effective Parent Education and Involvement Models and Programs; Contemporary Strategies for School Implementation. In M. J. Fine, ed., *The Second Handbook on Parent Education.* San Diego: Academic.

O'Connell, J. C., and D. C. Farran. 1982. Effects of Day Care Experience on the Use of Intentional Communicative Behaviors in a Sample of Socio-economically Depressed Infants. *Developmental Psychology* 18:22-29.

Okagaki, L., and R. L. Sternberg. 1993. Putting the Distance into Students' Hands: Practical Intelligence for School. In R. R. Cocking and K. A. Renninger, eds., *The Development and Meaning of Psychological Distance.* Hillsdale, N.J.: Lawrence Erlbaum and Associates.

Piaget, J. 1952. *The Origins of Intelligence in Children.* New York: International Universities Press.

———. 1972. *The Psychology of Intelligence.* Totowa, N.J.: Littlefield Adams.

Phillips, D., K. McCartney, and S. Scarr. 1987. Child-care Quality and Children's Social Development. *Developmental Psychology* 23:537-43.

Pollitt, E. 1990. *Malnutrition in the Classroom.* Lausanne: United Nations Educational, Scientific, and Cultural Organization.

Provence, S., and A. Naylor. 1983. *Working with Disadvantaged Parents and Children: Scientific Issues and Practice.* New Haven: Yale University Press.

Ramey, C. T. 1988. Early Intervention for High-risk Children: The Carolina Early Intervention Program. In R. H. Price, E. L. Cowen, R. P. Lorion, and J. Ramos-McKay, eds., *14 Ounces of Prevention: A Casebook for Practitioners.* Washington, D.C.: American Psychological Association.

Ramey, C. T., K. O. Yeates, and E. J. Short. 1984. The Plasticity of Intellectual Development: Insights from Early Intervention. *Child Development* 55:1913-25.

Rauh, V. A. , T. M. Achenbach, B. Nurcombe, C. T. Howell, and D. M. Teti. 1988. Minimizing Adverse Effects of Low Birthweight: Four-year Results of an Early Intervention Program. *Child Development* 59:544-53.

Rescorla, L. A., S. Provence, and A. Naylor. 1982. The Yale Child Welfare Research Program: Description and Results. In E. E. Zigler and E. W. Gordon, eds., *Day Care: Scientific and Social Policy Issues.* Boston: Auburn.

Reynolds, A. J., N. Mavrogenes, N. Bezruczko, and M. Hagemann. 1996. Cognitive and Family-support Mediators of Preschool Effectiveness: A Confirmatory Analysis. *Child Development* 67:1119-40.

Ricciuti, H. N. 1991. Malnutrition and Cognitive Development: Research-Policy Linkages and Current Research Directions. In R. J. Sternberg and L. Okagaki, eds., *Directors of Development.* Hillsdale, N.J.: Lawrence Erlbaum and Associates.

Riksen-Walraven, J. M. 1978. Effects of Caregiver Behavior on Habituation Rate and Self-efficacy in Humans. *International Journal of Behavioral Development* 1:105-30.

Roberts, J. E., S. Rabinowitch, D. M. Bryant, M. R. Burchinal, M. A. Koch, and C. T. Ramey. 1989. Language Skills of Children with Different Preschool Experiences. *Journal of Speech and Hearing Research* 32:773-86.

Royce, J. M., R. B. Darlington, and H. W. Murray. 1983. Pooled Analyses: Findings across Studies. In The Consortium for Longitudinal Studies, ed., *As the Twig Is Bent: Lasting Effects of Preschool Programs.* Hillsdale, N.J.: Lawrence Erlbaum and Associates.

Rutter, M. April 1996. Profound Early Deprivation and Later Social Relationship in Early Adoptees from Romanian Orphanages Followed at Age 4. Paper presented at 10th Biennial International Conference on Infant Studies, Providence, R. I.

Sameroff, A. J., R. Seifer, A. Baldwin, and C. Baldwin. 1993. Stability and Intelligence from Preschool to Adolescence: The Influence of Social and Family Risk Factors. *Child Development* 64:80-97.

Sameroff, A. J., R. Seifer, R. Barocas, M. Zax, and S. Greenspan. 1987. IQ Scores of 4-Year-old Children: Social-environmental Risk Factors. *Pediatrics* 79:343-50.

Sampson, R. J., and J. H. Laub. 1994. Urban Poverty and the Family Context of Delinquency: A New Look at Structure and Process in a Classic Study. *Child Development* 65:523-40.

Scarr, S., and M. Eisenberg. 1993. Child Care Research: Issues, Perspectives, and Results. *American Review of Psychology* 44:613-44.

Scarr, S., D. Phillips, K. McCartney, and M. Abbott-Shim. 1993. Quality of Child Care as an Aspect of Family and Child Care Policy in the United States. *Pediatrics* 91:182-88.

Scarr-Salapatek, S., and M. L. Williams. 1973. The Effects of Early Stimulation on Low-birth-weight Infants. *Child Development* 44:94-101.

Schliecker, E., D. R. White, and E. Jacobs. 1991. The Role of Day Care Quality in the Prediction of Children's Vocabulary. *Canadian Journal of Behavioral Science* 23:12-24.

Schnur, E., J. Brooks-Gunn, and V. C. Shipman. 1992. Who Attends Programs Serving Poor Children? The Case of Head Start Attendees and Nonattendees. *Journal of Applied Developmental Psychology* 13:405-21.

Schweinhart, L. J., M. V. Barnes, D. P. Weikart, W. S. Barnett, and A. S. Epstein. 1993. *Significant Benefits: The High/Scope Perry Preschool Study Through Age 27. Monographs of the High/Scope Educational Research Foundation 10.* Ypsilanti, Mich: High/Scope Press.

Schweinhart, L. J., and D. P. Weikart. 1980. *Young Children Grow Up: The Effects of the Perry Preschool Program on Youths Through Age 15.* Ypsilanti, Mich.: High/Scope Press.

———. 1988. The High/Scope Perry Program. In R. H. Price, E. L. Cowen, R. P. Lorion, and J. Ramos-McKay, eds., *14 Ounces of Prevention: A Casebook for Practitioners.* Washington, D.C.: American Psychological Association.

Scott-Jones, D. 1984. Family Influences on Cognitive Development and School Achievement. In E. W. Gordon, ed., *Review of Research in Education.* Vol. 11. Washington, D.C.: American Educational Research Association.

Scribner, S. 1984. Studying Working Intelligence. In B. Rogoff and J. Lave, eds., *Everyday Cognition: Its Development in Social Context.* Cambridge: Harvard University Press.

Seifer, R., and A. J. Sameroff. 1987. Multiple Determinants of Risk and Invulnerability. In E. J. Anthony and B. J. Cohler, eds., *The Invulnerable Child.* New York: Guilford.

Seitz, V. 1990. Intervention Programs for Impoverished Children: A Comparison of Educational and Family Support Models. *Annals of Child Development* 7:73-103.

Seitz, V., L. K. Rosenbaum, and N. H. Apfel. 1985. Effects of Family Support Intervention: A Ten-year Follow-up. *Child Development* 56:376-91.

Snow, C. E. 1983. Literacy and Language: Relationships During the Preschool Years. *Harvard Educational Review* 53:165-89.
Snyder, C., S. J. Eyres, and K. E. Barnard. 1979. New Findings about Mothers' Neonatal Expectations and Their Relationships to Infant Developments. *American Journal of Maternal and Child Nursing* 4:175-78.
Sternberg, R. J. 1977. *Intelligence, Information Processing, and Analogical Reasoning: The Componential Analysis of Human Abilities*. Hillsdale, N.J.: Lawrence Erlbaum and Associates.
———. 1984. *Mechanisms of Cognitive Development*. San Francisco: Freeman.
———. 1985. *Beyond IQ: A Triarchic Theory of Human Intelligence*. New York: Cambridge University Press.
———. 1988. *The Triarchic Mind: A New Theory of Human Intelligence*. New York: Viking.
———. 1990. *Metaphors of Mind: Conceptions of the Nature of Intelligence*. New York: Cambridge University Press.
———. 1996. *Successful Intelligence*. New York: Simon & Schuster.
Sternberg, R. J., and C. A. Berg. 1990. *Intellectual Development*. New York: Cambridge University Press.
Sternberg, R. J., and D. K. Detterman, eds. 1986. *What Is Intelligence? Contemporary Viewpoints on its Nature and Definition*. Norwood, N.J.: Ablex.
Sternberg, R. J., M. Ferrari, P. Clinkenbeard, and E. L. Grigorenko. 1996. Identification, Instruction, and Assessment of Gifted Children: A Construct Validation of a Triarchic Model. *Gifted Child Quarterly* 40:129-37.
Sternberg, R. J., and E. L. Grigorenko. 1996. *Intelligence, Heredity, and Environment*. New York: Cambridge University Press.
Sternberg, R. J., and J. S. Powell. 1983. Comprehending Verbal Comprehension. *American Psychologist* 38:878-93.
Sternberg, R. J., R. K. Wagner, W. M. Williams, and J. A. Horvath. 1995. Testing Common Sense. *American Psychologist* 50:912-27.
Stevens, J. H., Jr. 1984a. Black Grandmothers' and Black Adolescent Mothers' Knowledge about Parenting. *Developmental Psychology* 20:1017-25.
———. 1984b. Child Development Knowledge and Parenting Skill. *Family Relations* 33:237-44.
Tietze, W. 1987. A Structural Model for the Evaluation of Preschool Effects. *Early Childhood Research Quarterly* 2:133-53.
Tomasello, M., and M. J. Farrar. 1986. Joint Attention and Early Language. *Child Development* 57:1454-63.
Tuddenham, R. D. 1962. The Nature and Measurement of Intelligence. In L. J. Postman, ed., *Psychology in the Making*. New York: Knopf.
———. 1970. "Piagetian" Test of Cognitive Development. In W. B. Dockrell, ed., *On Intelligence, Contemporary Theories and Educational Implications: A Symposium, Toronto, 1969*. London: The Camelot Press Ltd.
Vandell, D. L., and M. A. Corasaniti. 1990. Child Care and the Family: Complex Contributors to Child Development. In K. McCartney, ed., *New Directions in Child Development*. San Francisco: Jossey-Bass.
Vartuli, S., and M. Winter. 1989. Parents as First Teachers. In M. J. Fine, ed., *The Second Handbook on Parent Education*. San Diego: Academic.
Wachs, T. D., W. Moussa, Z. Bishry, F. Yunis, A. Sobhy, G. McCabe, N. Jerome, O. Galal, G. Harrison, and A. Kirksey. 1993. Relations Between Nutrition and Cognitive Performance in Egyptian Toddlers. *Intelligence* 17:151-72.
Walberg, H. J., and S. Tsai. 1983. Matthew Effects in Education. *American Educational Research Journal* 20:359-73.
Wasik, B. H., C. T. Ramey, D. M. Bryant, and J. J. Sparling. 1990. A Longitudinal Study of Two Early Intervention Strategies: Project CARE. *Child Development* 61:1682-96.
Watkins, W. E., and E. Pollitt. n.d. "Stupidity of Worms": Do Intestinal Worms Impair Mental Performance? *Psychological Bulletin*. Forthcoming.
Wechsler, D. 1989. *Manual for the Wechsler Preschool and Primary Scale of Intelligence*. Rev. San Antonio: The Psychological Corporation.
Weikart, D. P. April 1996. Impact of Early Education on School Performance and Product. Paper Presented at World Bank Conference on Early Child Development: Investing in the Future, Atlanta, Ga.

White, K. R. 1985. Efficacy of Early Intervention. *Journal of Special Education* 19:401-16.
White, K. R., D. W. Bush, and G. C. Casto. 1985. Learning from Previous Reviews of Early Intervention. *Journal of Special Education* 19:417-28.
White, K. R., M. J. Taylor, and V. D. Moss. 1992. Does Research Support Claims about the Benefits of Involving Parents in Early Intervention Programs? *Review of Educational Research* 62:91-125.
Wood, D. 1980. Teaching the Young Child: Some Relationships Between Social Interaction, Language, and Thought. In D. R. Olson, ed., *The Social Foundation of Language and Thought*. New York: Norton.
Wood, D., Bruner, J., and G. Ross. 1976. The Role of Tutoring in Problem-solving. *Journal of Child Psychology and Psychiatry* 17:89-100.
Woodhead, M. 1988. When Psychology Informs Public Policy. *American Psychologist* 43:443-54.
Young, M. E. 1995. *Investing in Young Children.* World Bank Discussion Paper. Washington, D.C.
———. 1996. *Early Child Development: Investing in the Future*. Washington, D.C.: World Bank.
Zajonc, R. B. 1976. Family Configuration and Intelligence. *Science* 192:227-36.
Zigler, E., W. Abelson, P. K. Trickett, and V. Seitz. 1982. Is an Intervention Program Necessary in Order to Improve Economically Disadvantaged Children's IQ Scores? *Child Development* 53:340-48.
Zigler, E. F., and M. E. Lang. 1991. *Child Care Choices: Balancing the Needs of Children, Families, and Society.* New York: The Free Press.

II. Early Child Development: Program Options

Early Child Development: Investing in our Children's Future
M.E. Young, editor.

Fitting Early Childcare Services to Societal Needs and Characteristics

Moncrieff Cochran

Each nation's system of caring for and developing its young children is unique, responding to a distinctive combination of national needs mediated by a particular constellation of cultural beliefs, political and economic ideologies, resources, and social conditions. Such macrolevel factors help determine the need for early childcare and development programs and shape their form and content. Importation or imposition of other countries' early care and development models is counterproductive because the models may not result in policies and programs that meet the specific needs of a nation and reflect the values, beliefs, and social conditions in that society. Importation of a foreign model also is apt to replace a careful indigenous assessment of needs and cultural influences. Through such assessments, societies can make critical discoveries concerning the status of their children and families and factors affecting their vitality, a process essential to the long-term health of a nation and to development of public policies for improving its citizens' well-being.

The chapters in part I of this volume explored the importance and synergism of good health, adequate nutrition, and supportive psychosocial stimulation in early child development. The interrelationship of these microlevel factors has been demonstrated through studies in both industrialized and developing countries. In designing intervention programs for maximizing early child development, attention also must be paid to macrolevel factors affecting these programs. This first chapter in part II addresses these factors and provides a framework for describing and understanding their effect on early child development.

The chapter opens with a description of this organizing framework and two elements within the framework—identification of the *needs* and *circumstances* that might be addressed in developing childcare policies and programs. The subsequent section elaborates on another element within the framework—the *influences* in a particular country that mediate and legitimize the policies and programs initiated in response to needs and circumstances. The chapter then focuses on the dimensions ultimately involved in translating needs, circumstances, and influences into specific policies and programs. In closing, the framework is applied to two case examples in different societies, Colombia and Kenya.

The concepts and findings presented in this chapter are drawn heavily from the study which led to *The International Handbook of Child Care Policies and Programs* (Cochran 1993), reconsidered in light of the remarkable work by Myers, as compiled in his book, *The Twelve Who Survive: Strengthening Programs of Early Childhood Development in the Third World* (Myers 1992). Another especially valuable reference is the work by Lamb and others (1992).

Definition of Terms

In this chapter, *early care and education programs* are public programs that provide, alone or in combination, (a) childcare while parents are at school or employed (formal and informal sectors), (b) child development and early education experiences to preschool-aged children, and (c) child development-related information to the parents of preschool children. The term "public" simply distinguishes this care from childrearing activities normally carried out by parents in their home environments and from information provided informally through kinship and friendship networks (see Cochran 1993: 4-5). This definition emerged from a twenty-nine-country study of childcare policies and programs and is consistent with the concept of early child development used in this volume. This concept is expanded in this chapter to include early childhood care and development (ECCD).

A Framework for Matching Society's Needs and ECCD Services

Nations all over the world are investing in ECCD programs to supplement the childrearing activities of parents and other family members. These programmatic efforts differ from country to country. What accounts for these differences? Do they mask underlying similarities?

During the early 1990s a global comparison of public childcare policies and programs was conducted, called the International Comparison of Child Care Policies and Programs (ICCPP). This twenty-nine-country study was conducted on five continents, encompassing more than 80 percent of the world's population. The twenty-nine nations were: Australia, Brazil, Canada, China, Colombia, the Commonwealth of Independent States (now many countries, including Russia), Denmark, Finland, France, Germany, Hungary, India, Israel, Italy, Japan, Kenya, Mexico, Nicaragua, Norway, Peru, the Philippines, Poland, South Africa, Sweden, the United Kingdom, the United States, Venezuela, Vietnam, and Zimbabwe.

Results of the ICCPP were reported first in *The International Handbook of Child Care Policies and Programs* (Cochran 1993). One purpose of the study was to better understand the variety of public childcare policies worldwide, particularly the influences of cultural and religious beliefs about family function and gender roles. Analysis of the twenty-nine cases revealed a general framework for explaining the policies and programs of a given country. Figure 1 shows this framework in its simplest form.

The framework is composed of four basic elements. The first element is the historical changes of *urbanization and industrialization*, which have occurred or are occurring in every society, resulting in major restructuring of families and leading to the need for additional family supports. The second element is the *causal factors*, or present-day needs and circumstances in society that stimulate childcare policies and programs. Programs may differ from country to country because of differing societal needs. For example, in one country, employed mothers need other trustworthy adults to provide childcare while they are on the job, and in another country, children from low-income families may need to be prepared for success in primary school.

Even when two societies experience the same circumstances and needs for childcare, the programs they create differ significantly. This difference results from the third element

Figure 1. The General Framework

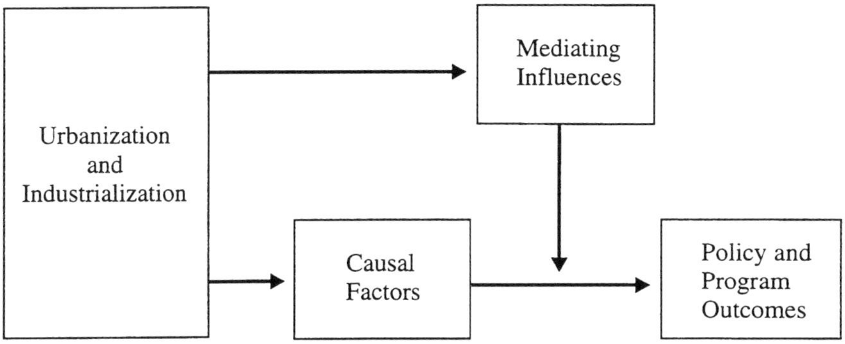

of the framework, a set of *mediating influences* that operates as a filter, legitimizing or making possible certain childcare responses while screening out others. Screening will shape public response to similar needs when mediating influences, such as cultural beliefs about appropriate childcare environments, are given expression in policymaking.

For example, cultural beliefs in Kenya include the importance of extended family and mutual assistance as well as the harambee, or self-help, ethos. These mediating influences support creation of a common public space for early childhood education in response to the need for enhancing childhood experiences and preparing children for primary school. In contrast, Latin American countries tend to have a strong nuclear family ethos, rooted partly in Catholicism. In some countries, for example, in Colombia, Venezuela, and to a lesser extent Ecuador and Peru (Myers 1992; Arango 1993), this mediating influence has contributed to developing home-based group care for young children needing extra stimulation and nutritional supplements (although center-based care also exists in these societies).

Finally, the fourth element of the framework is the childcare *policies and programs* resulting from circumstances and childcare needs of families in a given society and shaped by mediating influences such as religious beliefs, family values, the prevailing economic system, and available resources. A number of dimensions can be used to describe the policies and programs of each culture. The overall policy and program profile created by combining these various dimensions is unique for any given culture.

Figure 2 outlines the full range of causal factors, mediating influences, and outcome dimensions identified for the general framework in the twenty-nine ICCPP cases. It also indicates the screening process described earlier with an arrow from mediating influences that intersects the arrow linking causal factors to policy and program outcomes. Causal factors include all factors operating in the twenty-nine countries as a whole. Only a subset of these factors stimulates the need for childcare policies and programs in any particular country, as shown by examples later in this chapter.

Figure 3 applies the general framework to Kenya, illustrating how a particular nation is unique. For example, a comparison of figure 3 with figure 2 shows that only six of the nine causal factors from the general framework apply specifically to the Kenyan case. The

Figure 2. The Full Range of Factors, Influences, and Responses

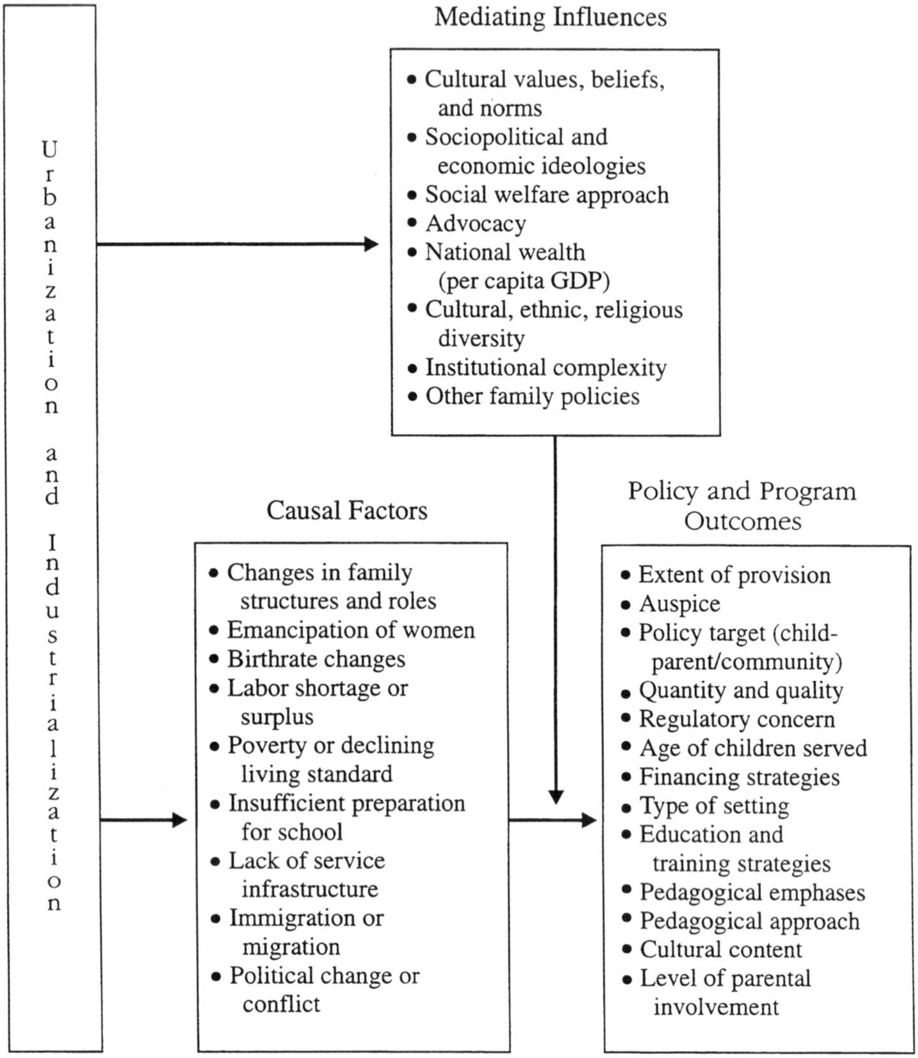

Note: GDP is gross domestic product.

mediating influences carry over more fully, but they are expressed in terms specific to Kenya. This combination of causes and mediating influences particular to Kenya results in unique policy and program responses, which are described in more detail later.

A danger with this type of framework is that it will be viewed as static, when in fact each of the countries from which it was derived was characterized by great dynamism. The word mediating was selected, in part, to convey this dynamism. In every society,

Figure 3. Early Childhood Programs in Kenya

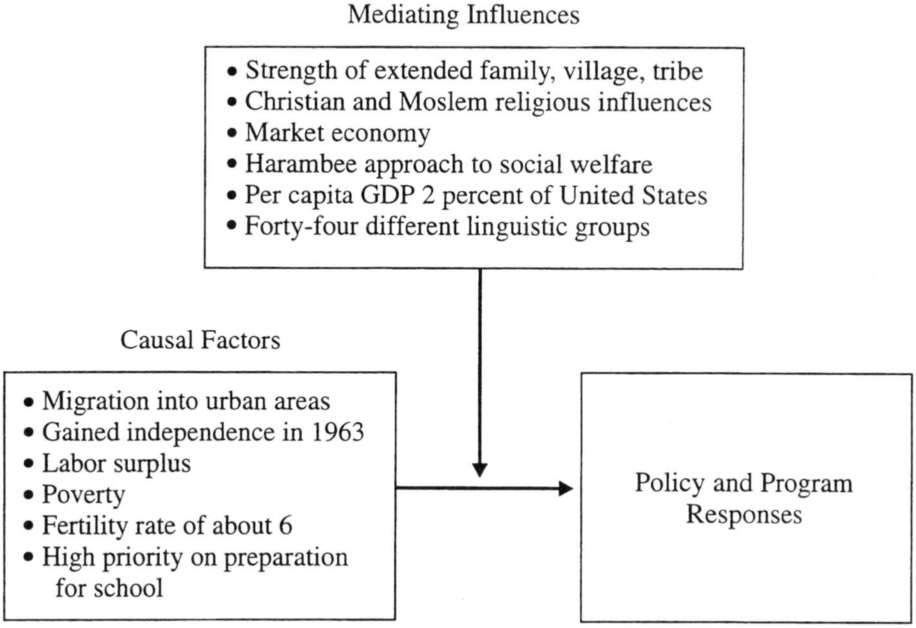

Note: GDP is gross domestic product.

factors affecting the need for childcare services evolve over time, as do some of the mediating influences. In Sweden, for instance, parental leave policies were expanded during the 1970s and 1980s, reducing the need for childcare services aimed at infants (Lamb and Sternberg 1992). This type of dynamism is difficult to capture in a two-dimensional framework.

Two elements of the framework, historical antecedents and contemporary causal factors, are explained briefly below. ICCPP case studies in industrialized and developing countries are used to illustrate the general applicability of the framework.

Historical Antecedents

The concentration of labor, capital, goods, and services necessary for trade and then industrial production contributes heavily to creation of the urban environment. In each of the twenty-nine ICCPP countries *industrialization and urbanization* have contributed to changes in family structures and roles. They have created nuclear family structures, separating parents from their own relatives and removing many of the childcare supports associated with the extended family and village.

Because men typically are given the heavy work associated with early stages of industrial development, movement of families from agrarian to industrial settings has led to increasingly specialized family roles. For example, men work outside the home while women remain in the household with more exclusive responsibility for childrearing than was the case on the farm, where production and childcare could be combined because children could help with production. (For a detailed exposition of these shifts within America and of the privatization of the family, see Hareven 1982a and 1982b.) As with large-scale or mechanized agriculture, industrial work changes the roles of parents, preventing them from supervising their children on the job.

The shift from agrarian to urban, industrialized economies began in Europe and North America during the second half of the nineteenth century with the onset of the Industrial Revolution (Degler 1980; Goode 1963; Greenfield 1961). Industrialization now is being supplanted in those and other parts of the world by the postindustrial information age. Many developing countries are still shifting from a rural, agrarian economic base to one that is organized largely around industry and the new technologies. For example, 80 percent of Kenyan families still live in rural farming and pastoral communities, although Kenya is the center of international capitalism in eastern Africa (Miller and Yeager 1994).

Demands of urban environments and industrial employment in developing countries (for example, in Cameroon, Kenya, Zimbabwe, Brazil, Mexico, Peru, the Philippines, and India) have disrupted childcare provision by extended families, friends, and neighbors. Traditionally, nonparental childcare in these and other countries included a child's grandparents and older siblings (especially sisters) and certain other members of the extended family. Such childcare obligations also may have extended beyond relatives to the neighborhood or village (Gill 1993; Palattio-Corpus 1993; Chada 1993; Kipkorir 1993; Anderson 1993; Rosemberg 1993; Tolbert and others 1993).

Contemporary Causal Factors

Besides identifying historical antecedents to ECCD policies and programs, the ICCPP study also illuminated more immediate, or contemporary, causal factors that trigger the need for new childcare alternatives. A number of interrelated economic and social changes in industrialized and developing countries continue to cause the family to adapt and change, stimulating demand for new forms of childcare. These changes are described below along with the effects of immigration and sociopolitical changes on childcare needs.

Cost of Living, Labor Shortages, and Women in the Work Force

One economic change in the industrialized countries of Europe and North America has been a steady increase in the cost of living, fueled by rising expectations and living standards as well as increasing costs to rear children and support a family. This post-World War II phenomenon has encouraged, and in many cases forced, one-earner families to consider increasing their earning capacity by having the mother enter the labor market. Mothers with young children also began entering the work force in response to labor shortages created by the world wars.

By entering the work force, women began to emancipate themselves from traditional role expectations. Increased educational opportunity, the right to vote, and labor demands resulting from growth in service jobs all contributed to a gradual change in social climate that enabled women to respond to labor shortages and increased cost of living by shifting successfully from a housework and childcare role inside the home to outside employment.

The Scandinavian countries of Sweden, Finland, and Norway became industrialized late by European standards, reaching full productivity in the late 1950s and early 1960s (Bø 1993; Huttunen and Turunen 1993; Gunnarsson 1993). Industrialization created a very strong demand for labor and resulted in labor shortages. Movements to emancipate women from exclusively domestic roles had progressed far enough in these countries to legitimize creation of public policies for bringing large numbers of women with young children into the labor force and developing comprehensive, national childcare systems. Leira (1987) points out that although childcare programs in Sweden and Denmark were developed to facilitate the taking of jobs by young mothers, in Norway the childcare system developed in response to the employment of mothers with very young children.

Low Birthrates

Another change contributing to the establishment of childcare programs in Scandinavia and creating pressure to develop high-quality programs was a low and falling birthrate. Such a birthrate indicated that the population was not replacing itself. Women of childbearing age needed to be drawn into the work force while being encouraged to have children. To do this, alternative childcare arrangements had to be of high enough quality to convince women and their partners that they could successfully combine childrearing with work outside the home. In Eastern Europe the combination of labor demand and falling birthrates was met with a more aggressive liberation ideology and more heavy-handed manipulation of labor supply and demand, creating somewhat different policy and birthrate outcomes (Korczak 1993; Nemenyi 1993).

One-Parent Families

As women have gained rights and roles not available to them previously, some functions of the marriage contract have ceased to exist or become less important. For example, women now are less financially dependent on a husband through eligibility for inheritance and access to the labor market. In the event of divorce, laws in a growing number of countries now guarantee mothers and children a significant proportion of the family assets. All of these changes have reduced the economic need for remaining in an unsatisfactory marriage.

The result of these changes has been a worldwide increase in divorce and a consequent growth in the number of one-parent families (see Cochran 1993). This change in family structure extends the shift from extended families to nuclear families one more step, reducing both childcare resources and the number of earners available inside the family still further. To function as primary sources of economic support for their families, through participation in the labor market, single parents need public childcare services. Because most of these parents work in relatively low paying jobs, services must be subsidized in order to make them accessible to parents with low incomes.

Poverty, School Preparation, and Service Delivery Infrastructure

A second group of economic and social factors stimulating the need for ECCD programs revolves around child poverty and focuses, although not exclusively, on developing countries. Concern for the large numbers of children living in poverty is a current stimulus for public childcare policies in societies as different as Brazil, Colombia, Mexico, India, South Africa, and Venezuela (Rosemberg 1993; Arango 1993; Tolbert and others

1993; Gill 1993; Mkhulisi and Cochran 1993; de Ascanio, de Orantes, and Recagno-Puente 1993; Myers 1992).

High birthrates are a major factor in the growing poverty in a number of developing countries. High birthrates cause concern and policy action, especially in Africa where more than thirty countries have total fertility rates above six live births for each woman (United Nations 1990). Rapid rates of population growth resulting from high birthrates overwhelm the carrying capacity of the agricultural land, leading to malnutrition, starvation, and mass movements of families from rural to urban areas where they continue to live in poor conditions (Miller and Yeager 1994; Harkness and Super 1992).

A consequence of living in poverty is a delay in the cognitive and behavioral development necessary for successful transition into primary school and successful performance in later school (see Martorell and Sternberg, this volume). The success of children in school is important to societies for a number of interrelated reasons (Myers 1992): reduced costs of schooling—fewer children repeat grades or require special educational services; better quality of available workers—higher skills result in better work; and reduced fertility rate—the fertility rate declines as the educational level of the general population increases (Zinn and Eitzen 1993).

In some societies a concern about population growth has led to emphasizing school preparation independent of poverty concerns, although the growth in population is likely to create more poor families throughout the next several decades. Policies developed in response to the more general concern about school preparation can be found in Brazil, Hungary (the Gypsies), India, Israel (the children of immigrants), Kenya, and Venezuela (Rosemberg 1993; Nemenyi 1993; Gill 1993; Sagi and Koren-Karie 1993; Kipkorir 1993; de Ascanio, de Orantes, and Recagno-Puente 1993).

The Head Start program in the United States provides medical, dental, and social services, in addition to preschool education, for children living in poverty. The program illustrates that childcare programs can deliver other services in countries without basic (or national) health, education, or social service infrastructures or in countries whose infrastructures are not sufficient to meet the needs of low-income families. Childcare programs that deliver other services are found frequently in developing countries (Zhengao 1993; Arango 1993; Gill 1993; Tran, Pham, and Dao 1993; Chada 1993). Myers (1992) also identifies this function of early education and care programs.

Immigration Policies

Immigration from one country to another, somewhat analogous to but more culturally complex than the migration from rural to urban areas discussed earlier, also affects the need for childcare services. The movement of families across national boundaries typically takes place because of employment opportunities in the receiving country or in response to persecution and discrimination in the country of origin. Childcare services provided for these families enable parents to be employed outside the home. The services also help children and their parents meet local families and learn the values, customs, and traditions of the new society. Combes (1993) offers an excellent discussion of parent-cooperative childcare centers in France designed to assist families that have immigrated from North African countries in adjusting to French culture. The Swedes have a great deal of experience developing bilingual childcare programs to serve a mix of native Swedish and immigrant families.

At the macroeconomic level, encouraging immigration may be viewed as an alternative to maximizing domestic labor potential (usually female homemakers or unskilled, unemployed persons). For example, believing immigration to be a less expensive solution to its labor needs, a nation may try to import workers from abroad rather than provide incentives (education, job training, childcare) to unemployed adult citizens. This action may dampen the demand for childcare services by using male immigrant workers to fill jobs that native women with young children might otherwise fill. However, hidden costs to society as a whole may result from higher levels of unemployment brought on by expanding the labor pool (through increased immigration) without corresponding growth in the labor market.

National Liberation, Expansionism, and Nation Building

Large-scale sociopolitical changes also affect childcare policies and programs. Such changes have stimulated major investments in childcare programs in a number of countries during the twentieth century. Childcare is used as a strategy for community development and renewal in many of the newly independent countries of Africa and Asia.

Historical examples of large-scale sociopolitical changes include Russia after the Russian Revolution, Poland and Hungary with the imposition of communism after World War II, Italy following World War II, and China after establishment of the People's Republic of China in 1949. More contemporary cases include Kenya (1963) and Zimbabwe (1980) after independence from Britain, Vietnam during and after the war of liberation (since 1970), Nicaragua following the 1979 revolution, and South Africa (since 1994) in response to apartheid and as part of the new nonracial democracy (Foteeva 1993; Korczak 1993; Nemenyi 1993; New 1993; Kipkorir 1993; Chada 1993; Tran, Pham, and Dao 1993; Torres 1993; Mkhulisi and Cochran 1993).

One goal of national liberation and nation building sometimes has been the emancipation of women from traditionally female roles and activities (reproduction) to production (paid work). Myers (1992) introduces a continuum for women's work, ranging from paid work outside the home to work at home for pay, unpaid support for other earners, unpaid production for family consumption (subsistence farming), and domestic chores (water, wood, laundry) and unpaid childcare within the household. He points out that in many countries, every kind of work included in this continuum is paid for and can be considered productive in economic terms.

In nation-building efforts, liberation often involves community-participation strategies. Myers (1992) lists twelve reasons why community participation in childcare and development programs is important, ranging from its intrinsic value for participants, to the amount of energy it harnesses and the value of indigenous knowledge and expertise. He also warns against exploiting community members in the name of self-reliance and reducing costs (Myers 1992).

Summary

Research has shown that two major combinations of factors impel societies to establish childcare policies and programs: (a) movement of mothers with young children into the work force (as a result of early labor shortages and currently rising costs of living), falling birthrates, and an increase in one-parent families; and (b) concerns about the effects of poverty on young children, the need to prepare them for success in school, and the desire to offer them health and nutritional services. Although the factors in (a) typify conditions in Europe, and the factors in (b) have driven childcare policy in many developing countries, generalizing the factors only to industrial and developing countries respectively would be inappropriate.

As urbanization and industrialization become more pronounced in developing countries, the number of mothers working for pay outside the home in those societies increases steadily and sometimes very rapidly, creating a growing need for programs that care for children 8 or more hours at a time. In the United States, a wealthy, postindustrial society, more than 20 percent of preschool children live in poverty. But the primary national investment in childcare and development (Head Start) focuses only on preparing those children for school. These contrasting examples illustrate that all societies are in a constant state of transition and that applying general rules often obscures more than it reveals.

Influences Mediating Translation of National Needs into Childcare Policies and Programs

How do nations respond to the need for new childcare alternatives once these needs become apparent? Analysis of the ICCPP case studies and profiles of childcare programs shows that nations each respond differently, a finding that confirms the conclusions of other investigators (Myers 1992; Lamb and Sternberg 1992). To some extent differences stem from the factors identified above that create the need for care. But other factors also are at work, and some influence the form and content of childcare programs more than any of the macrolevel demands discussed so far. These other influences are shown in figures 1 and 2 as mediating between perceived needs and outcomes.

Examples of interrelated mediating influences are discussed below. These include values and beliefs, sociopolitical and economic ideologies, social welfare, and advocacy. Other mediating factors that influence policies and programs independently are also described: national wealth; cultural, ethnic, and religious diversity; institutional complexity; and societal family policies.

Values, Ideologies, Social Welfare, and Advocacy

Because they have deep historical foundations, the values and prevailing beliefs of a society retain an underlying constancy despite being in a constant state of flux. The family and religion traditionally are the two primary institutions through which these values and beliefs about how the members of a society should relate to one another and to outsiders have been transmitted.

Spedding (1993: 536) identifies some basic beliefs passed on in the American family: "Citizens of the United States often characterize themselves as a nation of 'rugged individualists.' Ideals of individual freedom, personal and family privacy, self-sufficiency . . . and the responsibility of the less fortunate to help the more fortunate . . . are basic to the American culture." Spedding says that the immigrants' search for political and religious freedom in a new land of opportunity and the challenges they faced surviving the harsh demands of frontier life fostered and reinforced these basic beliefs. The nuclear family allowed immigrants to pack up and move on in search of greater opportunities, and alliances among families helped accomplish tasks too large for a couple and their children to perform (barnraising, harvesting, safety in emergencies).

The Christian religions that European settlers and immigrants brought with them to the new world taught a patriarchal system of relationships within the family: a dominant husband and father figure, a wife subordinate to the authority of the husband, and children subject to the authority and discipline of both parents. Sanday (1981) documents the relationship between orthodox Christianity and patriarchal relations between men and women.

Among ICCPP cases the influence of religion on beliefs about the family and role divisions within the family can be seen especially clearly in Italy and the Philippines. In some societies, the church defines public childcare as a charitable response to families who cannot support themselves in the traditional family form (an employed father married to a mother who cares for the children). This charity-based definition of childcare programs was the norm in Brazil as recently as the late 1970s and continues to be heard in U.S. congressional debates (New 1993; Palattio-Corpus 1993; Rosemberg 1993).

Nsamenang (1992) shows how a change in the value structure of the family, brought about by societal and religious influences, affected childcare. In precolonial Cameroon, children 11-15 years old cared for their siblings, making it possible for their mothers to work in the fields and carry out household chores. Nsamenang suggests that assigning this task to children promoted important cultural values such as a strong sense of responsibility for others, self-motivation, and appreciation for the collective effort to benefit the community as a whole. Colonialism and the arrival of Christian and Muslim missionaries introduced school enrollment for children to the Cameroonian family. This change in the family structure of values led to "one of the highest rates of school attendance in Africa" (Hodgkinson 1985). In examining the effect of school enrollment on childcare, Hodgkinson (1985: 319) concludes: "The net effect of the massive expansion of the school system was a disruption of the old social order, particularly child caretaking and patterns of network care. The difficulties in the child care scene were thus exacerbated by the increasing incidence of school enrollment. This implies that fewer children were available to provide day care when it was most needed, that is, when parents were at work, in the marketplace, or at the farm."

This observation raises a question about how the values prized by Cameroonian society (responsibility for others, self-motivation, and appreciation for the collective effort to benefit the community as a whole) will be instilled in young people who no longer learn them through providing childcare, the previous means of transmission. In addition to the importance of family and church in transmitting values and beliefs, several authors of ICCPP cases identified childcare programs as a means of passing culturally appropriate values and norms from one generation to the next [see Kipkorir's (1993) description of localized curriculum as a means of transmitting values manifested in community-based stories, poems, rhymes, games, dances, and songs.]

Values and beliefs, important mediating influences, are not static but evolve over time. Industrialization and urbanization are one powerful force that continues to shape values worldwide (see figures 1 and 2). Industrialization and urbanization not only established the conditions leading to a need for alternative childcare arrangements (by changing family structures and roles), but they also modified societal values and beliefs, two of the

unable or unwilling to pay the cost of necessary services. ICCPP countries in Scandinavia and Eastern Europe are well-established examples of more institutional approaches. More residual approaches are found in countries dominated by Anglo-Saxon traditions (especially the United States, but also Australia, Canada, and the United Kingdom) and in a number of Asian and Latin American countries.

A question that arises from the social welfare approach taken by a government or an outside agency is whether policies and programs will be imposed on families and communities without their being involved in their development, or whether a partnership will be adopted "in which communities work together *with* institutions from the larger society to solve common problems" (Myers 1992: 319). The institutional welfare approach typically has been designed and implemented from the top down, leaving little of the shaping power in the hands of program participants such as parents and teachers.

The residual welfare approach assumes that families who need assistance with childcar have demonstrated their inadequacy through an inability to look after themselves and therefore, must be incapable of contributing useful knowledge and ideas to program development. A parent-empowerment process has emerged recently in the United States and elsewhere partly as a reaction to this perspective (Cochran 1985, 1988, 1993, 1995; Cochran and Woolever 1983).

The partnership endorsed by Myers (1992) is neither an institutional or residual welfare approach. It requires rethinking the relationship between public institutions and local community members. Myers stresses that the success of a partnership depends on the participants, the form of participation, who controls the process, and the timing and duration of joint activities.

Some results of successful partnerships between the public sector and local community are: an important new understanding by community members of how to produce change and identify needs and rights, significant in-kind resource contributions by community members, a sense of ownership and responsibility for the service, a better fit between the welfare service and local values and norms, incorporation of time-tested local methods for delivering the service, and less dependence on outside professionals for skills not available in the local community (Myers 1992: 310-311). These advantages are also reflected in the author's studies of childcare and family support programs employing a parent-empowerment approach to program development, delivery, and evaluation (Cochran 1995). Such outcomes are important in any society, but they are especially critical in countries without substantial wealth per capita, which must rely heavily on local, nonmonetary resources for indoor and outdoor space, staff, food, and educational materials needed to provide a childcare and development program. This point is elaborated below in discussion of formal and informal program approaches.

Nations taking residual or institutional welfare approaches often use advocacy to stimulate awareness of need and highlight the negative consequences of inaction. Advocates in these societies rally specifically for childcare needs using larger issues such as children's or women's rights. In countries with more institutional approaches advocacy is used in efforts to turn ideological rhetoric into policy action.

In Kenya and Israel, for example, women's organizations have sponsored and run early childhood programs. In Italy, women organized to free themselves from a patriarchal system reinforced by the Catholic church. The resulting preschool and day-care legislation accompanied new laws related to family rights, equal pay for women, and abortion. In

Brazil, mobilization for childcare began as organized, neighborhood-level resistance to dictatorship. Women's organizations in China and Vietnam were influential in pushing communist and socialist regimes to deliver on promises of childcare programs necessary to free women for participation in education, employment, and government service on an equal basis with men (New 1993; Rosemberg 1993; Zhengao 1993; Tran, Pham, and Dao 1993; Sagi and Koren-Karie 1993; Kipkorir 1993; Campos 1992; Lee 1992; Rosenthal 1992; Corsaro and Emiliani 1992).

Advocacy for early childhood programs is especially important in the United States. Proponents such as the Children's Defense Fund have been concerned with the effects of poverty on children. Other advocates such as the National Association for the Education of Young Children lobby for improving the quality and expanding the amount of day care available to families with young children.

National Wealth

A factor that affects childcare policies and programs independently from the interrelated mediating influences described above is a nation's wealth. Even with equal commitment to childcare provision, a wealthy society is more capable than other societies of financing the necessary programs. Comparisons of wealth across nations often use as an index the annual gross national product (GNP) of a country divided by its population to produce a GNP per capita. The United Nations Department of International Economic and Social Affairs (1990) has published these data in U.S. dollars for 134 countries. Costly capital and human resource investments include building and equipping facilities, training and paying teachers and caregivers, and developing and disseminating educational materials.

A number of ICCPP cases demonstrate how resource limitations affect strategies for providing public childcare. Family-based childcare is especially attractive to policymakers in Venezuela and Colombia not only because it may be congruent with cultural tradition, but also because it is believed to be less expensive than center-based care. Some African and Latin American countries emphasizing center-based strategies (Kenya, Mexico, Nicaragua, Zimbabwe) have found ways to reduce costs to the states and municipalities by involving fathers and other men in building facilities and involving mothers and other women in helping staff the program. Vietnam is an interesting case example of transition from a relatively expensive, Soviet-style, exclusively center-based model to one that includes family day-care alternatives.

The wealth of a society is not necessarily a good predictor of its public and private investment in childcare, however. The United States is a powerful example of a very wealthy nation whose society as a whole invests very little in extrafamilial childcare. In this context, "society as a whole" refers to members of society (adults without children, parents without preschool children, private companies) who do not benefit directly from provision of the service. Parents pay more than 90 percent of the cost of American childcare, whereas the parental share is closer to 50 percent in Scandinavian countries and considerably less than that in a number of developing countries that are making major investments in childcare for low-income families.

In sharp contrast to the United States are countries like Colombia and Kenya that have far lower levels of average personal wealth (about 1/20th and 1/50th respectively) and yet major national programs, financed by public and private funds. Myers (1992: 93) notes:

"The economic feasibility of a programme . . . is only partly a matter of available funds—it is also a matter of *priorities* and of how funds are divided up. If a programme has been assigned a high priority, it can be afforded and made feasible by giving up something of lower priority." Myers (1992: 287) also concludes that "part of the cost complaints, then, are really a combined problem of social convention, weak political will, and the failure to recognize that early childhood care and development is a good investment."

Cultural, Ethnic, and Religious Diversity

National wealth may limit the number of children reached with a program, the location of the program, and the training and pay of teachers. However, cultural, ethnic, religious, or other types of diversity are more likely to affect the content of the program, the form and substance of ideas and experiences to which the children are exposed.

In the ICCPP study of Kenya, Kipkorir (1993: 348) describes the localized curriculum approach, which was developed in Kenya during the past decade because of recognition "that the centralized curriculum cannot adequately serve all the cultural patterns represented in Kenya." Kipkorir (1993) points out that by 1990 local collections of stories, poems, and riddles had been published in twenty-one different regional languages as a result of the localized curriculum approach, which emphasizes initiative taken by local teachers and parents. Writing about Australian childcare, Brennan (1993) tells of that system's inability to adapt to the needs of aboriginal people, paralleling the history of Canada and the United States.

Among the other multicultural societies included in the ICCPP study (for example, Brazil, Canada, China, France, India, Israel, Kenya, South Africa, the United Kingdom, and the United States), some have tried harder and been more successful than others at finding approaches to public childcare that are adaptable to local and regional differences (Cochran 1993). Even in the relatively homogeneous Scandinavian countries, the recent need to integrate large numbers of immigrant families from abroad requires childcare systems to adapt to a number of new issues that include developing multilingual settings and accommodating different beliefs about how teachers and parents should interrelate.

Rural-urban variation also is reflected in all the ICCPP cases. Another source of diversity in some of these countries results from their relatively decentralized political systems, in which the national government gives a great deal of policymaking authority to states, provinces, or other regional political structures. When power is decentralized and various local bodies are given regulatory control, policies related to training of caregivers, size of preschool groups, and caregiver-to-child ratios may vary considerably from one region to another.

Institutional Complexity

Institutional complexity refers to the distribution of a society's lines of authority for various aspects of a system such as childcare; that is, whether and to what extent authority is fragmented or streamlined. In many societies, three to six different national ministries, departments, or agencies have authority over different aspects of childcare provision. Sometimes the persons responsible for services to children 0-3 years old are not the same ones directing services to older children. This complexity reached absurdity in South Africa, where the policy of apartheid required different systems for each official racial designation and nonstate services had to be created to counter the deleterious effects of state provision (Mkhulisi and Cochran 1993). The consensus in the ICCPP study was that, in general, establishing overall authority in a single department or agency and streamlining the lines of responsibility result in less confusion and a higher quality of services provided at the local level.

Evidence also suggests that concentrating all decisionmaking authority at the top of the government, regardless of how streamlined, will likely lead to dense bureaucracy and institutional rigidity. For this reason, an international trend toward decentralization of regulatory authority is under way in order to better accommodate varying local conditions.

In the ICCPP study, Nemenyi (1993) uses historical analysis to document results of bureaucratic rigidity in Hungary, Rosemberg (1993) describes the impact of extremely large and complex administrative mechanisms on day care in São Paolo, Brazil, and Bø (1993) discusses the advantages and disadvantages of decentralization. To provide basic consistency within program types and ensure adequate levels of child development, the ICCPP study group supported addressing issues like caregiver qualifications, staff-child ratios, and group size in national regulations. However, the group also tended to favor leaving decisions about program content to the local level, with significant input from parents and other community members, ensuring that programs are responsive to local beliefs, traditions, and practices.

Other Family Policies

Finally, another independent mediating factor that may shape society's response to childcare needs is other family policies operating within that society. Other policies directly related to childcare include parental or maternity leave from employment immediately after a child's birth and allowances (called homecare allowance in Finland and childcare allowance in Hungary) that pay one parent to stay out of the work force and care for the child at home. As noted earlier, extending parental leave in Sweden to 12 months has nearly eliminated the need for infant day care. In contrast, the absence of paid parental leave in the United States places a heavy burden on public childcare provision, which sometimes must serve children as young as 6 weeks old.

Translating National Needs and Societal Influences into Policies and Programs

The framework adopted in this chapter suggests that a country's childcare policies and programs are responses to a set of perceived needs as mediated by various influences. Childcare outcomes will vary from country to country to the extent that perceived needs and mediating filters differ in each society. Based on analysis of the twenty-nine national ICCPP cases a number of dimensions can be specified for the variation in childcare policy and program outcomes.

Figure 4 highlights seven policy and five program dimensions. These dimensions are not exhaustive. They consist of policy and program elements common to the twenty-nine

Figure 4. Policy and Program Outcomes

Policy Outcomes

Provision	________	+	________	Nonprovision
Auspice Single	________	+	________	Multiple
Target Child	________	+	________	Parent and Community
Quantity	________	+	________	Quality
Regulated	________	+	________	Unregulated
Children Younger	________	+	________	Older
Financing Public	________	+	________	Private

Program Outcomes

Setting Center	________	+	________	Home
Staff Training Preservice	________	+	________	Inservice
Curriculum Goal Development	________	+	________	School Readiness
Pedagogy Child-directed	________	+	________	Teacher-directed
Parents Involved	________	+	________	Uninvolved

ICCPP cases that could be linked to needs and mediating influences. The distinction between policy and program dimensions, although admittedly crude, separates issues of general national intent from issues that define the actual shape and content of the programs operating in local communities. [See Lamb and others (1992) and Myers (1992) for additional ways of describing childcare policies and programs.]

Policy Outcomes

Policy outcomes start with the simple *extent of provision*. This parameter is an estimate of the proportion of children or families needing childcare services who actually receive them. Many countries provide little or no public childcare. Absence of childcare policy usually is explained, not by lack of need, but by mediating cultural influences that keep women in the home and childcare within the family. For instance, religious beliefs in Muslim countries exert powerful influence to keep women in traditional roles, mitigating policy interest in public childcare arrangements. National policies range from those in Scandinavia promising public childcare for all preschool children whose parents are employed or studying to those reluctant policies in the United States aimed primarily at 4-year-olds in low-income families.

The second policy dimension addresses *auspice*: the government ministry, department, or agency responsible for overseeing development of childcare capacity at the local level. Whoever receives this responsibility will decide how the need is perceived (for example, as educational, health related, social) and how responsibilities are assigned within existing government agencies. Myers (1992) argues very persuasively in favor of integrated programming, which is based on an integrated concept of the developing child. Commitment to such integration places even greater importance on the choice of a lead agency and on the cooperative agreements between the lead agency and those controlling complementary resources.

In Figure 4, *target* refers to whether policies are aimed at parents (as workers or childrearing agents) or directly at children. When freeing women for schooling or the work force creates the need for childcare, for example, the developmental needs of the child may become a secondary issue. At the other extreme, policies that exclusively emphasize preparing children for school in part-time programs do not take into account the needs of employed parents for full-time day care. In some African and Latin American countries the community is the target, with public childcare emerging as an entry point for community development.

The *quantity and quality* dimension is one of relative emphasis. In virtually every country the desire exists simultaneously for increased service coverage and improved quality of existing services. Choice of emphasis at the policy level depends on the stage of development of the national childcare initiative. Societies with a longer public childcare tradition tend to focus more on quality than societies entering the field of public childcare more recently (within the past 20 years) who are preoccupied with coverage. This conclusion reflects not only analysis of the twenty-nine national ICCPP cases (Cochran 1993) but also Myers' (1992) general concern with expanding the emphasis in the ECCD policies of developing countries from child survival to promotion of positive growth and development.

Governments use *regulation* to ensure child safety, monitor quality of care, and control the curricula of children's experiences. Controlling quality of care usually involves stipulating caregiver training and qualifications, adult-child ratios, group sizes, and characteristics of the care environments. Because regulations to improve the quality of public childcare also increase the cost of delivering that care, the need to reduce costs may result in program standards that do not demand increased expenditure for personnel or facilities. Pressure to prevent regulations that increase the cost of providing care can also come from market forces governed by parental ability to pay or from profit-making desires of proprietary programs.

The *age of children served* by public childcare in a particular society is determined partly by perceived need (for example, prepare for school, enable women to be employed, improve nutritional status) and partly by ideology regarding the age when children should be separated from their mothers. Full-time care for children 0-3 years old is much less common than care and education for 3-5 year olds. In Germany and Japan this variance results from the strong belief that mother and child should be together during the first 3 years of life. In countries where policies emphasize school preparation, the difference may stem from the belief that children are not ready for structured educational activities until they are 3 years old.

Finally, *financing* of childcare programs is determined by a nation's wealth and economic system. Less wealthy countries cannot afford to invest a large percentage of public funds in childcare even when their economic ideologies support public investment in social welfare. But even wealthy nations that can afford to raise substantial resources through public taxation of individuals and corporations tend to rely on private funding sources (parental fees, charitable contributions, direct support by private business), if they operate within free-enterprise economic ideologies.

Program Outcomes

The most visible dimension at the program level is the *setting and locale* for childcare provision. Formal provision usually takes place in homes or centers, and most countries use both settings, emphasizing one over the other. For example, Colombia, Venezuela, the United States, and Germany have childcare systems dominated by family-based care, but Kenya, Hungary, and the Scandinavian countries emphasize center-based care. Influences mediating choice of setting include societal values (collective-cooperative in contrast to individualistic-competitive), national wealth (centers may cost more to create and maintain than home settings, quality held constant), and age of the children (parents in many societies prefer home settings for their infants and toddlers).

Training strategies for educating childcare workers and preschool teachers range from college-based, preservice preparation in Europe (especially in Scandinavia) to almost exclusive reliance on inservice training in southeastern Africa. A primary determining factor is national wealth, because preservice training requires substantial investment in an educational infrastructure (teaching facilities, faculty salaries). But national priorities also are important. The United States is an example of a wealthy country that relies heavily on inservice training for center caregivers, in part because the status and salaries of preschool personnel are low, providing little incentive for college-educated adults to enter the preschool field.

At the level of *pedagogy*, parents in some countries (France, Kenya) apply considerable pressure to emphasize schooling or preparation for school, but in other countries (Norway,

Sweden, Zimbabwe) the strong emphasis is on supporting child development. Developmental stage of the child is a factor in determining program emphasis. In general, programs that provide more than custodial care for very young children have a developmental focus. Programs serving 3-6 year olds may or may not begin to take on the characteristics of a school.

Childcare pedagogies that emphasize preparation for school tend to stress *teacher-initiated* activities, whereas pedagogies with a heavy developmental focus tend to stress activities *initiated by the child.* Analysis of the twenty-nine ICCPP cases suggests that the international trend is away from didactic, teacher-dominated curricular approaches toward allowing children to take initiative in deciding what to investigate and how to engage with the environment.

National childcare approaches also show considerable variation on the final program dimension shown in figure 4, *level of parental involvement*, although ICCPP data suggest a global shift toward greater parental involvement. This shift is taking place for a number of reasons. In countries with long histories of public childcare and very centralized social welfare systems, the shift seems to signal a reaffirmation of parental rights and responsibilities (Eastern Europe) and a desire to forge closer ties between family and community (Scandinavia). Where public childcare and early education are part of broader, postindependence strategies of community development (Kenya, Nicaragua, Zimbabwe, Vietnam), the goals of parental involvement include developing trust, meeting parental expectations, respecting local teaching and childrearing traditions, and recruiting assistance to build and staff the childcare center. Community development is also a goal in a number of Latin American countries (Colombia, Mexico, Venezuela), partly as an employment opportunity for low-income parents and partly as a starting point of empowering women to take more control over their lives. Parental involvement also may be initiated by parents themselves in reaction to dissatisfaction with the childcare options available.

National wealth and social welfare orientation affect parental participation. Less wealthy nations may have to rely on parents and other community residents for everything from building construction to teaching assistance. As mentioned earlier, social welfare approaches that view early childhood services as efforts to compensate for parental inadequacies are unlikely to consider parents equal partners in program development and maintenance. Approaches that recognize and build on family strengths and potentials may provide a variety of ways for parents to contribute.

Two other aspects of childcare programs, *pedagogical approach* and *cultural content*, provide ways of understanding children and transmitting meaning. Pedagogical approach is the systematic manner for understanding and organizing the content of interactions between a child and the physical and social environment. Culturally specific content includes social, emotional, and intellectual subject matter.

ICCPP examples of culturally specific content range from the cooperative emphasis in Sweden to aesthetic education in Poland, folklore in Kenya, and intellectual competence in Israel. The loss of traditional family structures brought on by urbanization and industrialization has diminished avenues for transmitting cultural values and beliefs. Chada (1993) explains that the early childhood education and care program in Zimbabwe was conceived to transmit cultural traditions through stories, puzzles, proverbs, taboos, and songs, the manner previously used by grandparents and other elders.

Two Case Examples

When taken together, the fourteen policy and program characteristics described above will provide a reasonably complete picture of childcare goals and provision in a given country. Cross-national analysis of the ICCPP data indicates that the size, shape, and content of available childcare programs result from the macrolevel factors outlined earlier in this chapter: perceived needs as filtered by societal values, economic ideology, national wealth, and other mediating influences. Each society's unique combination of perceived needs, mediating influences, and policy and program outcomes operates as a dynamic whole, constantly evolving in response to internal domestic and external international pressures.

Two case examples illustrate how existing policies and programs reflect larger societal needs and characteristics, distinguishing one nation from another. Figure 5 places Colombian (C) and Kenyan (K) childcare policy and program outcomes on the twelve dimensions described earlier.

The Cs and Ks in figure 5 have been connected with dotted lines to create an outcomes profile for each country. Differences between the two profiles are explained largely by differing needs and mediating influences, as discussed below.

Colombia

The Colombian policy and program profile (figure 5) shows that childcare is provided to an estimated 50 percent of families needing the service, with more emphasis on reaching large numbers of children than on providing each with a stimulating environment organized by well-trained teachers and caregivers. The services are financed by a 3 percent public payroll tax, contributions of nongovernmental agencies, and parental fees. The policy focuses primarily on children, with particular concern for improving their nutritional status and compensating for the unstabilizing effects of poverty. Children rarely enter the home-based program before the age of 2, although infants and toddlers attend the urban centers.

At the program level, the nation is committed to "hogares de bienestar," or child welfare homes, which are run by women in private homes after a brief period of preservice training. During most of the day each mother is responsible for about fifteen preschool children, often in close quarters. Pedagogic emphasis is on child development, with little concern for school preparation or school. Originally parents were to volunteer to take turns supervising the children as a second adult, but most mothers are too involved with employment to make this commitment.

How does this outcomes profile reflect forces at work in the larger society? Basic components of the Colombian childcare system were developed in response to rapid urbanization between 1950 and 1985; the urban population increased from 30 to 70 percent of the population as a whole. This led to a high rate of urban poverty, and now 40 percent of the population lives in absolute poverty, including more than 2 million preschool children. Rapid urbanization also resulted in an increase in the number of families headed by women. Now about 25 percent of poor families are headed by women reporting incomes substantially below the minimum wage.

Figure 5. Policy and Program Outcomes: Kenya and Colombia

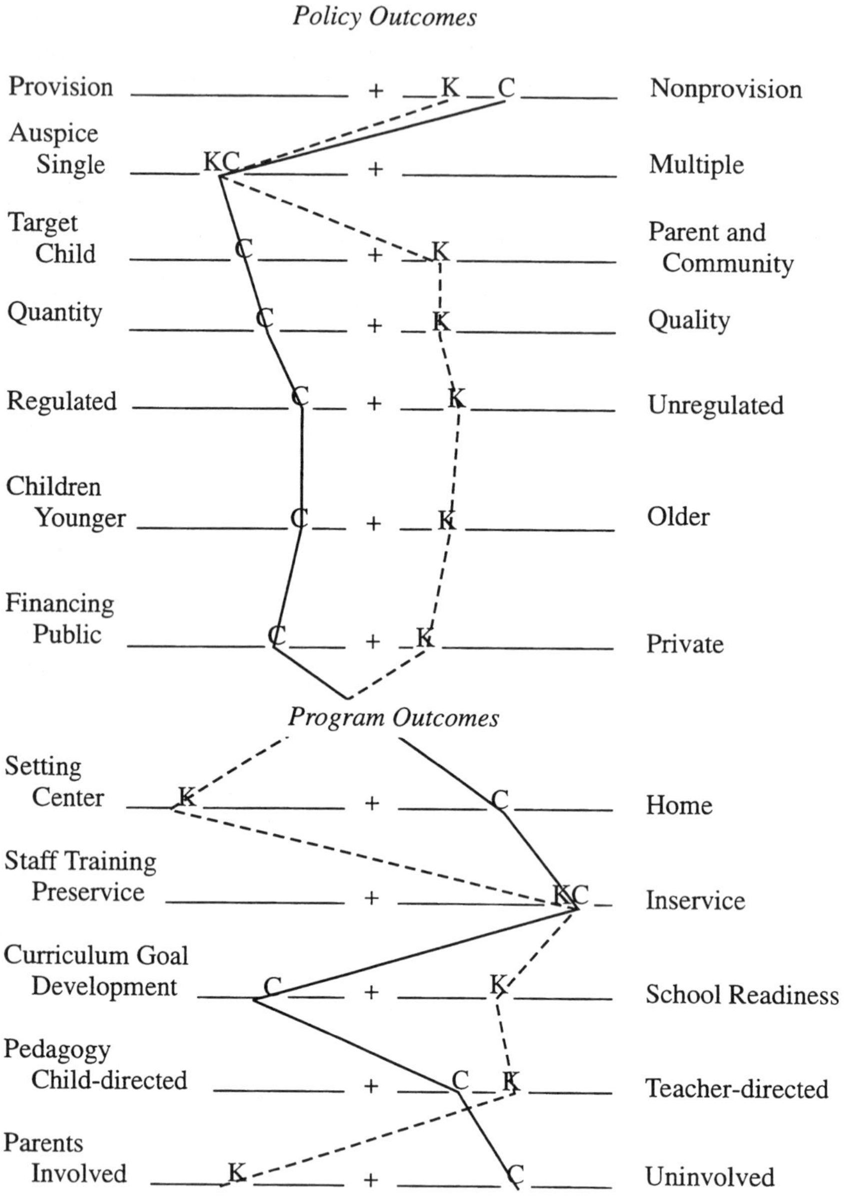

In response to this social crisis, the Child Welfare Homes program was established in 1987. The program was promoted from the national level by the National Institute of Family Welfare; it was financed with a 2 percent payroll tax on company salaries that was more recently increased to 3 percent. Participating homes receive housing loans and the national institute provides each home with equipment (stove, kitchen supplies, water filter) and nutritional supplement. The national system of family childcare homes was created to improve the nutritional status of poor children and provide them with secure environments while their parents were employed outside the home. Home, rather than center, settings were selected because they were less expensive to establish and reflected the strong family orientation of Colombian parents.

In Colombia a powerful correspondence exists between macrolevel forces and the characteristics of childcare programs at the microlevel. This correspondence is equally evident in Kenya, but it produces a rather different result.

Kenya

The Kenyan policy and program profile (figure 5) shows that childcare is provided to about 30 percent of the children estimated to need preschool services. Although this percentage has remained about the same for the past 5 years, a steady increase in the number of births has now increased the number of children receiving services. Although program quality is a concern, expanded coverage (quantity) is the highest priority because of high levels of unmet need. Because resources are extremely limited, regulations regarding indoor and outdoor spaces, caregiver preparation, group size, and ratio of adults to children are only guidelines, strongly encouraged but rarely achieved. Teacher salaries and local facilities are financed by parental fees and local community contributions (in the harambee tradition), and teacher training as well as development of curriculum guidelines and materials are financed by the state. Policies target both children (primarily 3-5 year olds) and parents, emphasizing preparing children for school and teaching parents about the importance of education.

At the program level, childcare services are exclusively center based and are usually offered for only part of the day, although some urban centers are offering full-day programs to accommodate mothers who are employed full-time. Teacher preparation is a 2-year period consisting of alternating 3-week residential sessions and four month-long periods of on-the-job teaching experience. This teacher preparation system is supported by a highly sophisticated network of district-level trainers and national training and curriculum specialists. As with the childcare service itself, demand still far outstrips supply, and many adults who staff preschools are untrained.

Pedagogic emphasis in the centers reflects strong parental concern for school preparation combined with a teacher training program grounded in developmental principles. Teachers are encouraged to organize their classrooms for hands-on play and creative manipulation of materials, but the constraints imposed by large adult-child ratios (average 30 to 1) and relatively small classrooms result in a great deal of didactic, teacher-directed learning. Children may learn as many as three languages: the local mother tongue, the national African language (Kiswahili), and English. A conscious effort has been made to organize learning around the history and culture of the local village and region through songs, poems, rhymes, games, and dances.

Parents are actively involved in Kenyan programs in a variety of ways: building and improving facilities, recruiting teachers, creating educational materials from found objects, and providing grain and vegetables for meals. They also attend parental education programs organized by teachers and district teacher-trainers.

As with the Colombian example, this profile of program characteristics in Kenya reflects the history, ideology, and economic conditions of the larger society. When Kenya became independent of Great Britain in 1963, early childhood education was seen as a locally targeted, nation-building strategy, invoking the traditional harambee process (translated "Let's all pull together") to mobilize local resources. With an income per capita of only about 30 percent of that found in Colombia and a fertility rate more than twice as high, very little revenue could be generated through taxation, and program development depended on in-kind contributions from parents and other community members of building supplies, labor, food, and teacher volunteers.

These same conditions exist today, although the fertility rate is dropping. Kenyan policymakers take seriously the cross-national data showing a relationship between increased educational levels and falling birthrates. This belief, combined with parental recognition that higher education leads to a higher standard of living for their children, results in policy that emphasizes school preparation.

Eighty percent of Kenyan families still live in rural areas (compared with less than 30 percent in Colombia), but growing migration into the cities is making demand for services in these areas increasingly acute. Combined with a commitment to development of the local community, the presence of more than forty-four separate linguistic groups and a growing Muslim population in an otherwise largely Christian society produces a significant investment in localizing childcare curriculum.

Conclusion

The organizing framework suggested in this chapter for matching ECCD programs to societal needs and characteristics is based on data from twenty-nine countries representing more than 80 percent of the world's population. These data highlight the unique needs and mediating influences operating in a given country and underscore the dangers of trying to transfer any particular ECCD model from one society to another.

The framework described and illustrated in this chapter will be useful to policy and program planners in any society engaged in self-study to prepare for creating or redesigning its ECCD system. Everyone with a stake in policy and program outcomes (parents, program providers, businesses, nongovernmental agencies and organizations, government, politicians, religious organizations, women's organizations, higher education institutions, and policymakers) must take part in identifying the needs that ECCD programs will address, understanding the societal forces that will shape the responses to these needs, and shaping the program characteristics that will result from these assessments.

Note

The author wishes to thank Robert Myers for his generosity with ideas and network contacts. Appreciation is also expressed to Lars Gunnarsson, Cassie Landers, and Alan Pence for their important roles in the research project that provided much of the basis for the content of this chapter. Sandy Rightmyer deserves much credit for preparation of the original manuscript. Special thanks are extended to the Bernard van Leer Foundation, the Mailman Family Foundation, and the Carnegie Corporation for financial support provided during the writing of this chapter.

References

Anderson, Jeanine. 1993. Peru. In Moncrieff Cochran, ed., *The International Handbook of Child Care Policies and Programs*. Westport, Conn.: Greenwood Press.

Arango, Marta. 1993. Colombia. In Moncrieff Cochran, ed., *The International Handbook of Child Care Policies and Programs*. Westport, Conn.: Greenwood Press.

Bø, Ingerid. 1993. Norway. In Moncrieff Cochran, ed., *The International Handbook of Child Care Policies and Programs*. Westport, Conn.: Greenwood Press.

Brennan, Deborah. 1993. Australia. In Moncrieff Cochran, ed., *The International Handbook of Child Care Policies and Programs*. Westport, Conn.: Greenwood Press.

Campos, Maria. 1992. Child Care in Brazil. In Michael Lamb, Kathleen Sternberg, Carl-Philip Hwang, and Anders Broberg, eds., *Child Care in Context*. Hillsdale, N.J.: Lawrence Erlbaum Associates, Inc.

Chada, Rosely. 1993. Zimbabwe. In Moncrieff Cochran, ed., *The International Handbook of Child Care Policies and Programs*. Westport, Conn.: Greenwood Press.

Cochran, Moncrieff. 1985. The Parental Empowerment Process: Building on Family Strengths. In J. Harris, ed., *Child Psychology in Action: Linking Research and Practice*. London: Croom Helm. Reprinted in *Equity and Choice* (Fall 1987) 4(1).

———. 1988. Parental Empowerment in Family Matters: Lessons Learned from a Research Program. In D. Powell, ed., *Parent Education and Support Programs: Consequences for Children and Families*. New York: Haworth Press.

———, ed. 1993. *The International Handbook of Child Care Policies and Programs*. Westport, Conn.: Greenwood Press.

———, ed. 1995. *Empowerment and Family Support*. Ithaca: Cornell University Media Services.

Cochran, Moncrieff, and Frank Woolever. 1983. Beyond the Deficit Model: The Empowerment of Parents with Information and Informal Supports. In I. Siegal and L. Laosa, eds., *Changing Families*. New York: Plenum.

Cohen, Bronwen. 1993. The United Kingdom. In Moncrieff Cochran, ed., *The International Handbook of Child Care Policies and Programs*. Westport, Conn.: Greenwood Press.

Combes, Josette. 1993. France. In Moncrieff Cochran, ed., *The International Handbook of Child Care Policies and Programs*. Westport, Conn.: Greenwood Press.

Corsaro, William, and Francesca Emiliani. 1992. Child Care, Early Education, and Children's Peer Culture in Italy. In Michael Lamb, Kathleen Sternberg, Carl-Philip Hwang, and Anders Broberg, eds., *Child Care in Context*. Hillsdale, N.J.: Lawrence Erlbaum Associates, Inc.

de Ascanio, Josefina, Maria de Orantes, and Ileana Recagno-Puente. 1993. Venezuela. In Moncrieff Cochran, ed., *The International Handbook of Child Care Policies and Programs*. Westport, Conn.: Greenwood Press.

Degler, Charles. 1980. *At Odds: Women and the Family in America from the Revolution to the Present*. New York: Oxford University Press.

Foteeva, Yekaterina. 1993. The Commonwealth of Independent States. In Moncrieff Cochran, ed., *The International Handbook of Child Care Policies and Programs*. Westport, Conn.: Greenwood Press.

Gill, Sukhdeep. 1993. India. In Moncrieff Cochran, ed., *The International Handbook of Child Care Policies and Programs*. Westport, Conn.: Greenwood Press.

Goode, William. 1963. *World Revolution and Family Patterns*. New York: Free Press.

Greenfield, Susan. 1961. Industrialization and the Family. *Sociological Theory* 67:312-22.

Gunnarsson, Lars. 1993. Sweden. In Moncrieff Cochran, ed., *The International Handbook of Child Care Policies and Programs*. Westport, Conn.: Greenwood Press.

Hareven, Tamara. 1982a. American Families in Transition: Historical Perspectives on Change. In F. Walsh, ed., *Normal Family Processes*. New York: The Guilford Press.

———. 1982b. *Family Time and Industrial Time*. New York: Cambridge University Press.

Harkness, Sara, and Charles Super. 1992. Shared Child Care in East Africa: Sociocultural Origins and Developmental Consequences. In Michael Lamb, Kathleen Sternberg, Carl-Philip Hwang, and Anders Broberg, eds., *Child Care in Context*. Hillsdale, N.J.: Lawrence Erlbaum Associates, Inc.

Hodgkinson, Harold. 1985. Cameroon: Economy. In *Africa South of the Sahara*. 15th ed. London: Europa Publications.

Huttunen, Eeva, and Merja-Maria Turunen. 1993. Finland. In Moncrieff Cochran, ed., *The International Handbook of Child Care Policies and Programs*. Westport, Conn.: Greenwood Press.

Kipkorir, Lea. 1993. Kenya. In Moncrieff Cochran, ed., *The International Handbook of Child Care Policies and Programs*. Westport, Conn.: Greenwood Press.

Korczak, Ewa. 1993. Poland. In Moncrieff Cochran, ed., *The International Handbook of Child Care Policies and Programs*. Westport, Conn.: Greenwood Press.

Lamb, Michael, and Kathleen Sternberg. 1992. Sociocultural Perspectives on Nonparental Child Care. In Michael Lamb, Kathleen Sternberg, Carl-Philip Hwang, and Anders Broberg, eds., *Child Care in Context*. Hillsdale, N.J.: Lawrence Erlbaum Associates, Inc.

Lamb, Michael, Kathleen Sternberg, Carl-Philip Hwang, and Anders Broberg, eds. 1992. *Child Care in Context*. Hillsdale, N.J.: Lawrence Erlbaum Associates, Inc.

Langsted, Ole, and Dion Sommer. 1993. Denmark. In Moncrieff Cochran, ed., *The International Handbook of Child Care Policies and Programs*. Westport, Conn.: Greenwood Press.

Lee, Lee. 1992. Day Care in the Peoples Republic of China. In Michael Lamb, Kathleen Sternberg, Carl-Philip, and Anders Broberg, eds., *Child Care in Context*. Hillsdale, N.J.: Lawrence Erlbaum Associates, Inc.

Leira, Arlaug. 1987. *Day Care for Children in Denmark, Norway, and Sweden*. Report #5. Oslo: Institute for Social Research.

Miller, Norman, and Roger Yeager. 1994. *Kenya: The Quest for Prosperity*. Boulder, Co.: Westview Press.

Mkhulisi, Mildred, and Moncrieff Cochran. 1993. South Africa. In Moncrieff Cochran, ed., *The International Handbook of Child Care Policies and Programs*. Westport, Conn.: Greenwood Press.

Myers, Robert. 1992. *The Twelve Who Survive: Strengthening Programs of Early Childhood Development in the Third World*. London: Routledge.

Nemenyi, Maria. 1993. Hungary. In Moncrieff Cochran, ed., *The International Handbook of Child Care Policies and Programs*. Westport, Conn.: Greenwood Press.

New, Rebecca. 1993. Italy. In Moncrieff Cochran, eds., *The International Handbook of Child Care Policies and Programs*. Westport, Conn.: Greenwood Press.

Nsamenang, Bame. 1992. Early Childhood Care and Education in Cameroon. In Michael Lamb, Kathleen Sternberg, Carl-Philip Hwang, and Anders Broberg, eds., *Child Care in Context*. Hillsdale, N.J.: Lawrence Erlbaum Associates, Inc.

Palattio-Corpus, Luz. 1993. The Philippines. In Moncrieff Cochran, ed., *The International Handbook of Child Care Policies and Programs*. Westport, Conn.: Greenwood Press.

Pence, Alan. 1993. Canada. In Moncrieff Cochran, ed., *The International Handbook of Child Care Policies and Programs*. Westport, Conn.: Greenwood Press.

Rosemberg, Fulvia. 1993. Brazil. In Moncrieff Cochran, ed., *The International Handbook of Child Care Policies and Programs*. Westport, Conn.: Greenwood Press.

Rosenthal, Miriam. 1992. Nonparental Child Care in Israel: A Cultural and Historical Perspective. In Michael Lamb, Kathleen Sternberg, Carl-Philip Hwang, and Anders Broberg, eds., *Child Care in Context*. Hillsdale, N.J.: Lawrence Erlbaum Associates, Inc.

Sagi, Abraham, and Nina Koren-Karie. Israel. In Moncrieff Cochran, ed., *The International Handbook of Child Care Policies and Programs.* Westport, Conn.: Greenwood Press.

Sanday, Peggy. 1981. *Female Power and Male Dominance.* Cambridge: Cambridge University Press.

Spedding, Polly. 1993. The United States of America. In Moncrieff Cochran, ed., *The International Handbook of Child Care Policies and Programs.* Westport, Conn.: Greenwood Press.

Tolbert, Kathryn, Elizabeth Shrader, Doroteo Mendoza, Guadalupe Chapela, Aurora Rabago, and Robert Klein. 1993. Mexico. In Moncrieff Cochran, ed., *The International Handbook of Child Care Policies and Programs.* Westport, Conn.: Greenwood Press.

Torres, Annabel. 1993. Nicaragua. In Moncrieff Cochran, ed., *The International Handbook of Child Care Policies and Programs.* Westport, Conn.: Greenwood Press.

Tran, Thi Trong, Mai Chi Pham, and Van Phu Dao. 1993. Vietnam. In Moncrieff Cochran, ed., *The International Handbook of Child Care Policies and Programs.* Westport, Conn.: Greenwood Press.

United Nations. 1990. Statistical Chart on Children, 1990. New York: United Nations Department of International Economic and Social Affairs, Statistical Office.

Zhengao, Wei. 1993. China. In Moncrieff Cochran, ed., *The International Handbook of Child Care Policies and Programs.* Westport, Conn.: Greenwood Press.

Zinn, Maxine Baca, and D. Stanley Eitzen. 1993. *Diversity in Families.* 3rd ed. New York: Harper Collins.

1997 Elsevier Science B.V.
Early Child Development: Investing in our Children's Future
M.E. Young, editor.

Programming in Early Childhood Care and Development

Judith L. Evans

As the twentieth century draws to a close, the importance of early childhood is eve. appreciated. This appreciation derives from a much greater understanding of the eff. child's early years have on subsequent growth and development and of the support required during early childhood to ensure a child's optimal growth. As Montessori notes: "The poor have not yet had proper consideration, and always there remains one class that is yet more completely ignored, even among the rich. Such is Childhood! All social problems are considered from the point of view of the adult and his needs. . . . Far more important are the needs of the child" (Montessori 1961: 120).

During the past 2 decades, strategies for programming early childhood have burgeoned, yielding a wide range of approaches to integrated programs for young children, from birth into the early primary school years. These programs, developed in response to new understanding of the ways in which children grow and develop, respond to both universal and specific developmental needs across a multitude of cultures. They result from attempts to find effective ways of using limited financial and human resources and from systematic evaluations of related ongoing efforts.

This chapter delineates the wide variety of complementary programming strategies currently available. The sections below present an historical overview and discussion of eight specific programming strategies. These strategies have different objectives, target different beneficiaries, and offer different program models. The strategies are complementary and can be effective as single or combined interventions initiated by public or private organizations. To achieve maximal effect, all eight approaches could be integrated into an overall, multipronged strategy of early childhood development.

Interventions to promote good nutrition and health, critical to children's physical, cognitive, and mental development, as presented in part I of this volume, are embedded in the eight approaches described. Cochran's framework for fitting early childcare services to societal needs and characteristics, presented in the preceding chapter, conveys some of the macrolevel factors and influences that impinge on the design and implementation of these programming strategies. As in Cochran's chapter, early childhood development is expanded here to include both early childhood care and development (ECCD).

Historical Perspective

Before the 1960s the predominant model of early childhood education programs was the *preschool*, offered to children from 3 to 6 years of age for a half-day, with a focus on *educating* children. Such preschool programs were attended predominantly by children from middle- and upper-middle-class families. These parents understood how the preschool experience could help prepare a child for school and had the resources to pay for this education. The preschool model was popular, predominating in all parts of the world. Myers notes (1995: 84), "For too many people, a child development . . . program immediately conjures up the image of twenty-five or thirty small children, ages 3 to 5, playing with blocks or fitting triangles and squares into brightly colored puzzle boards, supervised by a professional teacher in a 'preschool' classroom."

However, educators working in developing countries were all too aware of the limitations of the traditional preschool model. Myers continues (1995: 84), "it focuses narrowly on a child's mental development, is relatively expensive, and begins late in a child's life. It also involves a direct, 'institutional' approach, relying on creation of centers that 'compensate' for missing elements in the family and community environment while, too often, leaving parents and community members out of the program. This image seldom provides the most appropriate guide to programming for childcare and development in Third World locations."

As the limitations of preschool were identified and individuals realized that children who were not in preschool were the children who could benefit most from these programs, people sought to expand early childhood programming and began experimenting with alternative approaches. Alternatives were sought to replace the narrow definition of early childhood programs, the wait until a child is 3 years old before addressing the child's needs, a compensatory approach to early child education, the expensive infrastructure required for traditional preschools, and dependence on highly trained professional staff. Individuals sought models that would allow them to provide more services to a much greater number of people within resource constraints. Throughout the years a variety of strategies have been developed. Table 1 summarizes these complementary strategies.

The multipronged approach suggested by the complementary strategies in table 1 provides for support at all levels, beginning with children and extending to the family, community, society, and international arena. Strategy numbers 1 and 2 focus on programs that directly affect children. Number 3 addresses needs in the immediate environment. Number 4 provides examples of the technical and organizational support necessary to sustain ECCD programs, and numbers 5, 6, and 7 address the need for a supportive national ethos. Number 8 focuses on how international collaboration can strengthen early childhood programs. All these levels of support are necessary to sustain an emphasis on children and families that offers children maximal opportunities for realizing their potential. The sections below describe each type of strategy and highlight specific models and programs adopted in developing countries.

Deliver a Service Directly to Children

This approach focuses directly on children and includes activities from the time a child is born until the child enters the early primary grades (0-8 years of age). The immediate goal of this approach is to enhance a child's overall development. These programs promote child survival, childcare, socialization, child development, preparation for school, and rehabilitation. Although the programs may be offered in centers designed specifically as

Table 1. Complementary ECCD Programming Strategies

Program approach	Beneficiaries	Objectives	Models
1. Deliver a service directly to children	Children 0-8 years	Survival Health and nutrition Comprehensive development Socialization Rehabilitation Childcare School preparedness	Maternal and child health Home day care Center-based program Add-on centers Preschools (formal; nonformal) Comprehensive child development program Religious schools
2. Support and educate caregivers	Parents and family members Caregivers Teachers and other educators Siblings Elders	Create awareness Increase knowledge Change attitudes Improve and change practices Enhance skills	Home visiting Parent education Caregiver and teacher training Child-to-child Family life education
3. Promote community development	Community members Leaders and elders Community health workers Community organizers	Create awareness Mobilize for action Change conditions Take on ownership of program	Social marketing Social mobilization Technical mobilization Literacy programs School curriculum Media
4. Strengthen national resources and capabilities	Program personnel Supervisors Management staff Professionals Paraprofessionals Researchers	Increase knowledge Enhance skills Change behaviors Strengthen and sustain organizations Enhance local capabilities Increase local and national resources Develop local materials	Organizational development training Pre- and inservice training Experimental and demonstration projects Collaborative cross-national research projects Action research

Table 1.

Program approach	Beneficiaries	Objectives	Models
5. Strengthen demand and awareness	Policymakers General public Professionals Media	Create awareness Build political will Increase demand Change attitudes Create an enabling environment	Social marketing Multimedia dissemination of knowledge Advocacy
6. Develop national childcare and family policies	Policymakers Families with young children Society (over time)	Create awareness Assess current policy for families with young children Identify gaps Create supportive policy	Relate national and international efforts, such as the Education for All Initiative and the Convention on the Rights of the Child Participatory policy development
7. Develop supportive legal and regulatory frameworks	Policymakers Legislators Families with young children Society (over time)	Increase awareness of rights and resources Create supportive workplace Assure quality child care Implement protective environmental standards Institute maternal and paternal leave	Create alliances (women's groups, community groups, and so forth) Innovative public and private collaboration Tax incentives for private support of ECCD programs
8. Strengthen international collaboration	Donor agencies Bilateral agencies Foundations International nongovernmental organizations	Share experience Distill knowledge Maximize resources Increase awareness Increase resources Maximize impact and effectiveness	Consultative Group on Early Childhood Care and Development International Vitamin A Consultative Group Development for African Education Save the Children Alliance

Source: Adapted from Myers 1991.

preschools or childcare centers, they also are found in neighborhood homes, community centers, marketplaces, and even "under the trees." These programs can exist anywhere children are grouped together.

Historically a common way of categorizing these ECCD programs was in terms of *formal* and *nonformal* programs. In general, formal programs were in the public sector. They operated in special facilities that met a set of standards, were staffed by individuals with some training, and followed a set curriculum. As part of large bureaucracies, they were more rigid than nonformal programs. Nonformal programs were outside the public sector. They often had no special facility, were staffed by paraprofessionals (who may or may not have been trained), and used curriculum determined by the people creating the program. In the developing world, categorizing programs as formal or nonformal is no longer useful. Although ECCD programs sponsored and operated by governments exist, such as preschools operated by a Ministry of Education, formal and nonformal characteristics blur across the full range of ECCD efforts. Public- and private-sector efforts overlap and contain characteristics of both formal and nonformal programs.

Currently, ECCD programs are defined by how they are organized and where they are offered. In this chapter, programs that provide direct services to children are divided into neighborhood programs, workplace programs, center programs, and integrated, multipronged ECCD programs.

Neighborhood Programs

The most common example of a neighborhood ECCD program is *family day-care homes*. In their own homes, neighborhood women care for a small number of children (six to fifteen) between the ages of several months and school age. Older children commonly attend before and after school. Generally the mothers of these children work outside the home, the program runs for a full day, and the hours are based frequently on the needs of the working mothers. This model is found most commonly in urban and peri-urban areas where mothers can walk their children to a family day-care home.

The quality of care in family day-care homes depends on the training that day-care mothers receive. When the homes are sponsored by a nongovernmental organization (NGO) or the government, day-care mothers frequently receive preservice training for a minimum of 40 hours. To provide a quality experience for children, ongoing supervision, in the form of additional training, is required.

Generally children in family day-care homes sponsored by NGOs or the government receive a nutritional supplement, health checks, and activities to stimulate cognitive development. Depending on the program structure, the community may be greatly involved, for example, in determining who will serve as day-care mothers and/or paying the salary of these providers. In other instances, day-care mothers may simply be entrepreneurs who establish a program on their own, unconnected with any organization or external supports.

The family day-care home model has been supported by governments in several Latin American countries. Colombia, Venezuela, Peru, and Bolivia all have family day-care programs.

The *Colombian Community Child Care and Nutrition Project* is one of the largest systems of family day care in the world. This project supports *Homes for Well-being*, a community-based program providing services for children from birth to 7 years of age. Community mothers care for up to fifteen children in their home. They receive training in child development, family and community relations, nutrition, and health. The program provides food to ensure proper nutrition for the children and gives the mothers a loan for upgrading their homes to accommodate the children.

Homes for Well-being is operated and supported nationally by the Instituto Colombiano de Bienestar Familiar, in collaboration with the Ministry of Public Health, the National Apprentice Service, the Institute of Territorial Credit, and other governmental and private organizations. The program relies heavily on community involvement. Community members assess needs to determine the number of homes required and select the women who will be the care providers. Local associations manage the overall effort.

An evaluation of the program showed a positive effect on women's employment. Children in the program showed significant cognitive and social gains but no significant nutritional benefits, despite the high investment (Castillo, Ortiz, and Gonzalez 1993); the nutrition supplement for children accounts for half the costs of the program. As shown by other nutrition supplementation projects, the program may not improve nutritional status because parents believe that children receive their full daily nutritional requirements through the program and do not feed them at home. In reality the program provides only 50 to 70 percent of a child's nutritional needs. Parents need to be educated about the importance of continuing to feed children at home. Low nutrition moderates the program's positive effects on psychosocial development.

Workplace Programs

In some countries, childcare programs are provided at the workplace. Formal workplace programs are sponsored by businesses, industry, or the government, and nonformal workplace programs are initiated, and sometimes operated, by women workers.

Formal Workplace Programs

These ECCD programs generally are childcare centers sponsored by employers. Impetus for creating workplace childcare often comes from national legislation requiring employers with a certain number of women employees to provide childcare. Children in these centers range from infants to children just before school age. Depending on the legal enforcement of standards, these centers may provide only custodial care or a high-quality program. The full-day programs characteristic of workplace childcare usually provide meals, conduct a minimal health check, and keep the children clean. Parents participate little, if at all, in these programs.

The *Mobile Creches* program is an exemplary childcare program within the developing world. It is associated with the formal work sector in India, a country that has legislatively supported employer-sponsored childcare since 1964. Although for many years this legislation was not enforced, industries are continually pressured to comply. The Mobile Creches program was established to respond to particular concerns raised about the welfare of the numerous women workers and their children in India's construction industry. Construction sites are dangerous places for young children, yet the women cannot rely on extended family members to provide childcare. Also, the women and children are forced to relocate frequently as they and other workers complete buildings and begin construction on new ones.

To meet the needs of the women and children, a private voluntary organization, collaborating with India's construction industry, created the Mobile Creches work site ECCD program in 1969. This program is *mobile*; childcare centers and programs move as the population they serve moves. Mobile creches have since been established to serve the children of street cleaners, rag pickers, and other families who represent the lowest social status groups in India.

Staff within the Mobile Creches system is drawn from the lower-middle class. Soon after the program was initiated it became evident that traditional institutes for training teachers did not adequately prepare the care providers for meeting the unique needs of families and children served by mobile creches. Over time, the Mobile Creches program thus developed its own staff training. Because of the longevity of the program, women now teaching in mobile creches were once children in the creches.

The Mobile Creches training program also is offered to NGOs and government childcare programs serving young children in other settings. As the program has evolved, classes in adult education have been added, such as literacy programs, nutrition classes, and political discussion groups. What began as a childcare program has become a much larger development effort.

Nonformal Workplace Programs

Nonformal workplace programs usually are developed by local initiative. People within the community identify a problem and seek to solve it, with or without any form of organizational or government support. The care provided is generally custodial, and mothers contribute food for their children. Caregiving may be rotated among the mothers, and in-kind contributions are given to compensate the mothers who care for the children. With some assistance, such as caregiver training and provision of materials or food, these programs can provide a high-quality experience for young children.

Nonformal workplace programs are popular for women's work that is thought to be compatible with childcare. In this type of work children stay with their mothers as they work in the field, travel to market, or do piecework in their homes. Although the programs meet the unique needs of women in a given setting, they are flexible (they may be daily and seasonal) and address real needs.

The *Accra Market Women's Association* is an example of a nonformal work program in Ghana (Evans 1985). It began because the Accra Market Women's Association was interested in starting a childcare program for women involved in buying and selling. The association approached the Accra City Council, which agreed to fund the program. A committee was formed, consisting of members from the Women's Association, the City Council, the Department of Social Welfare (which is mandated to oversee early childhood programs), the Ministry of Health, and the Ministry of Water and Sewage. The program operated under the Administration of the Regional Medical Officer of Health and had a strong health and nutrition focus.

Mothers were encouraged to come to the center, a refurbished building near the market, to breastfeed their infants. Children were given a morning snack and a full lunch. To enter the program children were required to have a physical examination and appropriate immunizations. Once a month a public health nurse inspected the facilities, provided

nutrition, health, and social and economic development. This means that ECCD programs should provide *integrated* care. Although an integrated program that addresses the multiple needs of children and families would be most beneficial, few examples of fully integrated programs exist.

Summary

Programs that provide services directly to children are beneficial but must be approached with caution.

Benefits. Direct service programs have several benefits. First, direct attention allows program implementors to know what services children are actually receiving. When a program focuses on adults, the direct benefits for children are unclear. Second, monitoring health and nutritional status and providing safety are relatively easy when children are grouped together. It is also possible to monitor their physical, social, emotional, and cognitive development and plan activities accordingly and to identify children with special needs. Third, direct service programs give 3-7 year olds a chance to socialize with their peers in ways not possible at home. This activity prepares them for socializing within the larger culture and social environment. Fourth, center-based programs meet larger community needs. ECCD center-based programs can be an entry point to foster community development objectives, and the centers provide useful political visibility for organizing and sustaining programs.

Cautions. Two areas of caution relate to the development and implementation of programs in centers. First, centers can be expensive to build and maintain; the limited resources available to ECCD programs might be better used to train staff. Second and more importantly, center-based programs can distance children from families. A conflict may occur between the home and center in areas of language, values, and beliefs. Also, some parents may relinquish their children to the experts, abrogating the responsibility to support their child's growth and development. In both instances children are caught in the middle.

To avoid causing conflict between children and families, ECCD programs should support and educate adults, family members, and caregivers who influence the lives of children in the programs. Some examples of programs designed for these beneficiaries are described below.

Support and Educate Caregivers

In an international review of developments in ECCD programming, Paz (1990) notes that research in the 1970s increasingly showed the importance of parents in promoting children's development. Citing the work of Bronfenbrenner, Paz says that Bronfenbrenner "concluded that the family is the most effective and economical system for fostering and sustaining the development of the child, and that the involvement of the child's family is critical to the success of any intervention program. Moreover, evidence pointed to the fact that parents participating in programs for the sake of their children were themselves affected, even in spheres lying outside the parental role. The confidence gained by mothers was reflected in their increasing interest and participation in community affairs and in significant changes in their own life-style" (Paz 1990: 7).

Although some notable parent programs exist, this ECCD strategy is not nearly as well developed as programs directed toward children. Nonetheless, models have been developed that provide insight into involving parents more integrally in ECCD efforts.

In addition to parents, other persons who care and take responsibility for the growth and development of young children also are important. These persons include other family members and siblings, caregivers, teachers, and health care workers. The broad objectives of programs to reach these beneficiaries are to create awareness of the importance of a caregiver's role in supporting children's growth and development, to reinforce positive parenting practices, and to provide caregivers with additional knowledge and skills. Ultimately these programs empower caregivers to improve their care of and interaction with young children and to enrich the immediate living environment of the children. Three types of caregiver programs are discussed below: parent education programs, sibling education programs, and caregiver training.

Parent Education Programs

Parent education can be provided through home visits and organized group meetings.

Home Visiting

One way of working with parents is to provide one-to-one parent education through a trained home visitor. Home visiting programs frequently are used to serve hard-to-reach families where parents are isolated and unlikely to participate in a parent group. In the most common model, the home visit focuses on child development and ways the parents can promote that development. Home visitors are likely to be recruited from the population being served. With appropriate support and training, they can provide effective services that increase parental support of child development and enhance a mother's self-concept.

PRONOEI (Programa No Formal de Educación Inicial) is an example of a home-based initial education project in Peru. Created in the late 1970s, this project is an adaptation of the Portage Model developed in the United States. It was started on a pilot basis in 1977 in two urban settlements and four rural villages. The goal was to positively affect a child's development by teaching parents adequate childrearing and caretaking skills. Because the families being served were living in poverty, the program was designed to enhance the quality of interactions between children and their parents in the time available, not to create another demand on parents' already scarce time and energy resources (Jesien and others 1979).

In the PRONOEI program, nonprofessional community women were trained to provide weekly home visits to a mother and child. In Lima, home visitors ("animadoras") had a tenth-grade education on average; in rural areas, animadoras had a fifth-grade education. The home visitors were given 4 weeks of training in child development, teaching techniques, and construction of educational materials (Loftin 1979).

An animadora worked with ten families on a weekly basis and, with the aid of a supervisor, developed an individualized curriculum for children between the ages of 3 and

5 based on their developmental level. The animadora used a developmental profile with a child and mother, which provided the basis for determining activities and progress.

Research on the pilot project clearly indicated that children who participated in the program gained from the experience. In rural areas, children in the program were at age-appropriate developmental levels by the end of the year, while children in a control group faltered developmentally during the year (Loftin 1979).

Organized Group Meetings

Parent education frequently takes place in organized, periodic group meetings in the community. These organized programs can be developed as stand-alone efforts or be offered in conjunction with a center- or home-based program or as an activity within other groups, such as a literacy class or community development committee. Frequently parents determine topics for the periodic discussions, and the groups generally are led by a facilitator, who may or may not be a professional. The three examples below illustrate different ways of working with the parents of young children.

The *Mother-Child Education Program* (MOCEP) is an example from Turkey. This program began as a combination of home visiting and organized parent education. It included not only direct service but also research on the efficacy of training mothers in relation to a center program for children (Kagitcibasi, Bekman, and Goksel 1995).

MOCEP was developed to provide early enrichment to children from disadvantaged environments and to strengthen parenting skills. Program activities were designed to enrich a young child and train and support the mother. The parent education component, mother training, had two elements. The first, addressed through group discussions, was designed to increase a mother's sensitivity to her child's social and emotional needs and to help the mother support her child's personality growth. The second element, a Turkish adaptation of Israel's Home Instruction Program for Preschool Youngsters (HIPPY), was designed to support children's cognitive development. Home visits and group discussions were held on alternate weeks.

Evaluations of the program assessed short- and long-term outcomes. The short-term evaluation measured the cognitive, personality, and social development of a child. The evaluation showed significant differences in cognitive development (measured in a variety of ways) between children whose mothers had undergone training and those whose mothers had not. The program also had positive effects on the social and personality development of the children with trained mothers. These children displayed less dependency, less aggressiveness, better self-concept, and better school adjustment than children with untrained mothers.

The short-term evaluation also showed benefits of the program by measuring the mother's orientation to her child and direct effects of the program on the mother. Trained mothers were more verbal, less punitive, and more responsive to their children and had greater interaction with them than untrained mothers. Mothers who had been trained valued their child's autonomous behavior more and provided more cognitive stimulation than untrained mothers. The program directly affected trained mothers who became more likely than untrained mothers to share decisionmaking with their spouses on subjects such as birth control and child discipline. Trained mothers also enjoyed a greater degree of communication and role sharing with their spouses, demonstrated by husbands helping with household chores.

The long-term evaluation conducted in 1991, 6 years after completion of the intervention program, showed an important finding about children's school attainment. Of the young adolescents (13-15 years of age) in the mother-trained group, 86 percent were still in school, compared with 67 percent of adolescents with untrained mothers. Also, the children in the mother-trained group showed better school performance during the 5 years of primary school, had more positive attitudes toward schooling, and had a better self-concept than children in the group of untrained mothers.

Training also resulted in sustained positive changes for the mother. Mothers who had been trained reported better interactions and relationships with their children (for example, understanding the child, talking problems over with the child, and not beating the child) than untrained mothers. These results from interviews with the mothers agreed with findings from the adolescents' self-reports. Trained mothers also had better family relationships and had higher educational expectations for their children than untrained mothers. Overall the program enabled women to communicate more effectively with their children, prepare more positive environments for children's development and success, achieve better relationships with their family, and increase their status in the family (Kagitcibasi, Bekman, and Goksel 1995).

MOCEP became the basis of a major government educational policy. It also led to establishment of the Mother-Child Education Foundation (MOCEF) and served as the incentive for a new collaboration between the United Nations Children's Fund (UNICEF), the Ministry of Education, and MOCEF. For a more in-depth discussion of the value of parent education in child development, see the chapter by Kagitcibasi in this volume. In this chapter, Kagitcibasi elaborates on the Turkish experience with MOCEP. In a subsequent chapter, Lombard elaborates on the Israeli experience with HIPPY.

The *Programa de Padres y Hijos* (PPH) is a parent education program in Chile that does not have a home-visiting component. This program focuses on parent groups in poor communities. Although the ultimate goal is to support the personal growth of adults and the overall development of the community, the organizers began with childcare issues, which are primary for many parents. The program was begun in 1979 by the Centro de Investigaciónes y Desarrollo de la Educación (CIDE), a private research and development center. The program initially involved fifty groups of twenty families in Osorno and, later, an additional eighteen groups in Santiago. All families participating in the program had children ages 4-6.

Local persons are trained to lead the weekly parent meetings. At these meetings, and now through radio broadcasts, twelve themes are introduced during the year. Discussions and activities focus on one theme each month. At the weekly meetings a leader shows pictures depicting common incidents from the people's lives that offer opportunities to stimulate a child's learning. The leader guides discussion with the picture, showing what the child is doing developmentally and how parents can support the child's learning in that situation.

Also at the meetings parents discuss activities they can do with their child during the week. They suggest activities and games to use, and toys are available for them to take home for the week or use as models for making their own toys. Child development also is promoted by worksheets given to parents to use with their children.

The PPH program has been evaluated to determine its effects on children, parents, and the community. Teachers rated the school readiness of PPH children and children whose parents were not in the program, finding PPH children to rate higher. On the WISP (a Chilean version of the Wechsler's Intelligence Scale for Children), PPH children improved 6.2 points during a 4-month period compared with an increase of 3.4 points by the non-PPH children (Myers and Hertenberg 1987).

Adults in the PPH program exhibited different attitudes and actions than other adults, shown by the way they talked about the project, reached agreements, and acted on decisions. "The basic change identified was from apathy to participation in constructive activities as a sense of self-worth was strengthened" (Myers and Hertenberg 1987: 84).

The *Bina Keluarga Balita* (BKB) program in Indonesia adopts a quite different approach to parent education. The title of this program means "enhancing the role of women in comprehensive child development." Begun in 1981, it is targeted to disadvantaged families in urban and rural areas. The major objective in creating BKB was to develop a low-cost model that would deliver information to mothers, the first educators of children, enhancing their capacity to support their child's development.

The BKB project was upgraded to a national initiative by President Suharto in 1991. By early 1993 BKB reached more than 40,000 villages. In 1995 an estimated 2.7 million women were enrolled in BKB programs, with approximately 1.6 million women actually attending, which is one-third of all mothers in Indonesia with children under 5 years of age (UNICEF 1995).

Within the program, trained "kaders" (volunteers) hold monthly sessions with mothers who meet in groups based on the age of their child. During the sessions mothers learn about child development and the use of simple educational toys, language, songs, games, and storytelling in their interaction with their child. An evaluation of the BKB program conducted in 1992 showed that rapid expansion in 1991 decreased quality. In 1993 UNICEF supported the project to enhance quality, and in 1994 and 1995 sponsored activities to train kaders. UNICEF also has strengthened management capacity at all levels of the program.

Sibling Education Programs

Another group of individuals who can be educated to provide care to the youngest children is older siblings. The best known example of sibling education is the *Child-to-Child* approach, which emerged from two important events at the end of the 1970s. The first was the 1978 World Health Conference at Alma Ata where the international health community adopted the slogan "Health for All by the Year 2000." The second was the International Year of the Child in 1979. The slogan developed at Alma Ata provided the challenge. The International Year of the Child provided a focus on children, one avenue to meeting the challenge. Based on a naturally occurring situation in most developing countries, where older siblings commonly care for younger family members, Child-to-Child was formulated by an international group of health and education professionals as an approach to health education.

When Child-to-Child was launched it was promoted as a way to address health needs in a community by providing older children with appropriate health messages and practices that they would pass on to younger children. A core set of forty activity sheets was developed as a basis of the approach. The Child-to-Child book produced in 1979 also was a key resource. As people around the world create their own Child-to-Child programs they send materials back to the Child-to-Child Trust, located at the Institute of Education, University of London. The trust is a resource base for anyone interested in implementing Child-to-Child projects. Today more than eighty countries have Child-to-Child programs.

From the beginning Child-to-Child has integrated health and education. From the health perspective the emphasis has been on defining appropriate health messages for children regarding causes, symptoms, treatment, and prevention. The emphasis in education has been on using appropriate teaching methods that not only increase children's knowledge but also change their attitudes and practices.

Child-to-Child promotes an activity-based approach to teaching and learning. The child-centered, active learning approach of Child-to-Child programs is not limited to health education and can be used to teach any subject matter. The more it is seen as a way to "help teachers do their job better" and "help teachers teach things more easily that they had previously found difficult," the more readily the approach is incorporated into a teacher's repertoire of behaviors (Evans 1993b: 6).

The content of Child-to-Child programs has moved from health education to the *education of healthy children*. New topics for Child-to-Child materials include child stimulation and mental health. Child-to-Child programs also have begun stimulating educators to relate basic health messages in schools to health problems and resources in the community.

Caregiver Training

Critical to educating parents and family members of young children are the caregivers, teachers, and health care workers who work directly with the children. In fact, training these personnel is *the single most important factor* in creating quality early childhood programs.

A range of training and dissemination systems has been created to make early childhood programming available to a wider audience. Every early intervention strategy is accompanied by a training system. Figure 1 shows one way of mapping the various training systems on a grid.

Figure 1. Approaches to Training

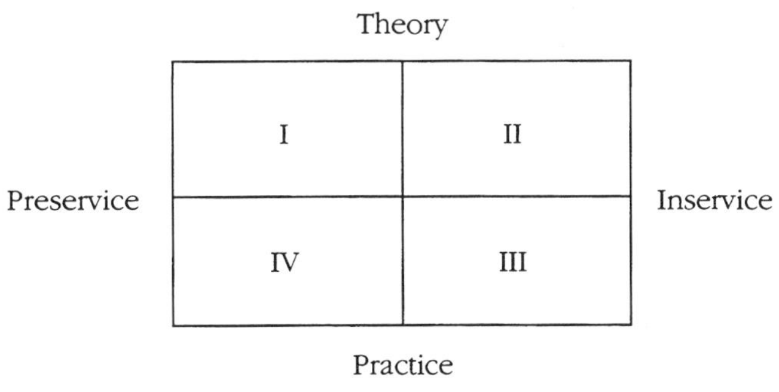

The horizontal axis shows preservice training in contrast to inservice training. The left side represents preservice training only; on the right side is on-the-job education of teachers (inservice). In between is every imaginable combination. The vertical axis represents the theory-to-practice continuum. Although preservice training with a highly theoretical focus (Quadrant I) is the predominant training model today, it does not begin to meet the needs or realities in most developing countries. Since the late 1980s, preference has shifted toward Quadrant III, which places greater emphasis on practical skills provided through inservice training.

The *District Centers for Early Childhood Education* (DICECEs) is a Quadrant-III (inservice training with an emphasis on practical knowledge and skills) training program for caregivers developed by the Kenya Institute of Education (KIE). During the past 20 years many community-based preschools have been established in Kenya. The impetus for these schools is Kenya's rapid population growth which has resulted in an inadequate number of openings in primary I education for all the children eligible. Recognizing that preschool education gives their children a better chance of obtaining placement in primary school, parents have created their own preschools. In the harambee, or self-help, tradition, these schools are built by the community, staffed by untrained parent-paid teachers, and operated with sparse equipment and materials.

KIE began to address training teachers for these community-based preschools in the late 1970s by creating district training centers. At these centers local teachers receive intensive training throughout a 2-year period during school holidays. During the school year they receive on-the-job training through periodic visits by training center staff. At the end of training, teachers receive a certificate in early childhood education.

In essence, KIE designed a training system to meet a very specific set of needs, and the system is solidly in place. KIE and related training experiences show that effective training programs can be created when the training is designed to meet the needs of trainees and the local communities they will serve.

Summary

A variety of adults and family members are integral to a child's daily life. An effective way to support children's growth and development is to improve the knowledge and skills of these individuals, providing them with new information and practices that enhance their role in the life of a child. The benefits and cautions of programs that support and educate caregivers are summarized below.

Benefits. Caregiver training as an ECCD programming strategy has several benefits. First, both caregivers and children benefit from programs involving family members and other adults. Second, improvements in a child's development are likely to be sustained because activities promoting this development are part of everyday life instead of being provided for only a few hours a day. Third, broad coverage can be achieved at relatively low costs. Child development information can be added to current programs, such as literacy programs, health centers, and women's groups.

Cautions. To be effective, information provided to caregivers must be timely to a child's developmental stage. The information also should be culturally appropriate, incorporating current beliefs and practices while adding to the caregivers' knowledge. The teaching-learning process of transmitting information should be participatory, allowing for interpersonal exchange and mutual support. The education of caregivers also must be recognized as an ongoing process; goals are unlikely to be achieved through one-time training.

Promote Community Development

For child-oriented strategies, the next step beyond the family is the community. Community development can be a powerful mechanism for creating early childcare programs.

The *Kushanda* Project in Zimbabwe, funded by the Bernard van Leer Foundation, is one example (Booker 1995). Following independence, former freedom fighters established a farming cooperative. The cooperative, known as "Shandisayi Pfungwa" ("use your brains") was headquartered on a resettlement farm. Its objective was to diversify and expand the economic base in the region. In addition to focusing on skills training for economic development, the cooperative had a social component that included adult literacy classes, extension courses on health and nutrition, and early child education.

The early childhood program evolved as women within the cooperative began complaining about their double workload. They were involved in agricultural production and also were responsible for childcare. Because women needed to be in the fields, children accompanied them and were largely unsupervised. The first step in developing an early childcare program was the designation of two women to play with the children. Subsequently parents requested that caregivers receive training so that children would receive the best possible care and education.

Under the Kushanda Project, two women from Shandisayi received a 2-year training course at St. Mary's Early Learning Center in Chitungwiza. Their training began at the same time that a preschool program for children 3-6 years of age was established at the cooperative, enabling trainees to combine practical experience with theoretical training.

As a result of the Kushanda training, the quality of the early childhood program that developed attracted the interest of parents who did not live on the farm, and they began sending their children to the Shandisayi center. This expansion facilitated an outreach program to promote the importance of ECCD to the broader community, which increased the demand for training. A shortened course was offered during 1987-88 to meet this demand.

Over time the Shandisayi center became a model for other communities. Satellite centers were created and received ongoing support from the Shandisayi cooperative early childhood program. Local government officials also requested that teachers in villages under their jurisdiction be trained by the Kushanda Project. By 1989 Kushanda expanded its staff and the scope of its training services, adding an adult and health education component "to increase the level of parents' knowledge of child health issues, and to increase their involvement in improving the health and sanitation environment of the community, particularly for their children" (Booker 1995: 68).

The Kushanda Project is a good example of an early childhood program that evolved from a community development project with economic and social development as primary objectives. Interestingly, the early childhood program eventually led back to addressing some basic health issues within the community at large.

Summary

Community development programs involving children emphasize changing conditions within a community to make a difference in the children's ability to survive and thrive. They also emphasize building on community initiative and empowering a community to define its needs and develop strategies to meet these needs. Community development programs can include water and sanitation projects or other efforts that improve the physical environment, all of which can affect the health, nutrition, and general development of children. Programs also can include projects to increase a community's knowledge and skills and its ability to organize to solve common problems. The benefits and cautions associated with community development programs are described below.

Benefits. The benefits of community development programs are far reaching. First, the programs affect the whole community, enhancing quality of life for all community members. Second, the effects are likely to be sustainable because the community defines its needs and takes the initiative at each step in the process. Third, community development programs can be the basis of efforts to empower the community to act on its own behalf socially and politically.

Cautions. Three areas of caution are relevant. First, it cannot be assumed that children will benefit directly from whatever program is developed. Without activities directed to children, benefits of the program may take a long time to, or may never, reach children. Also, community development programs offer no way to monitor the services children actually receive or children's health, nutritional, and developmental status. Second, the poorest children and families may not benefit directly from a community development program because they may not be considered part of the community or be involved in the community development process. Also, in some cultures women are not included in community organizations, and their voice is not heard when determining community activities.

Regardless of whether early childhood programs are designed to meet the specific needs of children, parents and other caregivers, or the community, these programs must operate within a larger context. To survive and thrive, they must be supported by local and national organizations within a political and socioeconomic context. The next five complementary strategies illustrate ECCD programs that can be implemented at these macrolevels.

Strengthen National Resources and Capabilities

Many individuals, agencies, and institutions implement the three strategies described above. To perform adequately, they need financial, material, and training resources to develop the capacity to plan, organize, implement, and evaluate ECCD efforts. Thus strengthened the individuals, agencies, and institutions serve as resources at the national level. They train those who support caregivers, those who work with parents, and those who work with the community. They also provide training for program and administrative staff and supervisors. In-country research capability through national and international training and exchanges also is necessary to support early childhood programs over time. The strengthening of national capacity further includes providing appropriate materials, equipment, and vehicles; upgrading physical facilities; and introducing new technologies.

Training Trainers

The *National Center for Early Childhood Education* (NACECE), established at the KIE in Nairobi, provides one example of efforts to strengthen national capacity. This center supports Kenya's inservice community training for caregivers in ECCD programs. When Kenya began training it was done by central staff from the NACECE. When the decentralized training model was developed for Kenya and the DICECEs were created to place trainers at the district level (see above), NACECE staff changed their roles. They were no longer directly training caregivers. Instead they became responsible for training trainers for DICECEs, managing an ever-growing training and credentialing system, overseeing expanded curriculum development efforts, and conducting program research and evaluations. To accommodate these new roles, NACECE staff received additional training to upgrade their knowledge and skills.

The infrastructure that supports this expanded training system could not have been developed if donors had been willing to fund only direct services. Several organizations supported Kenya's effort to strengthen its national capacity for ECCD. The Bernard van Leer Foundation funded development of the national curriculum and overall training system as well as creation and maintenance of NACECE. The Aga Khan Foundation and UNICEF participate in development and support of various DICECEs, and the government of Kenya pays the salaries of NACECE and DICECE staff.

Another example of strengthening national capacity is an international training of trainers project, *More and Better*. A primary concern throughout the world is supporting and enhancing effective training systems. As ECCD programs have developed, people learned by doing, by gathering information from a variety of sources, and by developing their own training systems. The challenge today is using the effective training programs to create cadres of trainers who can disseminate this training to a wider audience. Africa is experimenting with one approach to accomplish this.

In 1992, the Bernard van Leer Foundation in collaboration with the United Nations Educational, Scientific, and Cultural Organization (UNESCO), UNICEF, and Save the Children USA, developed a system for training national ECCD trainers. In February 1995 two or more trainers from each of nine Sub-Saharan African countries met for 3 weeks of training. Upon completion of their training these individuals returned to their home countries and began teaching other trainers.

A training pack, "Enhancing the Skills of Early Childhood Trainers," was developed to support the effort (Bernard van Leer Foundation/UNESCO 1995). The pack consists of five separate booklets. The first introduces the philosophy and training approach of the training pack. The second focuses on strategies for effective training. The third gives the trainer more in-depth information on the development of young children and is to be used as a resource when the trainer develops a training scheme. The fourth presents the rationale for experiential and participatory training methods, and the fifth contains a list of resources for the trainer.

Enhancing Formal Education

Another way of building institutional capacity is enhancing formal education to meet the needs of children entering the system. The link between early childhood programs and children's experience in early primary school has increasingly been recognized as important. Part of the impetus for this recognition comes from the "Education for All Initiative" which linked the early years with basic education. This link was based on an understanding of the continuity of children's development from birth through early primary school. Extending this link, policymakers and programmers acknowledge a relationship between early childhood experiences and later school attainment and performance.

A further impetus for linking early childhood programs and primary school is the high rates of school dropout and repetition in many developing countries. These rates are particularly high during the first 3 years of primary school. Because the predominant response to these high rates is that children are not ready for school, readiness programs have been created. For example, in the *Bridging Program* in South Africa, children have a year of schooling within the formal school system before they are admitted into the first primary grade. In India's *Promoting Primary and Elementary Education* program, children ages 3-6 spend 2 hours a day in centers designed to help prepare them to enter school.

These particular readiness programs assume that children will perform better and stay in school longer if they are better prepared when they begin school. However, children's school experiences involve not only the children per se but also their interaction with the school. Therefore, the readiness equation must include the school's readiness to receive a child. For example, many schools assume that children are empty vessels to be filled and they are not aware of children's developmental differences and the experiences they bring with them as they enter school.

The importance of a school's readiness to receive children is illustrated by the experience of NGOs in implementing high-quality preschools and then discovering that children have negative primary school experiences despite being well prepared for learning. Readiness for learning is not always the same as readiness for school. A high-quality preschool prepares children to continue learning, but it may not prepare them to survive some of the stultifying experiences they may have in primary school. These experiences cause people to question the value of early childhood programs if the benefits are lost when children enter a primary school of questionable quality.

Without ways to work with primary school teachers and provide continuity between preschool and primary school experiences, the argument could be made quite legitimately that investing in preschool is not worthwhile. Although he does not argue against investments in preschool if primary schools are not adequately prepared to receive children, Myers (1988: 2-3), in a review of research on the relationship between preschools and primary school performance, concludes that "program decisions about early childhood intervention and about improvements in primary schooling should be considered together, not separately."

Although few in number, some programs address both children's readiness for school and the school's readiness to receive children (Subaran, forthcoming). One example is the *Joint Innovative Project* sponsored by UNESCO in China. Four major actions were taken within the project. One increased preschool provision; a second focused on improving teaching methods and teaching materials at the primary level; a third improved teacher training; and a fourth attempted to increase parent and community involvement.

Another example of a program designed to bridge the gap between preschool and primary school is a preschool program in South Africa, developed as part of larger school reform within the Bophuthatswana school system. As in the China project, this program focused on increased preschool provision, curriculum continuity, teacher training, and community involvement. Both programs address readiness by focusing on children and all the essential elements in a child's environment: family, community, and school.

Summary

The benefits and cautions associated with this strategy are similar to those for the next four macrolevel strategies. Basically these strategies are designed to make a difference in children's environment and in the cultural and political ethos that surrounds families as they raise their children. The effect of these strategies on the lives of specific children is difficult to see. However, without these macrolevel supports, the services provided directly to children and the work with parents and other caregivers are unsustainable and children will have difficulty maintaining the gains they achieved through early childhood initiatives.

Strengthen Demand and Awareness

This strategy focuses on disseminating information about the importance of early years to a broad audience to raise their awareness, increase the demand for ECCD services, and create an enabling environment for young children and their families. The potential audience includes policymakers, politicians, the general public, and families and communities who could benefit directly and immediately from ECCD programs.

Social marketing can increase awareness and demand. Methods include working with the media (radio, television, videos, and films) to promote understanding of early childhood and family issues, coalition building, and advocacy. Linking national efforts to international ones, such as the "Education for All Initiative" and the "Convention on the Rights of the Child" (CRC), further strengthen awareness.

Use of Media

Enhancing ECD, a video-based child development program sponsored by UNICEF, is one effort to strengthen awareness and increase demand by using the media. This effort assumes that positive child outcomes that result from child development programs cannot be sustained without parental involvement. The program to help caregivers provide an optimal learning environment for children is designed for a general audience and parents.

The videos provide essential child development knowledge, strategies, and resources for enhancing parents' ability to support their child's development during the first 6 years of life. Each one of the four animated videos is accompanied by a "Facilitators' and Parents' Guidebook" that includes basic information on normal child development, activities to enhance early child development, and suggestions for creating effective home learning environments.

Animation is used to achieve a relatively culture-free portrayal of basic child development concepts. The materials can be used in multiple ways with a wide variety of audiences; the animation can be combined with country-specific live action or be used as a stand-alone animated series. To facilitate a country's adaptation, a "Production Guidebook" suggests ways to add materials that are appropriate for each country.

The animation series also has been designed for national television broadcast, an important step in using videos to raise awareness. The broadcast quality of the series and its availability in a range of convenient videocassette formats appeal to commercial broadcasters and enable service providers to use the series in a variety of group settings, including community-based parent discussion groups, training courses for professionals and paraprofessionals, and health care centers. The video-based strategy will complement, and be integrated into, existing UNICEF-assisted programs designed to provide care and education directly to young children (Landers and Sporn 1994).

International Initiatives

International initiatives also can raise awareness. For example, the Jomtien World Conference on Education for All (EFA), convened in 1990 by the World Bank, UNESCO, UNICEF, and the United Nations Development Programme, focused international attention on education. Its basic message was that developing countries and international agencies should confront the problems of illiteracy and educational decline by concentrating energies and investment in basic education. According to the "Framework for Action to Meet Basic Learning Needs" developed at the EFA conference, national basic education is composed of four pillars:

- A 4-year concentrated, primary cycle for all children that provides basic reading, writing, numeracy, and life skills (both family and environmental)
- Nonformal education for children and adults (especially women) not reached by schools
- Expansion and improvement of early child development, care, and education services
- Further teaching of basic knowledge and life skills to the population through various communication channels.

The EFA designation of early childhood programs as a pillar in the pursuit of basic education has forced some governments to address their role in provision of ECCD programs. A few governments have taken action. For example, this international initiative affected ECCD programming in Mexico, which is "undertaking a US$100 million nonformal education project aimed at boosting the efficiency and quality of preschool education in ten of the poorest states of the country. By preparing children from poor families for their entrance to primary school and introducing parent education, Mexico hopes to help 1,200,000 children under the age of four to learn better" (Bennett 1993/1994: 10).

In addition to increasing action on behalf of young children and their families, increased awareness also may lead to changes in policies and legislation.

Develop National Childcare and Family Policies

National policies that support the development and implementation of ECCD programs are necessary to assure the sustainability of these programs over time. Policies must encourage social service delivery systems and employment that are family sensitive. Activities to develop national childcare and family policies include analyzing current policies, getting involved in creating new policies if necessary, and facilitating implementation of current supportive policies. Policies can be influenced by internal and external pressures, which include international influences and pressure from donors, and by other strategies.

The Accra Declaration is an example of policy changes resulting from internal pressures in Ghana. This recent initiative provided a new perspective and approach to the country's focus on young children. The declaration places highest priority on children who are at greatest risk. It calls collectively on relevant government departments, agencies, NGOs, individuals, and other partners in early child development to broaden Ghana's scope and vision for young children.

The Accra Declaration has provided the impetus for greater cooperation among government, donors, and NGOs. It also sets the stage for a different kind of programming for young children and offers official sanction for a greater variety of activities to receive attention and funding. Shifting from the more traditional emphasis on preschools as preparation for formal schooling, the declaration calls for ECCD programs to offer a range of community-based services for children in the most need.

Because the Accra Declaration arose from a National Seminar on Early Childhood Development held in 1993, it represents the collective thinking on young children and their needs by diverse stakeholders in ECCD. As the Ghana government adapts its education and social strategies to this new perspective, it will be supported by these ECCD stakeholders who helped focus attention on children.

Policies also can be influenced by international pressure. Two types of international pressures are common. The first is pressures from international initiatives that generate a set of principles which countries formally agree should be implemented. Good examples of this phenomenon are the EFA initiative described above and the CRC. Countries respond to these international initiatives by setting new goals for themselves, establishing different priorities, amending current policies, and creating new policies.

The second type of external pressure comes from donors. Many international donors establish conditions for receipt of their funds and loans, which may involve implementation or revision of policies. For example, some countries must make structural adjustments to their economic policies to receive funds from donors like the World Bank. To better evaluate a donor's offer, countries increasingly are realizing the need to make adjustments before collaborating with donors. One way is for countries to establish policies so they have a clear agenda when approached by donors. With relevant policies a government can more readily facilitate coordination among donors and reduce duplication of services.

Creation of or change in policy does not have to be from the "top down," resting solely in the hands of lawmakers and ministry personnel. Because policy is not created in a vacuum, each local solution, successful research project, or advocacy effort also can influence decisionmakers about the best support for young children and their families. For example, because of longitudinal research results showing the benefits of parent education, MOCEP in Turkey led to changes in government policy, increasing government support for early childhood programs through the Ministry of Education (Kagitcibasi, Bekman, and Goksel 1995).

Policy reviews, as well as research, can argue for appropriate policy. In recent years, Malaysia, Namibia, and South Africa have undertaken policy reviews, and each time the review led to a new or renewed focus on early childhood and set the stage for increased government involvement in such programming.

Another strategy is monitoring the National Plans of Action that have been developed by governments that are signatories to the CRC. In some instances NGOs have reviewed a government's assessment of its compliance with the CRC. Such reviews have been completed in the Philippines and other countries. It is an effective strategy for holding a government accountable for its actions.

Summary

Regardless of the impetus for change, policymaking is a process. This process should help a government formulate ECCD policies linked to overall national development priorities. It also should lead to effective implementation, monitoring, management, and coordination of ECCD programs and subsequent identification of policies and strategies for strengthening the contribution of ECCD to national development.

Develop Supportive Legal and Regulatory Frameworks

Activities to develop supportive legal and regulatory frameworks are designed to increase people's awareness of their rights and legal resources and to increase the use and monitoring of, and compliance with, international regulations and conventions, such as International Labor Organization regulations and the CRC. The objective of these activities is to institute provisions that allow families to support the growth and development of their children and that improve the quality of the work environment. Regulations that help meet this objective, for example, are maternal and paternal leave policies and breastfeeding policies. Some countries include the rights of children in their constitutions; children's rights were included in the new constitutions of Brazil in 1990 and Colombia in 1993.

Legislation and regulations to promote implementation of high-quality early childhood programs are needed and must be supportive. Sometimes regulations can inhibit rather than support original intentions. For example, as early childhood programs proliferate, governments may determine they cannot afford to operate ECCD programs. Instead, they may decide to provide guidelines for the programs and register them, letting people know what programs are being offered and where. Regulations developed by a government for the establishment of centers (generally based on standards from industrial countries) often are so restrictive that most ECCD programs cannot comply and thus operate illegally. In effect, the government limits the availability of high-quality ECCD programs rather than supporting a diversity of approaches appropriate to the setting.

The *Guidelines on Pre-Primary Education* issued by Nigeria in 1987 illustrate the need for supportive regulations in contrast to prohibitive ones (Nigeria 1987). The section of the guidelines on Requirements for Pre-Primary Institutions addresses the following areas: physical facilities, playground, furniture, fees, teacher qualifications, and other miscellaneous items. The physical facilities section states that a "building must conform to the following standards: (i) The classroom size should be 12 m by 6.5 m to accommodate about 25 children; (ii) Each classroom should be cross-ventilated and well lighted; (iii) Each classroom must have storage facilities and built-in cupboards for items of equipment; (iv) The classroom should have two access doorways to serve as alternative exits, and a veranda on either side of the classroom; (v) There must be a cloakroom, toilets and wash hand basins of appropriate height" (Nigeria 1987: 5).

Few early childhood programs in Nigeria could meet these criteria. Such prohibitive regulations restricted the growth of registered preprimary programs, leading to an increase in the number of unregistered clandestine programs.

In recent years UNICEF has been working with the Nigerian government to create a more realistic set of guidelines for establishing early childhood care, development, and education (ECCDE) centers (UNICEF 1994). Some of the differences in the new guidelines illustrate a shift from using standards of industrialized countries to creating programs within a context that is appropriate for local children. For example, new guidelines begin by identifying different types of centers that can be developed. Requirements for physical facilities now state that "(a) [The] building must be safe, strong and in good condition; (b) [the] classroom must: be spacious . . . be located on the ground floor if a storied building . . . be equipped with age appropriate seats and mats" (UNICEF 1994: 4). Today the policies and derivative laws and regulations support development of a range of ECCD alternatives within Nigeria, and most programs can now be registered.

As well as being supportive, legislation and regulations should mandate and offer incentives for the private sector to provide programs supporting young children and their families. Examples of such regulations include taxation programs in Colombia that earmark funds to support early childhood programs and the Children's Trust Fund developed in Mauritius to subsidize ECCD programs. Legal structures also are being created to support the increase in partnerships among governments, NGOs, and private agencies.

Strengthen International Collaboration

Most major international and bilateral donor agencies and many private foundations currently fund ECCD programs. To exchange lessons learned, cooperate in development of programs, and mitigate duplication of efforts, formal and informal mechanisms have been established that encourage collaboration. The direct beneficiaries of this strategy include donor agencies, UN agencies, international NGOs, foundations, policymakers, and researchers.

Examples of such collaborative models are the Consultative Group on Early Childhood Care and Development, the Association for the Development of Education in Africa, the Save the Children Alliance, the International Vitamin A Consultative Group, and the International School Health and Nutrition Network. All of these groups are important in strengthening an understanding of issues that need to be addressed, in bringing forward the latest theoretical and practical experience, and in fostering a synergism within the field that is not possible through individual efforts.

Conclusion

No single model for ECCD programs prevails. However, despite multiple factors influencing a child's life (health, education, social services, community development, agriculture, and so forth), a variety of cultural contexts, and the different skills and knowledge of local practitioners, ECCD programs tend to look alike. There are several reasons for this.

First, some needs, such as those for food, safety, security, and protection from the elements, are basic to humankind. And some goals are common across cultures, such as producing healthy, productive adults to perpetuate the culture. Programs designed to meet these needs and objectives will have some commonalities.

Second, in designing the first early childhood programs for developing countries, Western models of early childhood programs were introduced, primarily in the form of preschools. Although this model has been adapted, the basic structure and premise of Western-based preschool education still predominates in most countries. Third, the world has grown smaller through shared knowledge and technologies, and experiences gained in one part of the world can be instantly shared with another part of the world.

For some time people worldwide have been creating alternative early childhood programs, learning about what works and what does not. This experience could create an arrogance in the imposition of models except that, through constant learning, respect has been gained for local communities and the need to build onto existing systems and structures.

Much has been learned about how to support families and the development of young children and yet there is much more to learn (Evans 1994). The challenges ahead include:

- Development of a better understanding of the economics of creating, implementing, and sustaining early childhood programs and becoming bolder about the level of resources needed for investments to pay off.

- Encouragement of early childhood educators to work more closely with governments, ensuring that appropriate policies are established to support the development of programs for young children and their families.

- Assessment of the rapidly expanding set of approaches, techniques, and methodologies designed to affect children's development in their early years and determination of which methods should be disseminated based on demonstrated effectiveness.

- Increased focus on developing appropriate programs for children under the age of 3. Children within this age group are relatively invisible. Yet, research indicates that this period is critical for health, nutrition, and cognitive stimulation. Specific experience is needed in developing effective programs for the youngest children and their families.

- Continued experimentation with more flexible inservice training models whose substance and form should be developed from identified needs and sound educational practice. The threshold between theory and practice must be established. Teachers need practical skills to involve children actively in the learning process and a solid theoretical base to invent new activities that support children's learning.

- Creation of linkages between preschool and primary school. For example, (a) development of curricula that provide a continuity of experience for children, (b) provision of upgraded and ongoing teacher training that prepares teachers to work with children 3-8 years of age, and (c) increased involvement of parents and the community in children's education at the beginning and throughout the school years.

- Continued definition of "integration." Expecting to use only one model of integration is unrealistic; integration is defined differently in different situations. The challenge in creating integrated projects is for all participants to agree on a definition of the term in a given context. Perhaps over time clusters of programs can be created to exemplify how sectors can work together and to demonstrate clearly the effects of different integrated models.

- Continued development of programs with parents that meet their needs. Although programs that educate and enable parents have grown dramatically in some countries, they are virtually nonexistent in others.

The primary challenge is to continue to explore development of partnerships among and between governments, NGOs, donors, and the private sector. Organizations must shift their approaches from competition to cooperation, a difficult task for organizations that have been competitive historically. As organizations and governments work together, however, to break down the barriers between them, greater advancement will be possible on all fronts.

References

Bennett, J. 1993/1994. Educating Young Children: A Broader Vision. *Coordinators' Notebook.* No. 14.

Bernard van Leer Foundation/UNESCO (United Nations Educational, Scientific, and Cultural Organization). 1995. *Enhancing the Skills of Early Childhood Trainers.* Paris: UNESCO.

Booker, S. 1995. *We Are Your Children: The Kushanda Early Childhood Education and Care Dissemination Program, Zimbabwe 1985-1993.* The Hague: Bernard van Leer Foundation.

Castillo, C., N. Ortiz, and A. Gonzalez. 1993. *Home-based Community Day Care and Children's Rights: The Colombian Case.* Florence, Italy: International Child Development Center.

Evans, J. L. 1985. The Utilization of Early Childhood Care and Education Programs for Delivery of Maternal and Child Health/Primary Health Care components: A Framework for Decision-making. A Paper Commissioned by the World Health Organization. Geneva: WHO.

———. 1989. Developing an Early Childhood Care and Development Strategy for the 90s. Paper presented at Childhood in the 21st Century: International Conference on Early Childhood Education and Development (0-6 years), July 31-August 4. Hong Kong.

———. 1993a. Health Care: The Care Required to Survive and Thrive. *Coordinators' Notebook.* No. 13.

———. 1993b. *Participatory Evaluations of Child-to-Child Projects in India.* Geneva: Aga Khan Foundation.

———. 1994. Early Childhood Care and Development: Where We Stand and the Challenges We Face. Paper presented at the National Consultation on ECCD, organized by the National Inter-agency Committee on Early Childhood Care and Development, November 11-12. Quezon City, Philippines.

Evans, J. L., and K. Ismail. 1994. *Malaysian Early Childhood Development Study.* Kuala Lumpur: UNICEF (United Nations Children's Fund).

Jesien, G., J. Aliaga, and M. Llanos Zuloaga. 1979. A Home-Based Non-formal Program: Context and Description Validation of the Portage Model in Peru. Paper prepared for the InterAmerican Congress of Psychology, July. Lima, Peru.

Kagitcibasi, C., S. Bekman, and A. Goksel. 1995. A Multipurpose Model of Nonformal Education: The Mother-Child Education Program. *Coordinators' Notebook.* No. 17.

Landers, C., and M. Sporn. 1994. Enhancing Early Child Development: A Video-Based Parent Education Strategy. Paper presented at the Second UNICEF Animation Summit, November 14-18. Orlando, Fla.

Levinger, B. 1992. *Promoting Child Quality: Issues, Trends and Strategies.* New York: UNDP (United Nations Development Programme).

Loftin, C. 1979. Manual de Entrenamiento para Programas no Escolarizados con Base en el Hogar. Unpublished manuscript. Cooperative Educational Service Agency, Portage, Wis.

Mauras, M., C. L. Latorre, and J. Filp. 1979. Alternativas de Atencion al Preescolar en America Latina y el Caribe. Santiago, Chile: UNICEF (United Nations Children's Fund).

Montessori, M. 1961. *To Educate the Human Potential.* Adyar, Madras 20, India: Kalaksheta Publications.

Myers, R. G. 1988. Effects of early childhood intervention on primary school progress and performance in the developing countries: An update. Paper presented at a seminar on The Importance of Nutrition and Early Stimulation for the Education of Children in the Third World, April 6-9. Stockholm.

———. 1991. *Toward a Fair Start for Children.* Paris: UNESCO (United Nations Educational, Scientific, and Cultural Organization).

———. 1995. *The Twelve Who Survive: Strengthening Programs of Early Childhood Development in the Third World.* Ypsilanti, Mich.: High/Scope Press.

Myers, R. G., and R. Hertenberg. 1987. *The Eleven Who Survive: Toward a Re-Examination of Early Childhood Development Program Options and Costs.* Report No. EDT69. Washington D.C.: World Bank.

Nigeria, Federal Ministry of Education. 1987. *Guidelines on Pre-Primary Education.* Lagos: Government of Nigeria.

Paz, R. 1990. *Paths to Empowerment: Ten Years of Early Childhood Work in Israel.* The Hague: Bernard van Leer Foundation.

Pollitt, E. 1984. *Nutrition and Educational Achievement.* Nutrition Education Series. Issue 9. Paris: UNESCO (United Nations Educational, Scientific, and Cultural Organization).

Pollitt, E., K. S. Gorman, P. L. Engle, R. Martorell, and J. Rivera. 1993. Early Supplementary Feeding and Cognition. *Monographs of the Society for Research in Child Development* 58:7.

Subaran, Ida. n.d. Links between Early Childhood Development and Primary Education. Paris: UNESCO (United Nations Educational, Scientific, and Cultural Organization). Forthcoming.

UNICEF (United Nations Children's Fund). 1994. Guidelines for the Establishment of Early Childcare Development and Education (ECCDE) Centres. In line with the Federal Government of Nigeria and UNICEF Cooperation Agreement on Basic Education. Nigeria: UNICEF.

———. 1995. *Progress Report Enhancing the Role of Women in Comprehensive Child Development Project, July 1994-June 1995.* Jakarta, Indonesia: UNICEF.

Early Child Development: Investing in our Children's Future
M.E. Young, editor.

Early Childhood Programs: Elements of Quality

Lawrence J. Schweinhart

Childcare and educational programs influence children's development. High-quality programs that meet children's needs and emphasize positive outcomes can help assure a child's optimal development. Studies conducted throughout the world point to certain elements of quality common to effective programs. By acknowledging these elements and incorporating them into existing and new programs, countries can enhance the development of their children, enabling them to become productive, responsible adults.

This chapter identifies and describes seven elements of quality for early childhood programs focused on childcare and education. The discussion includes the rationale for selecting each element and the implications of incorporating it in programs around the world. Preceding this discussion is a definition of key terms related to assessing a program's quality. Also included is a description of an international project now under way, the Preprimary Project of the International Association for the Evaluation of Educational Achievement (IEA). In this multinational, 10-year project, researchers are identifying and describing the settings, processes, and effects of early childcare and education. The project already is advancing understanding of the importance of high-quality programs for early childhood.

Quality is an essential concept that must be addressed when considering different program options for early child development. The two previous chapters in this volume present other useful conceptual frameworks. Cochran offers a general framework for understanding societal factors that influence policy and program options, and Evans suggests a multipronged approach consisting of eight complementary strategies for promoting early childcare and development. Both authors emphasize the need for high-quality programs. Because quality is the critical link between program design and effective outcomes, the components of quality are explored in this chapter.

Definitions

Children spend their early years growing from infancy (birth to 1 year) to toddlerhood (1-3 years), to preschool age (3-6 years), to primary school age (6-8 years). Throughout the world, almost all young children live in homes with their families who introduce them to other settings, such as neighborhoods, homes of friends and relatives, stores, churches, playgrounds, and program settings.

Program Settings

Program settings for young children include schools, childcare centers, and childcare homes. In all these settings, adults maintain elements of quality that they believe will positively influence children's development. The quality of these programs can be observed in the present, but usually is measured by a program's effect on children's development, an effect that may extend throughout a child's lifetime. Because early childhood programs occupy many waking hours of young children, they must not be regarded as providing only custodial care; their contribution to children's futures must not be denied. Because *all* programs for young children have the capacity to contribute to their futures, the quality of *all* early childhood programs is important.

Ideal and Relative Quality

In developing plans for early childhood programs within the policy frameworks of various countries and political contexts, program quality must be specified in ideal and relative terms. *Ideal* program quality includes program elements that optimize young children's development. *Relative* program quality involves dimensions on which programs at least surpass the settings in which young children would otherwise spend their time. Although all programs should strive for ideal quality, limitations of money and caregiver education may require planners to settle for a relative level of quality.

Specifying program quality in relative terms in a specific situation is difficult, however, because some observers usually will not want to accept the specifics of that situation as given. Also, a given situation at one time or place often is not the same as an apparently similar situation at another time or place. For example, one element of optimum, or ideal, program quality is for one adult to serve no more than ten 4-years-olds. Yet the Aga Khan Foundation, to maximize its reach in populous countries throughout the world, has a standard of one adult serving twenty 4-year-olds; this relative level of program quality is clearly less than optimum. Although such a policy cannot be justified as *optimizing* children's development, it may be the position that best balances competing demands for child development and service to the largest number of children. In contrast, the Head Start program in the United States has opted for the ideal ratio of one adult serving no more than ten 4-year-olds, sacrificing service to the largest number of children.

The question in balancing ideal and relative quality is how far programs can deviate from standards of optimum quality and still be worthwhile. Certainly a "do-no-harm" rule must apply to all publicly supported programs. No publicly funded program should harm young children's development, that is, make it worse than it would have been without the program. This rule is important particularly when early childhood programs are adjunct to policies with other primary purposes, such as child nutrition or family welfare assistance. The rule is obviously too weak for early childhood programs whose primary purpose is contributing to child development. As a rule, for such programs, the economic and intangible returns on investment should be sufficient to justify making the investment. Indeed, a strong case can be made that this tougher rule be applied to all early childhood programs.

Essential Elements of Quality for Early Childhood Programs

From the time of Frederich Froebel (1782-1852), early childhood educators have strived to specify the elements of quality for early childhood programs and communicate them to other early childhood educators (Evans 1975; Epstein, Schweinhart, and McAdoo 1995; Goffin 1993). These elements are the same for formal or informal programs, although there are some differences.

Formal programs specify many elements, rely primarily on professionally prepared and certified staff, and usually are conducted in dedicated facilities, such as schools and childcare centers. *Informal programs* specify fewer elements, rely primarily on parents or other adults without professional preparation and certification, and usually are conducted in homes. Informal programs differentiate less than formal programs between staff and parents, which can be valuable, but for informal programs to contribute to child development, they must still excel in the key elements of program quality. The research findings pertaining to quality and the essential elements of quality are described below.

Research Findings

Research in the United States and other countries indicates that high-quality preschool programs for young children have important short- and long-term benefits for children and families. These programs are especially valuable for children living in poverty, improving their school success and opportunities and saving taxpayer dollars by preventing later problems. Researchers have identified and validated these effects (for a brief review of this research, see Schweinhart, Barnes, and Weikart 1993).

Several experimentally designed studies address the effectiveness of various curriculum models (Powell 1986). Studies of childcare in the United States have assessed the value of several basic program features to make policy recommendations about them (Ruopp and others 1979; Travers and Goodson 1980; Whitebook, Howe, and Phillips 1989; Child Care Study Team 1995).

In other countries, researchers have examined the effects of early health and nutrition programs and early education programs on children's age of enrollment, progress, and performance in primary school (Myers 1992). Four studies focusing on health and nutrition programs began in Latin America in the 1970s; two were in Colombia (Herrera and Super 1983; McKay 1982), one was in Mexico (Chavez and Martinez 1981), and another was in Guatemala (Klein 1979). These were prospective studies—all but one beginning prenatally, all following children into primary school, and one following children beyond third grade. The studies were fairly rigorous, randomly assigning children to groups. The four studies showed the effects of nutritional supplements, and some involved maternal tutoring.

In addition, thirteen studies of preschool education, some including a parent education component, have been conducted in Brazil (Feijo 1984; Brazil 1983), Chile (Filp and others 1983; Richards 1985), Colombia (Nimnicht and Posada 1986), Peru (Myers 1985), India (Chaturvedi and others 1987; Lal and Wati 1986), Turkey (Kagitcibasi, Sunar, and Bekman 1987), and Morocco (Wagner and Spratt 1987). These studies varied in rigor (some used random assignment to groups, some were prospective, and some were retrospective), but all compared children who participated in preschool programs with those who had not.

Myers (1992) summarizes the findings of all seventeen of these studies of the effects of early health and nutrition and education programs. Children who participated in these programs enrolled in school at earlier ages and made better progress in school, in some cases dramatically better than children who did not participate. Participants had higher rates of promotion and lower rates of grade repetition and school dropout than nonparticipants. Children who participated in most of the preschool education programs but not the health and nutrition programs performed better in school than children in the comparison group. In one nutrition program, two preschool education programs, and one parent education program, participating children received higher ratings for their social behavior than children in the comparison group.

Myers' review of the findings from these studies provides valuable comparative evidence that has broad applicability, as already noted by Cochran in this volume. According to Myers (1992: 252), "These conclusions are encouraging. When placed alongside the results from the United States and Europe, they suggest that similarly positive effects for early interventions are not only possible [throughout the world], but that the potential for bringing about improvements is greatest where social or economic conditions prejudice entrance, continuation, and performance in primary school."

Relevant findings from these other countries indicate that the elements of quality for early childhood programs identified in U.S. research may be applied judiciously to all programs for young children throughout the world. Various associations on early childhood in the United States (for example, the National Association for the Education of Young Children 1984 and the National Association of Elementary School Principals 1990) have endorsed such elements of quality. Research also indicates that high-quality early childhood programs can take place in any setting with adequate resources and qualified staff. These settings include private nursery schools, public schools, Head Start programs, day-care centers, and day-care homes.

Standards of Quality

Table 1 lists seven standards of quality for early childhood programs (Schweinhart 1988, 1990, 1992; Schweinhart, Koshel, and Bridgman 1986; Schweinhart and Weikart 1993). Every element addressed in table 1 is important to the operation of a high-quality early childhood program. Striving for a high-quality program is possible even when obstacles prohibit the full realization of certain standards. For example, despite a ratio of children to teachers that is less than optimal, a kindergarten class with twenty-five or thirty children can maintain a curriculum based on child-initiated learning activities. Obstacles such as large class sizes must still be overcome, but should not become an excuse to stop striving for high quality.

The development of high-quality early childhood programs, particularly for children living in poverty, has become a priority on the policy agendas of many nations. To justify increased public expenditure, services delivered must be of the quality necessary to be counted a wise investment in children and families.

Table 1. Seven Standards of Quality for Early Childhood Programs

1. The program offers a validated child development curriculum.
2. The program uses a validated child development assessment strategy.
3. The number of young children for each teacher is low enough to enable staff to positively influence young children's development.
4. Staff are trained to know how to positively influence young children's development and support families to do the same.
5. Staff receive systematic inservice training and supervisory support to positively influence young children's development.
6. Families are partners with teachers in positively influencing young children's development.
7. The program meets child health and family needs.

Source: Schweinhart 1988.

The seven elements of quality (listed in table 1) essential for early childhood programs that contribute to the development of young children are described below. These elements are: a validated child development curriculum; a validated child development assessment strategy; low enrollment limits; trained staff; supervisory support and systematic inservice training; families as partners with teachers; and meeting child health and family needs.

A Validated Child Development Curriculum

The child development curriculum is key to an effective early childhood program. A good curriculum is based on children's intellectual, social, and physical development and encourages youngsters to initiate their own learning activities within a supportive environment. Programs throughout the world use several validated models of child development curriculum; the High/Scope Curriculum (Hohmann, Banet, and Weikart 1979; Hohmann and Weikart 1995) and the Montessori method (Montessori 1964) are the best known. The distinctions, levels, and models of early child development curriculum are discussed below.

Curriculum Distinctions

Curriculum distinctions can be made by type of educational approach and type of child activity. Regarding educational approach, early childhood educators must make distinctions among teacher-centered education, learner-centered education, and custodial care.

In teacher-centered education, teachers communicate lessons to groups of students. Using this approach to teach groups of infants or toddlers is absurd, as Elkind (1987) notes when he calls use of teacher-centered education the "miseducation" of young children. All education often is equated with teacher-centered education, however, resulting in some early childhood caregivers who do not consider themselves teachers in educational programs because they do not use, or believe in, a teacher-centered approach to young children.

As noted previously, educational programs for young children take place in community agencies, childcare centers, and homes as well as schools. In these settings, teachers can use learner-centered education, leading students to learning by designing the settings and creating the circumstances for students to learn lessons on their own or with individual assistance from teachers. Early childhood programs that adopt a learner-centered approach *are* educational, for without a learner-centered approach, these programs would be merely custodial.

Early childhood educators also must distinguish between child-initiated activity and other forms of play. Child-initiated activity is purposeful. With an effective child development curriculum, children have many opportunities to initiate their own activities and take responsibility for completing them. The adults help children make decisions, but do not make all the decisions for them. Teachers also do not rely on a precisely sequenced set of lessons and workbooks in reading, writing, and arithmetic and do not attempt to maintain strict control. Instead, they create a framework, or learning environment, that frees children to choose activities and carry them out as the children see fit. By emphasizing decisionmaking and problem solving, this learning environment prepares children for academic learning and for the work demands of the real world that they will face eventually.

Any early childhood program in the world can and ideally should be learner-centered and based on child-initiated activity. However, this approach may be countercultural in authoritarian cultures. Indeed, the case can be made that all education, at least in the liberal arts, is countercultural in this sense. As outsiders, dealing with this situation by making no attempt to change people's attitudes toward young children or by insisting that people change immediately will not improve anything. The best alternative is an interactionist approach.

The *interactionist approach* begins with accepting people as they are and encouraging them toward gradual, developmental change while respecting their culture and personal autonomy and being open to the possibility of development in one's own beliefs. For example, showing people discrepancies with their belief that teacher-centered education will help children become independent problem solvers may encourage them to resolve the discrepancies themselves. Their gradual progress toward the ideal standard of a learner-centered approach based on child-initiated learning activities will yield relative standards along the way. This progress depends on the effectiveness of the curriculum training that they receive and on their own openness to change.

Curriculum Levels

Early childhood educators approach curriculum on three levels: general principles, curriculum models, and specific practices. At the level of general principles, they assume or strive for widespread consensus that certain curriculum principles should apply in every early childhood program. These general curriculum principles also might be called good practice. Some early childhood education textbooks implicitly adopt this position without identifying it (for example, Hendrick 1988).

In recent years, the National Association for the Education of Young Children (NAEYC) has strived toward recognition and widespread consensus for general curriculum principles called *developmentally appropriate practice* (Bredekamp 1987). However, critics have challenged the claim that consensus exists on developmentally appropriate practice, raising questions about whether the approach is sufficiently sensitive to individual and cultural differences (Mallory and New 1994). An NAEYC panel is currently struggling to accommodate these criticisms.

At the level of curriculum models, early childhood educators each may adopt a specific curriculum model as their own from various available models. The number of early childhood curriculum models increased dramatically in the 1970s when the U.S. government began to support their development and dissemination (in Planned Variation Head Start in the preschool years and Follow Through in the primary grades).

Because it tolerates and even encourages diversity, this level of curriculum models has political advantages over the level of general principles. Early childhood educators can combine the two levels easily by applying general principles, such as the principles of developmentally appropriate practice, in selecting acceptable curriculum models. Epstein, Schweinhart, and McAdoo (1995) use this combined approach by adopting developmentally appropriate practice as part of their criteria for comparing curriculum models.

At the level of specific practices, early childhood educators adopt discrete activities or actions, such as providing blocks in the classroom, encouraging children to make choices, or using a particular assessment tool. Specific practices may result from general principles, curriculum models, or both. If they do not come from these sources, the educational approach is called *eclectic*, selecting what appear to be the best practices from a variety of sources. Eclectic approaches may even include curriculum models as sources of specific practices, but not as guiding frameworks.

Curriculum Models

Early childhood educators who adopt curriculum models may use them as exclusive sources of their educational practices or as frameworks to guide their selection of practices from various other sources, even from other curriculum models. For example, some early childhood educators adopt the Creative Curriculum as their principal model but also use the Kamii-DeVries Curriculum as a supplement or source of educational practices they consider consistent with their principal approach.

To assist educators in selecting a curriculum model, Epstein, Schweinhart, and McAdoo (1995) reviewed and compared six widely used early childhood models of curriculum and training. They built on the work of several authors and editors over the past two decades (DeVries and Kohlberg 1990; Evans 1975; Goffin 1993; Roopnarine and Johnson 1993). The following six models were reviewed:

- Bank Street College of Education's Developmental Interaction approach (Biber 1984)

- The Creative Curriculum developed by Diane Trister Dodge at Teaching Strategies, Inc. (Dodge 1988)

- The Direct Instruction model developed by Carl Bereiter and Siegfried Engelmann (Bereiter and Engelmann 1966)

- The High/Scope Curriculum developed under the guidance of David Weikart at the High/Scope Educational Research Foundation (Hohmann and Weikart 1995)

- The Kamii-DeVries constructivist approach developed by Constance Kamii and Rheta DeVries (DeVries and Kohlberg 1990)

- The Montessori method based on the work of Maria Montessori (Montessori 1964).

These six curriculum models are used throughout the world. Although other comprehensive models of early childhood curriculum may exist, these six, reviewed below, are the most well known and widely used.

Distinctions. The six most common curriculum models have various distinctions. For example, the Direct Instruction model is teacher-centered, and the other five curriculum models are learner-centered. In the terms of Kohlberg and Mayer (1972), the Direct Instruction model also is *behaviorist*, and the other five curriculum models are *cognitive-developmental* to some extent. The High/Scope Curriculum and Kamii-DeVries constructivist approach are fully cognitive-developmental, whereas the Developmental Interaction approach, Creative Curriculum, and Montessori method have been influenced by the maturationist approach as well.

Further distinctions give each of these six curriculum models their unique identities. The Developmental Interaction approach encourages teachers to be highly responsive to children's choices. The Creative Curriculum focuses on arranging the learning environment into ten interest areas. Direct Instruction features high-paced, scripted sessions of questions and answers between teachers and small groups. The High/Scope Curriculum emphasizes a daily routine in which children plan, carry out, and review their own activities. In the Kamii-DeVries constructivist approach, teachers involve children in group games to foster their cognitive development. The Montessori approach places great emphasis on prescribed Montessori materials, each designed to teach children certain lessons.

Documentation, Validation, and Dissemination. Epstein, Schweinhart, and McAdoo (1995) reviewed the documentation, validation, and dissemination of these six early childhood curriculum models. *Documentation* clarifies the model's definition of curriculum and training goals, objectives, practices, content, and processes, enabling the definitions to be communicated to and used by others. *Validation* gives evidence of how well a model works, how well it achieves its goals and objectives, and whether its claims of effectiveness can be trusted. *Dissemination* is the process and the result of communicating the model to others through documentation and training; it involves the model's generalizability to diverse populations and settings.

Successful validation and dissemination depend on and complement successful documentation. Successful dissemination ought to, but does not necessarily, require successful validation. For users of the curriculum model, documentation provides available materials; dissemination provides available training and study materials; and validation gives assurance that the curriculum model is effective.

Although all six models scored high on documentation because they documented all of their approaches to working with children and training teachers, some of the documentation had limitations. For example, the Direct Instruction model is purposely neither comprehensive nor developmentally appropriate by NAEYC's criteria. Three models do not use the full range of effective adult learning strategies: The Kamii-DeVries constructivist approach provides little documentation on observation and feedback; the Creative Curriculum has little presentation of theoretical rationale; and the Direct Instruction model does not encourage reflection and sharing during training.

In validation, the High/Scope Curriculum scored high; the Montessori method, Developmental Interaction approach, Kamii-DeVries constructivist approach, and Direct Instruction model scored medium; and the Creative Curriculum scored low. Validation scores were based on the availability of reliable and valid assessment tools for specific models and on evidence for effectiveness of curriculum and training models. Table 2 summarizes evidence for the effectiveness of curriculum models and their training systems, as reviewed by Epstein, Schweinhart, and McAdoo (1995).

Table 2. Research Findings on Effectiveness of Early Childhood Curriculum Models

Curriculum model	Finding	Sources
High/Scope	Considerable evidence of the effectiveness of its curriculum and its training program	Schweinhart and others, 1986, 1993; Epstein 1993
Montessori	Some evidence of reaching its goals for children	Boehnlein 1988; Karnes and others 1983; Miller and Bizzell 1983
Developmental Interaction	Evidence of its effectiveness with primary-grade children	Bowman and others 1976; Gilkeson and others 1981
Kamii-DeVries	Short-term positive effects in some areas of child development	Gulub and Kolen 1976; DeVries and others 1991
Direct Instruction	Intellectual and language effects of preschool programs diminishing in the primary grades; no evidence of positive social or emotional effects; some evidence of long-term negative effects on social conduct	Burts and others 1992; Gersten and Keating 1987; Schweinhart and others 1986; Hyson and others 1989; Karnes and others 1983

The High/Scope Curriculum offers psychometrically acceptable measures of both children and teaching, and the Developmental Interaction approach has a psychometrically acceptable measure of children. The Kamii-DeVries constructivist approach has developmental measures of children and teaching. The Montessori approach has no measures of child development but is currently assessing the psychometric characteristics of a measure for teacher competencies. The Creative Curriculum and Direct Instruction offer model-specific measures without evidence of reliability or validity, although Direct Instruction relies on standardized achievement tests with known psychometric characteristics.

In dissemination, the Montessori method, Developmental Interaction approach, High/Scope Curriculum, and Creative Curriculum scored high; the Kamii-DeVries constructivist approach and Direct Instruction model scored medium. Direct Instruction scored only medium because it lacks implementation records, and so far Kamii-DeVries has been used only in Missouri and a few other places. High/Scope, Direct Instruction, Montessori, and Creative Curriculum appear to have excellent or good capacity for dissemination.

High/Scope and Montessori, which have field-based associations supported by face-to-face training, cost more than Creative Curriculum and Direct Instruction. Creative Curriculum and Direct Instruction, which are primarily publication-based without face-to-face training, cost less, but evidence of their effectiveness without face-to-face training is lacking. The two higher-education approaches, Developmental Interaction and Kamii-DeVries, are more costly than the other four models, and training lasts 2 years.

A Validated Child Development Assessment Strategy

Because evaluation compares observed learning with intended lessons and a curriculum is a plan of intended lessons, everything noted above for curriculum also applies to evaluation. Validated assessment strategies also require valid and reliable evaluation plans, assessment tools, and assessment methods. For a related discussion of evaluation issues, see Kagitcibasi in this volume.

Evaluation Plans

Evaluation plans should take into account teachers' general curriculum principles, the curriculum model(s) they use, and their specific practices. If teachers support developmentally appropriate practice, their evaluations should be developmentally appropriate; if teachers use specific curriculum models, their evaluations should fit these curriculum models; and if teachers' practices are eclectic, their evaluations should be eclectic in the same way. Of course, evaluations of purely eclectic programs never can be generalized to other eclectic programs because, by definition, each eclectic program is unique.

Assessment Tools

Valid and reliable evaluations depend on valid and reliable assessment tools. For the most part, existing assessment tools with demonstrated validity and reliability have assessed teacher-centered rather than learner-centered education, or teaching that communicates information rather than creates settings and circumstances for student learning. Because most early childhood curriculum models, which contrast with traditional teacher-centered education, have existed for only about 3 decades, most tools to assess them do not yet have demonstrated reliability and validity. However, tools for assessing today's learner-centered education are key to future evaluation of early childhood programs.

Assessment Methods
Assessment of early childhood education will define the success of that education. The challenge of assessing early childhood education is applying the methods of assessment to the process and outcome goals of early childhood education. Although some standard assessment practices that are developed for older children, adolescents, and adults may conflict with some process goals, early childhood education must not surrender its process goals to resolve this conflict; surrendering would irreparably harm early childhood education and the young children it serves. Rather, new assessment practices must be developed that are consistent with the process goals of early childhood education.

Assessment defines the goals of education, and there are two types of assessment for early childhood education: screening and progress assessment. Screening determines who should enter a program by examining a child's performance (Meisels 1985, 1987). Progress assessment clarifies program objectives and determines how well children, teachers, and programs are reaching these objectives. In either case, misassessment is a serious concern that results from incorrectly defining the process and outcome goals of early childhood education.

Testing. The prevalent approach of testing young children, especially group testing, often constitutes misassessment. Current testing gives young children a series of questions to answer immediately, although they may not have the experience or inclination to do so. Each test question has one right answer, although a child may not understand the question or may give a creative answer that is considered incorrect. Such testing gives children the underlying message that the teacher is in charge and they must do exactly what the teacher says. Ironically, such testing also undermines a teacher's authority; tests are designed to be teacher proof and achieve high reliability by removing teacher judgment from the assessment process.

Like teacher-directed instruction, the testing described above presents prescribed, virtually scripted, behavioral sequences. It guarantees that children are observed performing various skills but sacrifices the initiative that is central to good early childhood programs. The test's interaction style has few parallels in children's lives beyond school and, thus, lacks ecological validity; children may reject or grow tired of the respondent role. The goal is to use a benign, unobtrusive process to assess children's knowledge, but such testing is neither benign nor unobtrusive because it is foreign to children's experience.

Many tests focus narrowly on numbers, letters, shapes, colors, simple language, and basic logic while ignoring initiative, creative representation, social relations, and music and movement. Many tests are inappropriate to children's various cultures and day-to-day experience (National Center for Fair and Open Testing 1991). Test results also may be misused to make important placement decisions, sometimes mislabeling children as disabled. A child who has a bad day when tested could be placed unnecessarily in special education classes for years.

Systematic Observation. The principal assessment alternative to testing is systematic observation of children's activities in their day-to-day settings. Observation fits an interactive style of curriculum, in which give and take between teacher and children is the norm. Although careful observation requires effort, the approach has high ecological validity and presents minimal intrusion into what children should be doing in early childhood classrooms (Goodwin and Driscoll 1980). Children's activities naturally integrate all dimensions of their development—intellectual, motivational, social, physical, aesthetic, and so on.

One method of assessing young children by systematic observation is taking anecdotal notes on their activities. But anecdotal notes alone are not enough for good assessment because they do not offer criteria for judging the developmental value of activities, nor do they provide evidence of reliability and validity. A better method is using anecdotal notes to compile developmental scales of proven reliability and validity.

Combining anecdotal notes with developmental scales permits children to engage in activities anytime and anywhere that teachers can see them. This method defines categories of acceptable answers rather than single right answers. It expects teachers to set a framework for children to initiate their own activities. This method embraces a broad definition of child development that includes not only logic and language, but also initiative, creative representation, social relations, and music and movement. It also is culturally sensitive when teachers as trained observers focus on objective, culturally neutral descriptions of behavior (for example, "Pat hit Bob") rather than subjective, culturally loaded interpretations (for example, "Pat was very angry with Bob"). Finally, this method empowers teachers by recognizing their judgment as essential to assessment.

The High/Scope Preschool Child Observation Record (COR) is one example of an observational assessment tool (High/Scope Educational Research Foundation 1992). This assessment tool, although developed for use in the High/Scope Curriculum, can be used in all early childhood programs regardless of the curriculum model used, as long as the model has such goals for children. A 2-year study of sixty-four Head Start teaching teams found that the COR is a feasible, valid, and reliable assessment tool (Schweinhart and others 1993).

To use the COR, a trained teacher assesses each child's behavior and activities in six categories of development: initiative, social relations, creative representation, music and movement, language and literacy, and logic and mathematics. Throughout several months, the teacher writes brief notes describing episodes of each child's behavior in these six categories. The teacher then uses these notes to rate a child's behavior on thirty 5-level COR items within these categories. Teachers score the COR two or three times a year, obtaining initial ratings 6-8 weeks into the program year. Trained outside observers, assessing sets of four children during three program sessions, also have used the COR to evaluate programs (Epstein 1993).

The COR and similar efforts are examples of assessing early childhood education that respects both methods of assessment and process and outcome goals for this education. Without such assessment tools, early childhood education may become distorted by tests that embody a style of education inconsistent with developmentally appropriate practice. With such assessment tools, early childhood educators can understand the children they serve and the great promise that society hopes and expects early childhood education to accomplish.

Low Enrollment Limits

Low enrollment limits are essential to maintaining the high staff-child ratio and small group sizes that are hallmarks of high-quality early childhood programs. Facts about enrollment size based on research can help policymakers decide appropriate class sizes for the children whom programs serve. Table 3 presents research findings of staffing and staff development in early childhood programs.

Table 3. Research Findings on Staffing and Staff Development of Early Childhood Programs

Finding	Source(s)
Staffing	
Three- to five-year-olds develop best in classes of sixteen to twenty children with two adults present. When compared with children in larger groups, children in small groups receive more staff attention; engage more frequently in reflection, verbal initiative, and cooperation; engage less frequently in aimless wandering and noninvolvement in free play; and experience greater improvement in knowledge and skills.	Ruopp and others 1979; Travers and Goodson 1980; Child Care Study Team 1995
General educational level of adults is not strongly related to desirable child outcomes. However, in programs with a greater percentage of staff who had child-related training or day-care experience, children more often have a good relationship with the lead caregiver; are more likely to finish whatever projects they start; talk more during free play; are more involved in classroom activities in general; and show significant improvement in knowledge and skills.	Ruopp and others 1979; Travers and Goodson 1980
Staff development	
Systematic training and supervision in a curriculum model that emphasizes child initiative significantly improves the effectiveness of early childhood programs that have already achieved a high degree of quality in other ways.	Epstein 1993
Systematic inservice curriculum training is most successful in promoting program quality when an agency has a supportive administration that includes a trained curriculum specialist on staff who provides teachers with hands-on workshops, observation and feedback, and follow-up sessions.	

According to the U.S. National Day Care study, 3-5 year olds develop best in classes with enrollment limits of sixteen to twenty children and with two adults present, a teacher or caregiver and an assistant. The study found that, compared with those in larger groups, children in these groups received more staff attention; engaged more frequently in reflection, verbal initiative, and cooperation; engaged less frequently in aimless wandering and noninvolvement in free play; and experienced greater improvement in knowledge and skills (Ruopp and others 1979; Travers and Goodson 1980). Although enrollment limits must be set according to a country's available resources for the program and temperaments of young children may differ, these empirical findings have some applicability in other nations.

The National Day Care study also found that an enrollment limit of twenty with two adults present is best for children of normal or average intellectual ability and socioeconomic circumstances. However, study findings suggest that an enrollment limit of sixteen with two adults present is best for a Head Start or prekindergarten program that primarily serves children who live in poverty or are otherwise at special risk of school failure (Ruopp and others 1979).

In addition, the study recommends a 1-4 adult-child ratio for infants and toddlers through age 2 (1-1 for infants under 6 weeks). The study recommends that enrollments be limited to eight babies (up to 18 months) and twelve toddlers (19-36 months) (Ruopp and others 1979). The Cost, Quality, and Child Outcomes in Child Care Centers study (Child Care Study Team 1995) also affirms the importance of high staff-child ratios for quality care at childcare centers, but has yet to specify the ideal ratios found for program quality and optimum child outcomes.

Because staff-child ratio, along with staff compensation, determines the cost of early childhood programs, tradeoffs may occur between program quality and other goals; that is, relative standards may replace ideal standards. When the program's only goal is to contribute to child development, having a staff-child ratio of more than ten 4-year-olds to each teacher makes contribution to child development unlikely. However, if the program has other goals, such as providing childcare for families, the tradeoffs become more complicated. Lack of a childcare program may place children in physical danger because the alternative for many of them is to remain unsupervised at home or elsewhere. These cases present ethical dilemmas that can be resolved only on a case-by-case basis, striving to provide the greatest good for the greatest number and to avoid harm to anyone.

Trained Staff

Not just anyone can teach young children. The care and education of young children is a teaching specialty. Like other teachers who specialize in lower or upper elementary school, middle school, or high school education, teachers of young children must specialize, understanding early child development and education. Successfully teaching children at one age level does not qualify a teacher to work with children at another level. For example, a teacher changing from working with 12-year-olds to working with 4- or 5-year-olds must shift to a more appropriate nurturing, nondirective teaching style and set of expectations.

Several U.S. childcare studies establish the value of child-related training, such as courses and practice in childcare, early childhood education, child development, child psychology, and elementary education. Surprisingly, studies show that the general educational level of adults is not strongly related to desirable outcomes (Ruopp and others 1979; Travers and Goodson 1980). In comparing programs, those with a greater percentage of staff who had child-related training or day-care experience more often showed a good relationship between children and the lead caregiver and had children more likely to finish whatever project they started and to be more talkative during free play. Children in these programs also were more involved in classroom activities and showed significant improvement in knowledge and skills.

Research does not support ideas that anyone can teach young children well and that credentials or other evidence of child development training are unnecessary. These ideas do not recognize the special teaching and caregiving style required to work successfully with groups of young children, skills that incorporate and go beyond parenting skills. Imagine a parent who had to single-handedly take care of ten 4-year-olds. Although some persons are naturally gifted with this style, most develop it through training and experience.

In the long term, to provide quality education for young children, adequately trained teachers and caregivers throughout the world should be given professional status and receive compensation that reflects such professionalism. To attract talented young people to early childhood education, they should be offered salaries equal to those of elementary school teachers. Unfortunately the average annual salary of experienced early childhood educators in the United States today is several thousand dollars less than the average annual salary of new elementary school teachers (Grubb 1986). Administrators and policymakers must recognize the problem of low wages in early childhood education and try to rectify it at the local level. Policymakers and administrators can make a difference by treating preschool teachers as fully qualified teachers and by encouraging others to do so as well.

In the short term, providing high-quality early childhood programs relies on training in early childhood curriculum rather than teaching credentials and professional status. Indeed, probably the single, most effective way to improve the quality of early childhood education around the world is to offer curriculum training to program providers, regardless of their background in early childhood education or related areas of knowledge. In many countries, not enough credentialed early childhood educators are available to staff a large-scale program, and the only available alternative may be relying on people who receive targeted, inservice training in early childhood curriculum.

Supervisory Support and Systematic Inservice Training

Supervisory support and training of early childhood staff, including educators and caregivers, are essential for assuring the effectiveness of an early child development program.

Supervisory Support

Agency directors and other program administrators must understand and actively support the goals and operation of an early childhood program and its child development curriculum. They should be prepared to:

- Explain and defend the curriculum to parents, teachers, staff, other administrators, and community leaders

- Assure that staff, children, and the program are evaluated by developmentally appropriate measures and standards

- Provide the program with equipment and resources necessary for a child development curriculum

- Hire qualified staff and see that they receive adequate compensation, encouraging teamwork among staff in each classroom

- Allocate staff time for daily planning

- Allocate staff time for monthly inservice training sessions and ensure that these sessions lead to systematic application of child development principles in the classroom

- Work with staff and parents to resolve childcare needs of employed parents by part-day or full-day programs.

Types of Training

Three types of training are needed: initial training, inservice training, and training of trainers.

Initial Training. As mentioned earlier, the key to developing or improving the quality of many early childhood programs is providing intensive early childhood curriculum training to program providers, who may have no background in early childhood education. This initial training program is provided best by on-site educators, enabling the training to be systematic and results-oriented and to combine theory and practice.

Inservice Training. Program administrators especially are responsible for providing inservice training for early childhood staff. Such training should take place at least monthly and address issues that arise in day-to-day classroom activities. Besides promoting professionalism, inservice training gives staff the opportunity to receive emotional support from administrators and other teachers for their efforts to implement the curriculum.

Various approaches may be taken to inservice training. Some inservice training is systematic and results-oriented while other training is unsystematic and not results-oriented. The typical large early childhood conference falls into the latter category, consisting of numerous 1- or 2-hour sessions on topics unrelated to each other beyond their focus on some aspects of early childhood. A conference attendee may learn useful lessons, but these lessons are unrelated to each other. This conference approach sometimes is extended to all inservice training, which becomes a jumble of ideas that do not lead anywhere. In contrast, inservice training can be systematic with sessions logically related to each other, leading to specific results, such as teachers who are able to apply a specific curriculum approach in their classrooms.

Early childhood inservice training also may be theoretical, practical, or a combination of both. Clearly, combining the theoretical and the practical has the greatest advantage. A purely theoretical approach may not be applicable to practice or may require participants to make very speculative translations into practice. A purely practical approach may become a cookbook approach, in which participants mindlessly and perhaps incorrectly follow rules without understanding the reasons for doing so. A combined approach, which alternates between inservice training sessions and classroom practice, brings theory to the practical level, permitting theory and practice to correct and modify each other and participants to integrate a theoretical approach into their day-to-day practice.

Training Trainers. Training in early childhood and adult education also must be provided for trainers. The High/Scope Foundation pioneered Training of Trainers programs during the past decade, and evaluation (Epstein 1993) showed that systematic training and supervision in the High/Scope Curriculum significantly improves the effectiveness of even high-quality early childhood programs. The evaluation found that systematic inservice curriculum training promotes program quality most successfully in agencies with a supportive administration that includes a trained curriculum specialist who gives teachers hands-on workshops, observation and feedback, and follow-up sessions. Effective trainers focus on coherent, validated, developmentally appropriate curriculum models.

The evaluation also showed that each certified High/Scope trainer worked with an average of twenty-five teachers and assistant teachers in thirteen classrooms. The teachers they trained scored significantly better than comparable teachers without such training, not only in their understanding of the High/Scope Curriculum, but also in their actual implementation of the approach. Children in the High/Scope classrooms scored significantly higher than children in comparison classrooms in initiative, social relations, music and movement, and overall development.

Families as Partners with Teachers

A high-quality early childhood program involves parents and is sensitive to their needs. Administrators and staff should form partnerships with parents, recognizing their crucial importance in child development. Administrators and staff should be able to explain child development principles to parents, applying them to children. They should realize that parents can help them understand children and family backgrounds better. If parents ask a staff member how they can help their 4-year-old learn to read, staff should be able to focus on the most appropriate language skills for children at this age.

Teachers who form partnerships with parents should not be too authoritarian, claiming to know what is best for a child regardless of parental perceptions, or too accommodating, placing inappropriate academic demands on young children as a result of parental pressure. Although staff members, as qualified early childhood professionals, are experts on principles of child development, parents are the long-term experts on their children's behavior, traits, and family background.

Staff members provide a valuable service when they help parents see a child's behavior in developmental terms, perhaps helping identify inappropriate expectations that parents may hold. Parents of any socioeconomic level may hold inappropriate expectations for their children. Some parents' expectations are too low; they do not always perceive the value of early childhood education in helping children develop the knowledge, skills, and positive attitudes of which they are capable. Parental expectations for other children are too high or inappropriately academic. By working together, staff and parents can achieve balance.

Educators have the responsibility and opportunity to help parents in many other ways. Parents should be encouraged to come to the classroom in a meaningful capacity to learn, as either informed observers or volunteer teaching and caregiving assistants. If parents drop off and pick up their children at school, teachers can seize the opportunity to talk with them about their child's progress. Ideally, they also would meet with parents, individually or as a group, at least monthly, and they may have to reach uninvolved parents by scheduling home visits. Also, when parents are employed, parent-staff communication is more difficult to maintain and must be pursued more vigorously.

Teachers should try to schedule evening conferences, possibly in parents' homes, to accommodate the schedules of working parents.

Because many parents are eager to learn more about child development and child rearing techniques, teachers can present material at parent-staff meetings on relevant topics, such as disciplining children properly, forming developmentally appropriate expectations for children, child-initiated learning, promoting development through parent-child activities, and assessing children's developmental status and progress. Administrators who actively participate in these meetings can contribute greatly to the success of their programs.

Lessons on involving parents with teachers are applicable throughout the world. Effective early childhood programs should support parents rather than undermine their authority. Working with parents enhances understanding of the relationship between curriculum and indigenous culture. When an authoritarian culture, for example, does not include a learner-centered approach to early childhood programs, teachers may respond in three ways. They may adopt: the indigenous approach, making no attempt to influence parents' authoritarian attitudes toward young children; an aggressive approach, totally rejecting and overriding parents' authoritarian ways; or an interactionist approach, accepting parents' authoritarian ways but encouraging them to shift gradually toward a more learner-centered approach to young children.

Meeting Child Health and Family Needs

Families throughout the world wrestle with many issues in addition to helping their young children develop educationally in appropriate ways. Policymakers, administrators, and teachers must be aware of parents' problems and be prepared to help them find solutions, for example, by being familiar with the various community services available to these families.

In many countries, early childcare and education are best offered as components of integrated, collaborative services associated with community development programs. Particularly in extreme poverty conditions, the noneducational needs of children and families must be met if an educational program is to work at all. Young children living in poverty may need meals at the early childhood program site. Often, poor families need assistance in finding or employing agencies to help them. Because parents who are poor often lack education and may be illiterate, literacy training can be combined with early childhood programs.

Early childhood education programs also create opportunities for child development within other programs that serve children and families. For example, in some places children must travel great distances to receive nutritious food or medical care and may spend long hours waiting for these services. Such situations present excellent opportunities for programs that contribute to children's development, rather than letting the children wait for services in unstimulating settings. For example, some Head Start programs in the United States provide educational programming on school buses because children spend so much time in transit.

Because meeting the other needs of children and families is the element of program quality most sensitive to context, it is the element most likely to reach relative rather than ideal standards. Although the ideal standard is simply meeting children's and families' needs, early childhood educators can only meet needs to the extent that available resources will allow. Early childhood programs cannot always meet all the needs of families, but early childhood educators can always be counselors and friends to children and their families who live in poverty and experience other social problems.

A major project under way that will shed considerable light on this and other elements of quality in early childhood programs is the IEA Preprimary Project, described below.

The IEA Preprimary Project

The IEA Preprimary Project is a 10-year study of early childhood in eleven to fifteen countries around the world. The aims of the project are to identify and describe the types of early childcare and education settings used by families with 4-year-old children in these countries; describe processes occurring within these settings; and examine differential effects of the settings on later child development. The project has three phases.

Phase 1

Phase 1 was conducted from 1987 to 1991 and consisted of a household survey of representative samples of families with 4-year-old children. National project coordinators collaboratively developed the survey instrument, called the Parent/Guardian Interview. Also at the beginning of the project, national study directors produced profiles on childcare and education in eleven participating countries (Olmsted and Weikart 1989). The eleven countries in phase 1 were Belgium, China, Finland, Germany, Hong Kong, Italy, Nigeria, Portugal, Spain, Thailand, and the United States.

Project researchers from the eleven countries wrote the phase 1 report (Olmsted and Weikart 1994). The report describes each country's sampling and data collection methodology and each country's sample characteristics (parents, households and families, and child health). Chapters describe each country's findings for families' weekly use of early childhood services, the use of organized facilities, and children's daily routines. A nation-by-nation examination of the findings also is presented along with a summary and commentaries by four international experts in early childhood programs.

The study shows a worldwide trend toward extraparental childcare and education, especially in urban areas. Extraparental childcare and education settings are virtually universal among 4-year-olds in Hong Kong (100 percent) and Belgium (98 percent) and serve a clear majority of 4-year-olds in Italy (85 percent), Germany (82 percent), Spain (79 percent), Finland (75 percent), Portugal (71 percent), and the United States (61 percent); they also serve significant numbers of 4-year-olds in the more rural countries of China (45 percent), Thailand (37 percent), and Nigeria (35 percent).

Most of the care and education in most of the countries is provided in organized facilities rather than homes, but Finland, Portugal, and Thailand have more children in home-based programs than in programs in organized facilities. In Belgium, Finland, Germany, Hong Kong, Italy, and Portugal, government agencies or religious organizations sponsor a majority of group childcare settings, in contrast to China or the United States where they do not.

The 4-year-olds who receive extraparental care and education spend an average of 34-55 hours a week in these settings in eight of the countries. Children spend less time in these settings in the United States (28 hours), Germany (25 hours), and Hong Kong (17 hours) due to a significant amount of part-day preschool programs in these countries. At least 92 percent of the parents in each of the eleven countries said that they were either "somewhat satisfied" or "very satisfied" with the extraparental settings in which their 4-year-olds spent their time. In all of the countries, mothers (as opposed to fathers or both parents) assumed principal responsibility for parental childcare, ranging from 58 percent of the total parental-care time in Belgium to 89 percent in Hong Kong.

Phase 2

Phase 2 of the IEA Preprimary Project, called the Quality of Life study, is a multinational observational study of the characteristics of settings experienced by 4-year-olds and the relationship between children's experiences in these settings and their concurrent developmental status. It began in 1989 and will produce reports through 1998. As part of phase 2, the international coordinating center prepared fifteen videotapes illustrating the variety of early childhood settings encountered in each of the fifteen countries participating in phase 2. These countries are Belgium, China, Finland, Greece, Hong Kong, Indonesia, Ireland, Italy, Nigeria, Poland, Romania, Slovenia, Spain, Thailand, and the United States. Countries who participated in phase 1 observed the major settings identified in phase 1, including children's own homes if feasible.

Across most of the countries studied, teachers agreed that the most important skills for 4-year-olds are social skills with peers, self-sufficiency skills, and language skills. The least important are self-assessment skills, social skills with adults, and preacademic skills. In most countries, at least 75 percent of the lead teachers or caregivers are certified in some way, with the exception of Thailand (10 percent), Hong Kong (36 percent in kindergartens, 22 percent in day nurseries), and China (37 percent in rural kindergartens). Teachers' average years of schooling range from 10.2 years (in Thailand's childcare centers) to 16.7 years (in the public school prekindergarten programs of the United States). Median class sizes range from fourteen children (in Ireland and among other group settings in the United States) to thirty-three and one-half children (in China's rural kindergartens). Median numbers of children served by each adult range from a low of six (in Ireland's disadvantaged preschools) to a high of thirty (in China's rural kindergartens and Thailand's educational programs).

Phase 3

Phase 3 of the IEA Preprimary Project is a follow-up study of the children observed at age 4. It began in 1993 and will produce reports through 2000. The 4-year-olds selected for observation and assessment in phase 2 are being reassessed at age 7, the age when children from all participating countries will have completed at least 1 year of primary school. The assessment at age 7 gathers information on the children from many sources, including interviews with teachers and parents and tests and observations of children. Phase 3 will show the effects of children's experiences in various preschool settings.

Defining quality in early childhood settings ultimately depends on the influence of these settings and their elements on child development during and after children's experience in these settings. As data on children's developmental status are collected in phase 2 and phase 3, researchers will identify which setting elements in countries around the world most strongly influence children's development; that is, which elements constitute quality and contribute to effectiveness. The IEA Preprimary Project offers rich data for testing (to confirm or improve) currently accepted definitions of the elements of quality for early childhood programs.

Implications for Countries Around the World

The implications of assuring quality in early childhood programs are applicable to all countries. These implications, identified previously, are summarized below.

Ample evidence from various countries shows that selected early childhood programs help children enroll in school at earlier ages and make better progress. This progress is indicated by higher rates of promotion and lower rates of grade repetition and school dropout for children participating in early childhood programs. Findings from long-term studies of impoverished children in the United States suggest that high-quality, early childhood programs in other countries will help children achieve greater educational success, followed by greater economic success and social responsibility in adulthood.

Program providers can assess the quality of existing early childhood programs through questionnaires and other means. Table 4 presents an example of the type of questionnaire available.

Early childhood programs throughout the world should use a well-defined, learner-centered curriculum model that includes curriculum-specific assessment procedures. Early childhood teachers and caregivers should have adequate training, be accorded professional status, and receive commensurate compensation. Adequate training does not refer only to teaching credentials, but also to systematic, results-oriented inservice training that combines early childhood theory and practice. Parents and other nonprofessionals employed in informal early childhood programs should serve under the guidance of educated professionals who offer inservice training and supervisory support.

High-quality early childhood programs should support parents rather than undermine their authority. If parents have an authoritarian approach, teachers should adopt an interactionist approach, working with parents as partners and encouraging them to shift gradually toward a learner-centered approach to their young children.

In many countries, early childcare and education are best offered as components of integrated, collaborative services associated with community development programs. To the extent that resources allow, such services might include adult literacy education, meals, medical care, and referrals to other agencies. The time children spend in a center to receive services, such as meals or health care, is an opportunity to provide high-quality early childhood education.

The seven essential elements of quality for early childhood programs described in this chapter identify an ideal standard that maximizes young children's development. Governments not able to attain this ideal may need to adopt a relative standard of program quality, or the best they can afford under the circumstances. Of course, public money should not be invested in early childhood programs that harm or contribute little to young children's development. Early childhood programs that attain the levels of quality defined in this chapter will contribute substantially to the lives of children and families and will provide societies with a healthy return on investment.

Table 4. Quality Questionnaire for Early Childhood Programs

A. Enrollment and Staffing

1. How many children are enrolled in the program group?

2. Given the number of adults assigned to work with this group, what is the adult-child ratio?

   _____ to _____

3. What is the extent of child development or early childhood education training for each adult assigned to work with the group?

__ Graduate school	__ Graduate school	__ Graduate school
__ Bachelor's degree	__ Bachelor's degree	__ Bachelor's degree
__ Some college	__ Some college	__ Some college
__ Professional credential	__ Professional credential	__ Professional credential
__ Inservice training:	__ Inservice training:	__ Inservice training:
______________	______________	______________

B. Supervisory Support and Inservice Training

4. How much time does the program administrator spend discussing educational curriculum and program operation with teaching staff?

   __ Minutes each day, week, or month (circle one)

5. How much time does the teaching staff have for team planning, on the job but not in contact with children?

   __ Minutes each day, week, or month (circle one)

6. How many hours of inservice training have the teaching staff had this school year (or during the past 12 months)?

   __ Hours

7. Do the sessions of inservice training all support the same curriculum approach?

Table 4.

C. Parent Involvement

8. How much time does the teaching staff spend in informal discussions about children with parents?

   __ Minutes each day, week, or month (circle one)

9. How many meetings with parent groups have the teaching staff held this school year (or during the past 12 months)?

   __ Meetings

10. Did the topics of these meetings all support the same curriculum approach?

    ____

11. How many meetings with parents in individual families, at the program site or in the parents' homes, have the teaching staff held during the past 12 months?

    __ Meetings with each family

D. Noneducational Needs of Children and Families

12. Do the teaching staff know what other early childcare and educational arrangements their children have?

    __ No __ Yes

13. Have staff met during the past 12 months with other caregivers?

    __ No __ Yes

14. Do the staff know how to make referrals to social agencies for families who live in poverty or face other problems?

    __ No __ Yes

15. Do the staff know how to refer children with special needs, and are they sensitive to children's special needs?

    __ No __ Yes

Table 4.

E.	*Child-initiated Learning*
16.	Is the room arranged in interest areas?
	__ No __ Yes
17.	Does the room have a variety of materials, both designed for children and not designed specifically for children, that are accessible to the children and have a variety of uses?
	__ No __ Somewhat __ Yes
18.	Do children spend a substantial portion of each day engaged in activities that they initiate themselves with teacher support?
	__ No __ Somewhat __ Yes
19.	In group activities, are children given opportunities to make choices about activities?
	__ No __ Somewhat __ Yes
20.	Do the staff spend substantial time talking to children as individuals and in small groups?
	__ No __ Somewhat __ Yes

Source: Schweinhart 1988.

Note

Thanks to David Weikart, Patricia Olmsted, and the staff of the IEA Preprimary Project for providing information on this important worldwide study; to Mary Young for ably representing the World Bank's interest in early childhood programs as an ideal means of investing in people; and to the World Bank for providing financial support to write this chapter.

References

Bereiter, C., and S. Engelmann, 1966. *Teaching Disadvantaged Children in the Preschool.* Englewood Cliffs, N.J.: Prentice-Hall.

Biber, B. 1984. *Early Education and Psychological Development.* New Haven: Yale University Press.

Boehnlein, M. 1988. Montessori Research: Analysis in Retrospect. *The NAMTA Quarterly* 13(3):1-119.

Bowman, G. W., R. S. Mayer, H. Wolotsky, E. C. Gilkeson, J. H. Williams, and R. Pecheone. 1976. *The BRACE Program for Systematic Observation.* New York: Bank Street Publications.

Brazil, Ministério da Saúde y Instituto Nacional de Alimentação e Nutrição. 1983. *Analição do PROAPE/A lagoas com enfoque na área econômica.* Brasilia.

Bredekamp. S., ed. 1987. *Developmentally Appropriate Practice in Early Childhood Programs Serving Children from Birth through Age 8: Expanded Edition.* Washington, D.C.: National Association for the Education of Young Children.

Burts, D. C., C. H. Hart, R. Charlesworth, P. O. Fleege, J. Mosley, and R. H. Thomasson. 1992. Observed Activities and Stress Behaviors of Children in Developmentally Appropriate and Inappropriate Kindergarten Classrooms. *Early Childhood Research Quarterly* 7:297-318.

Chaturvedi, E., B. C. Srivastava, J. V. Singh, and M. Prasad. 1987. Impact of Six Years Exposure to ICDS Scheme on Psycho-social Development. *Indian Pediatrics* 24:153-60.

Chavez, A., and C. Martinez. 1981. School Performance of Supplemented and Unsupplemented Children from a Poor Rural Area. In A. E. Harper and G. K. David, eds. *Nutrition in Health and Disease and International Development: Symposia from the XIIth International Congress on Nutrition, 77, Progress in Clinical and Biological Research.* New York: Alan R. Liss, Inc.

Child Care Study Team. 1995. *Cost, Quality, and Child Outcomes in Child Care Centers Executive Summary.* Denver: University of Colorado.

DeVries, R., J. P. Haney, and B. Zan. 1991. Sociomoral Atmosphere in Direct-instruction, Eclectic, and Constructivist Kindergartens: A Study of Teachers' Enacted Interpersonal Understanding. *Early Childhood Research Quarterly* 6:449-71.

DeVries, R., and L. Kohlberg. 1990. *Constructivist Early Education: Overview and Comparison with Other Programs.* Washington, D.C.: National Association for the Education of Young Children.

Dodge, D. T. 1988. *A Guide for Supervisors and Trainers on Implementing the Creative Curriculum for Early Childhood.* 2nd ed. Washington, D.C.: Teaching Strategies, Inc.

Elkind, D. 1987. *Miseducation: Preschoolers at Risk.* New York: Knopf.

Epstein, A. S. 1993. *Training for Quality: Improving Early Childhood Programs through Systematic Inservice Training.* Ypsilanti, Mich.: High/Scope Press.

Epstein, A. S., L. J. Schweinhart, and L. McAdoo. 1995. *Models: A Comparison of Curriculum-based Training Models in Early Childhood Education.* Ypsilanti, Mich.: High/Scope Press.

Evans, E. D. 1975. *Contemporary Influences in Early Childhood Education.* 2nd ed. New York: Holt, Rinehart and Winston.

Feijo, M. 1984. Early Childhood Education Programs and Children's Subsequent Learning: A Brazilian Case Study. Unpublished doctoral diss., Stanford University, Department of Education, Stanford, Calif.

Filp, J., S. Donoso, S. Cardemil, E. Dieguez, J. Torres, and E. Schiefelbein. 1983. Relationship between Pre-primary and Grade One Primary Education in State Schools in Chile. In K. King and R. Myers, eds., *Preventing School Failure: The Relationship between Preschool and Primary Education.* Ottawa: International Development Research Centre.

Gersten, R., and T. Keating. 1987. Improving High School Performance of "At-risk" Students: A Study of Long-term Benefits of Direct Instruction. *Educational Leadership* 44(6):28-31.

Gilkeson, E. C., L. M. Smithberg, G. W. Bowman, and W. R. Rhine. 1981. Bank Street Model: A Developmental-Interaction Approach. In W. R. Rhine, ed., *Making schools More Effective: New Directions from Follow Through.* New York: Academic Press.

Goffin, S. G. 1993. *Curriculum Models and Early Childhood Education: Appraising the Relationship.* New York: Merrill.

Golub, M., and C. Kolen. 1976. Evaluation of a Piagetian Kindergarten Program. Manuscript based on paper presented at Sixth Annual Symposium of The Jean Piaget Society, Philadelphia, Penn.

Goodwin, W. L., and L. A. Driscoll. 1980. *Handbook for Measurement and Evaluation in Early Childhood Education.* San Francisco: Jossey-Bass.

Grubb, W. N. 1986. *Young Children Face the States: Issues and Options for Early Childhood Programs.* New Brunswick, N.J.: Rutgers University, Center for Policy Research in Education.

Hendrick, J. 1988. *The Whole Child: Developmental Education for the Early Years.* Columbus, O.: Merrill.

Herrera, M., and C. Super. 1983. *School Performance and Physical Growth of Underprivileged Children: Results of the Bogota Project at Seven Years: Report to the World Bank.* Cambridge: Harvard University, School of Public Health.

High/Scope Educational Research Foundation. 1992. *High/Scope Child Observation Record.* Ypsilanti, Mich.: High/Scope Press.

Hohmann, M., B. Banet, and D. P. Weikart. 1979. *Young Children in Action: A Manual for Preschool Educators.* Ypsilanti, Mich.: High/Scope Press.

Hohmann, M., and D. P. Weikart. 1995. *Educating Young Children: Active Learning Practices for Preschool and Child Care Programs*. Ypsilanti, Mich.: High/Scope Press.

Hyson, M. C., K. L. Van Trieste, and V. Rauch. November 1989. NAEYC's Developmentally Appropriate Practice Guidelines: Current Research. Paper presented at the preconference sessions of the meeting of the National Association for the Education of Young Children, Atlanta, Ga.

Kagitcibasi, M. B., D. Sunar, and S. Bekman. 1987. *Comprehensive Preschool Education Project: Final Report to the International Development Research Centre*. Istanbul: Bogazic University.

Karnes, M. B., A. M. Schwedel, and M. B. Williams. 1983. A Comparison of Five Approaches for Educating Young Children from Low-income Homes. In Consortium for Longitudinal Studies. *As the Twig Is Bent: Lasting Effects of Preschool Programs*. Hillsdale, N.J.: Lawrence Erlbaum Associates, Inc.

Klein, R. 1979. Malnutrition and Human Behavior: A Backward Glance at an Ongoing Longitudinal Study. In D. Levitsky, ed., *Malnutrition, Environment and Behaviour*. Ithaca: Cornell University Press.

Kohlberg, L., and R. Mayer. 1972. Development as the Aim of Education. *Harvard Educational Review* 42:449-96.

Lal, S., and R. Wati. February 1986. Non-formal Preschool Education: An Effort to Enhance School Enrollment. Paper presented at the National Conference on Research on ICDS. New Delhi: National Institute for Public Cooperation in Child Development.

Mallory, B. C., and R. S. New. 1994. *Diversity and Developmentally Appropriate Practices*. New York: Teachers College Press.

McKay, A. 1982. Longitudinal Study of the Long-term Effects of the Duration of Early Childhood Intervention on Cognitive Ability and Primary School Performance. Unpublished doctoral diss., Northwestern University, Evanston, Il.

Meisels, S. J. 1985. *Developmental Screening in Early Childhood: A Guide*. rev. ed. Washington, D.C.: National Association for the Education of Young Children.

———. 1987. Uses and Abuses of Developmental Screening and School Readiness Testing. *Young Children* 42(2):4-6, 68-73.

Miller, L. B., and R. P. Bizzell. 1983. The Louisville Experiment: A Comparison of Four Programs. In Consortium for Longitudinal Studies. *As the Twig Is Bent: Lasting Effects of Preschool Programs*. Hillsdale, N.J.: Lawrence Erlbaum Associates, Inc.

Montessori, M. 1964. *The Montessori Method*. New York: Schocken.

Myers, R. 1985. Preschool Education as a Catalyst for Community Development: A Report Prepared for the U.S. Agency for International Development. Lima, Peru.

———. 1992. *The Twelve Who Survive: Strengthening Programmes of Early Childhood Development in the Third World*. New York: Routledge.

National Association for the Education of Young Children. 1984. *Accreditation Criteria & Procedures of the National Academy of Early Childhood Programs*. Washington, D.C.: National Association for the Education of Young Children.

National Association of Elementary School Principals. 1990. *Early Childhood Education and the Elementary School Principal: Standards for Quality Programs for Young Children*. Alexandria, Va.: National Association of Elementary School Principals.

National Center for Fair and Open Testing. 1991. *Standardized Tests and Our Children: A Guide to Testing Reform*. Cambridge, Mass.

Nimnicht, G., and P. E. Posada. 1986. *The Intellectual Development of Children in Project Promesa: A Report Prepared for the Bernard van Leer Foundation*. Medellin, Colombia: Centro Internacional de Educación y Desarrollo Humano.

Olmsted, P. P., and D. P. Weikart. 1994. *Families Speak: Early Childhood Care and Education in 11 Countries*. Ypsilanti, Mich.: High/Scope Press.

Powell, D. R. September 1986. Effects of Program Models and Teaching Practices. *Young Children* 41(6):60-67.

Richards, H. 1985. *The Evaluation of Cultural Action*. London: Macmillan.

Roopnarine, J. L., and J. E. Johnson, eds. (1993). *Approaches to Early Childhood Education*. 2nd ed. New York: Macmillan.

Ruopp, R., J. Travers, F. Glantz, and C. Coelen. 1979. *Children at the Center: Summary Findings and Policy Implications of the National Day Care Study*. Cambridge, Mass.: Abt Associates.

Schweinhart, L. J. 1988. *A School Administrator's Guide to Early Childhood Programs*. Ypsilanti, Mich.: High/Scope Press.

———. 1990. How Policymakers Can Help Deliver High-quality Early Childhood Programs. In *Early Childhood and Family Education: Analysis and Recommendations of the Council of Chief State School Officers*. New York: Harcourt Brace Jovanovich.

———. 1992. Early Childhood Education. In M. C. Alkin, ed., *Encyclopedia of Educational Research*. 6th ed. New York: Macmillan.

Schweinhart, L. J., H. V. Barnes, and D. P. Weikart, with W. S. Barnett, and A. S. Epstein. 1993. *Significant Benefits: The High/Scope Perry Preschool Study through Age 27*. Monographs of the High/Scope Educational Research Foundation, 10. Ypsilanti, Mich.: High/Scope Press.

Schweinhart, L. J., J. J. Koshel, and A. Bridgman. 1986. *Policy Options for Preschool Programs*. Ypsilanti, Mich.: High/Scope Press, in collaboration with the National Governors' Association. ERIC Document Nos. PS 016 196 and ED 276 515. Revised for *Phi Delta Kappan* 68 (March 1987):524-29.

Schweinhart, L. J., S. McNair, H. Barnes, and M. Larner. 1993. Observing Young Children in Action to Assess their Development: The High/Scope Child Observation Record Study. *Educational and Psychological Measurement* 53:445-55.

Schweinhart, L. J., and D. P. Weikart. 1993. Success by empowerment: The High/Scope Perry Preschool Study through Age 27. *Young Children* 48(7):54-58.

Schweinhart, L. J., D. P. Weikart, and M. B. Larner. 1986. Consequences of Three Preschool Curriculum Models through Age 15. *Early Childhood Research Quarterly*, 1:15-45.

Travers J., and B. D. Goodson. 1980. *Research Results of the National Day Care Study*. Final Report of the National Day Care Study. Vol. 2. Cambridge, Mass.: Abt Associates.

Wagner, D., and J. Spratt. 1987. Cognitive Consequences of Contrasting Pedagogies: The Effects of Quaranic Preschooling in Morocco. *Child Development* 58:1209-19.

Whitebook, M., C. Howes, and D. Phillips. 1989. *Final Report of the National Child Care Staffing Study*. Oakland, Calif.: Child Care Employee Project.

Early Child Development: Investing in our Children's Future
M.E. Young, editor.

Parent Education and Child Development

Cigdem Kagitcibasi

The relationship between parent education and child development has been studied and documented for more than 2 decades. Bronfenbrenner (1974) was one of the first to emphasize the importance, and cost-effectiveness, of family involvement in both fostering and sustaining children's development. Parent education, in particular, has been shown to be an effective way of intervening to enhance early child development. Parent education not only affects children directly, but also improves mothers' attitudes and behaviors and enriches the entire family environment.

The three preceding chapters presented conceptual frameworks for matching childcare services to societal needs, programming early childcare and development, and assuring quality in early childhood programs. The involvement of family, and particularly parents, is an important component of each of these frameworks. Specifically, support and education of caregivers, especially parents and family members, is one of eight complementary programming strategies for early childhood care and development highlighted by Evans in one of these chapters.

Despite increasing evidence and recognition, the value of parent education for child development continues to be debated. To help resolve this debate, this chapter focuses on the effects of parent education in child development interventions. The chapter opens with a definition of parent education and a consideration of effects documented from early and recent reviews of studies conducted in the United States and developing countries. For a more in-depth examination, a case study of the Turkish Early Enrichment Project (TEEP) is provided. This project included a specific parent education component.

Based on the experience gained from TEEP, seven essential ingredients for parent education and child development interventions are then described in relation to planning, implementing, and evaluating child development programs. In the next chapter, Lombard further explores the value of parent education by describing two home-based programs from Israel.

Definitions

Parent education has several different meanings and is used interchangeably with parental involvement, parental participation, family involvement, home visiting, and family support. On one hand, the various terms reflect differences in the disciplinary approaches and services rendered, such as child health and nutrition, social services, and child and parent education. On the other hand, the terms reflect the target of intervention, children, parents, families, and communities.

The diversity of meaning behind parent education is apparent in the different concepts guiding child development programs. For example, Marfo and Kysela (1985) isolate three distinct approaches to characterizing the role of parents in early intervention programs for children with disabilities: (a) the parent therapy model, in which counseling or support groups help parents cope with stress; (b) the parent training model, which emphasizes the role of parental behavior in teaching skills to children; and (c) the parent-child interaction model, which focuses on sensitizing parents to their children's needs. The selected outcome will reflect the model chosen, although the immediate goal of each model is parental change.

From the perspective of social support, programs typically are distinguished according to the following domains: providing information, for example about child health and development and parenting; providing emotional and appraisal support, such as empathy, reinforcement, feedback regarding parental roles, and access to other parents; and providing instrumental assistance, such as referrals to services and material benefits (Weiss and Jacobs 1988).

Concepts for parent education and support programs focusing on early child development commonly are developed according to the following criteria:

- Type and purpose of service (health care, informational support and education for parenting and child development, emotional support, educational day care)
- Target of service (children, mothers, parent-child interaction, families)
- Location of service (home visits, childcare center, community center, group settings)
- Providers of service (teacher, health professional, paraprofessional, social worker, psychologist)
- Length and timing of service (one-time service, short- or long-term service; beginning of service in infancy, early childhood).

Programs tend to combine different aspects of these criteria. For example, family support and educational models of early intervention (that is, different types of services) may be combined and are not mutually exclusive, both involving parent support and early education (commonly at a center). Because programs typically combine different approaches, distinguishing the effects of a specific approach often is difficult. The reviews of child development programs summarized below describe some of the known effects of parent education on early child development.

Effects of Parent Education in Child Development Interventions

Research and evaluation of child development interventions have broadened over time, shifting from a focus on children's cognitive development to include program effects on parents and the community. The summary below, of early and recent reviews of programs in the United States and developing countries, demonstrates this shift and emphasizes the effects of parent education. The lessons learned from research on child development programs in both the United States and developing countries also are summarized.

The U.S. Experience

Most longitudinal research and careful evaluation of child development programs have been conducted in the United States. Other industrialized countries, such as the United Kingdom, often refer to these efforts (Ball 1994). For this reason and because of space limitations, only the U.S. experience is reviewed below.

Early Reviews

The roots of U.S. intervention programs targeting child development are found in the War on Poverty initiative of the Johnson era and especially in the Head Start program (Zigler and Berman 1983; Zigler and Weiss 1985; Woodhead 1988; Halpern 1990; Zigler and Muenchow 1992; Zigler and Valentine 1979). Head Start and other early child development interventions focused mainly on children and typically did not involve parent education. Nevertheless, they form the basis for current concepts and programs of early child development interventions.

Most early interventions focused on providing direct cognitive training to children at a center and on measuring child outcomes. Early evaluations, in particular the Westinghouse Report (Cicirelli, Evans, and Schiller 1969), concluded prematurely that Head Start had failed, and a subsequent report prepared for the World Bank (Smilansky 1979) also was very critical of early intervention programs. Numerous methodological problems in the Westinghouse Report cast doubt on its results (Campbell and Erlebacher 1970; Smith and Bissell 1970; White 1970). The Smilansky report referred mainly to the first wave of negative evaluations based on research in the 1960s; it did not use later information that showed positive, longer-term effects. Despite their flaws, these reports influenced public opinion and policy.

In addition to being negative, early evaluations had other problems: vague criteria for success; exclusive dependence on intelligence quotient (IQ) measures, which convey a unidimensional concept of child development based on cognitive competence defined narrowly in psychometric terms; abstraction of children from their environment and a focus on individual child outcomes; and the short time period covered by the evaluations. An unrealistic and unnecessary goal, raising IQs, which was attributed to Head Start and reinforced by the media (Woodhead 1988), lay beneath these problems. IQ was singled out as a magic yet concrete target, excluding other beneficial outcomes.

Later evaluations were more positive. A major effort was a meta-analysis of more than 1,500 studies of the Head Start program, forming the basis for the Head Start Evaluation, Synthesis, and Utilization Project. One report on cognitive effects documented in seventy-one studies (Harrell 1983) showed gains in cognitive competence, school readiness, and school achievement. Evidence also was shown of positive effects on children's socioemotional development and health (McKey and others 1985). However, IQ gains of Head Start participants, in comparison with control group members, tended to dissipate over time.

Smaller-scale interventions typically used experimental designs, which often were lacking in Head Start programs. Some of the smaller-scale projects involved costly interventions, often starting in infancy. Among them were the Early Training Project (Klaus and Gray 1968; Gray, Ramsey, and Klaus 1983), the Milwaukee Project (Garber and Heber 1983; Garber 1988), the Abecedarian Project (Ramey, Yeates, and Short 1984), the Perry Preschool Project (Schweinhart and Weikart 1980; Berrueta-Clement and others 1984, 1987), and the Mother-Child Home Program (Levenstein, O'Hara, and Madden 1983).

Longitudinal studies of these projects showed better school performance and social adjustment for children in experimental groups compared with those in control groups. Results included lower rates of grade retention and referral to special classes, higher rates of high school completion and employment, and lower incidence of crime and teenage pregnancy. Higher achievement motivation, higher occupational aspirations and expectations, and a more positive self-concept among children in the experimental groups indicated motivational gains and psychological well-being.

Findings from other studies showed positive parental outlooks. Parents had higher aspirations and expectations for their children and indicated more satisfaction with their children's school progress, even when the study controlled for grade retention and referrals to special classes. These findings came from evaluations of single studies, especially of the Perry Preschool Project. They also came from pooled findings of eleven high-quality studies evaluated by meta-analyses conducted by the Consortium for Longitudinal Studies (Royce, Darlington, and Murray 1983; Lazar and Darlington 1982), which was formed in 1975 in response to the negative public image created for preschool effectiveness by the reports mentioned above.

Recent Reviews

A number of recent reviews examined several characteristics and comparative effects of early U.S. interventions targeting child development. A main question is whether the interventions provided early education, family support, or a combination of the two. Early education is defined as direct education provided to children, mainly at a preschool or childcare center. Family support may include parenting education, mostly conducted through home visits.

The following topics are addressed in these reviews: goals of program evaluation, parental changes, family functioning, direct education vs. family support, and social competence and juvenile delinquency. The main points emphasized in the reviews are described below to give an overview of common findings and highlight important issues.

Goals of Program Evaluation. In an analysis of education and family support programs, Weiss (1988) examines the goals of program evaluation and the dependent measures used to assess them in nineteen different studies, covering more than a dozen programs conducted between 1978 and 1984. Some of these evaluations are meta-analyses of several programs, such as the Consortium for Longitudinal Studies mentioned above (Lazar and Darlington 1982), and one is a long-term follow-up of the Perry Preschool Project. Weiss (1988) summarizes the programs' effects on children, parents, parent-child interaction, and family functioning.

As a general trend, evaluations of intervention projects are shifting from exclusively emphasizing a child's cognitive development to including changes in parents and parent-child interaction and, more recently, changes in formal and informal social support to the family. Alongside this shift in evaluations from children to the larger context is an explicit effort in more recent studies to determine a program's effect on parents and the family, and thus indirectly on a child. For example, the Head Start experimental programs [Parent Child Development Centers (PCDC) and Child and Family Resource Programs (CFRP)] are designed to assess early childhood programs that are oriented toward parents and family.

Parental Changes. A number of studies promoting enhanced child development show a variety of parental changes. Changes in parents include increased knowledge of child development (Rodriguez 1983; Rodriguez and Cortez 1988); increased recognition of their role as their child's teacher (Travers and others 1982; Slaughter 1983); better caregiving, illustrated by better control techniques, more elaborate verbal communication, better maternal teaching strategies, and more initiation of contact with their child's teacher (Andrews and others 1982; Gray and Ruttle 1980; Slaughter 1983; Hauser-Cram 1983); and less restrictive, less punitive orientation toward their child (Olds and others 1986a, 1988; Rodriguez 1983).

These studies also show direct effects on parents. These changes in the adults' characteristics, which are considered to indirectly benefit children, include gaining a greater sense of control (Travers and others 1982), enhanced self-esteem and coping (Travers and others 1982; Slaughter 1983), and better problem-solving skills (Andrews and others 1982).

Parent-oriented programs also result in more straightforward and policy-relevant gains for adults. For example, the Rochester Nurse Home Visitation Program (Olds and others 1986a, 1986b, 1988) and the CFRP (Travers and others 1982) promoted further education and employment for mothers and families. Similarly, a longitudinal evaluation of the Yale Child Welfare Research Project (Provence and Naylor 1983; Rescorla, Provence, and Naylor 1982; Seitz, Rosenbaum, and Apfel 1985) showed adult improvement in residence, further education, economic self-sufficiency, and quality of life.

Family Functioning. Although evaluations of child development programs have not included family functioning, parental changes that involve better general functioning can be expected to promote better overall family functioning. Gradually, programs are giving more specific attention to variables affecting couples and families. For example, a survey of 217 education and family support programs (Maciuika and Weiss 1987) showed that 75 percent of the programs addressed family communication skills and 72 percent addressed family management and problem-solving skills.

Farran (1990) reviewed thirty-two intervention programs for socioeconomically disadvantaged children, the results of which were published between 1977 and 1986. Many of the programs also were reviewed by Weiss (1988). Farran groups the studies according to four factors: time of the intervention's onset (within the first year of a child's life, between 12 and 36 months, and between 37 and 60 months); location of intervention (home- or center-based); length of follow-up (short, moderate, or long); and the service provider (staff or parents). Farran also notes some general problems of longitudinal research, such as attrition. For example, Slaughter (1983) lost almost one-half of the original sample during the 2 years of the study, and the Early Training Project (Gray and Ramsey 1985) followed only fourteen girls out of ninety children to completion of high school. The final and original samples clearly differ in such cases.

Results from Farran's review of home-based programs were mixed. Gray's Home Visit Program (Gray and Ruttle 1980) and the Project CARE Parent Education Program (Ramey and others 1985) showed no positive effects of home visits. The Field program (Field and others 1982) showed positive effects for the home visit group, but less than those obtained for the center-based group. Slaughter's study (1983) showed positive effects on some of the measures. Only the earlier projects by Gordon (Gordon, Guinagh, and Jester 1977; Jester and Guinagh 1983) and Levenstein (Levenstein and others 1983) and a later one by Slater (1986) produced unequivocally positive intervention effects.

As for long-term effects evaluated in four programs (Epstein and Weikart 1979; Gray and Ruttle 1980; Jester and Guinagh 1983; Levenstein and others 1983), only Levenstein's showed sustained impact. On the basis of these mixed results, Farran (1990) questions the effectiveness of home-based intervention and single-shot, center-based programs without continued intervention, although he admits that long-term effects may surface later.

In their review of intervention programs, Seitz and Provence (1990) take a more positive outlook toward parent-focused programs. They distinguish between programs focused on cognitive development with parents as teachers and programs with health and social outcomes. The home visit programs of Levenstein (1970) and Gordon (Gordon, Guinagh, and Jester 1977) are successful examples of the former. The Rochester Nurse Home Visitation Program (Olds and others 1986a, 1986b, 1988), the Montreal Home Visitation Study (Larson 1980), and the Yale Child Welfare Research Project (Provence and Naylor 1983; Rescorla and others 1982; Seitz, Rosenbaum, and Apfel 1985) are examples of the latter.

In the programs with health and social outcomes evaluated by Seitz and Provence (1990), various effects on parents were obtained. Effects of the Rochester program included better childcare (less child abuse and neglect; fewer child injuries); better self-care (less smoking during pregnancy); and further education and employment. The Montreal program showed better home environments, improved responsiveness, and provision of early stimulation. The Yale program showed, for parents, further education and employment, as well as increased spacing between children and lowered fertility and, for children, improved language ability at 30 months of age, as well as better school attendance and adjustment for boys. Many effects were more notable in the follow-up assessment than in the immediate results of the interventions.

Direct Education vs. Family Support. In a separate review, Seitz (1990) compares the educational and family support models of intervention. Early and intensive programs using the educational model include the Milwaukee Project (Garber and Heber 1983; Garber 1988) and the Abecedarian Project (Ramey, Yeates, and Short 1984; Ramey and others 1985). Later preschool programs include the Perry Preschool Project (Schweinhart and Weikart 1980; Berrueta-Clement 1984). Programs using the family support model are the Yale Child Welfare Research Project (Provence and Naylor 1983; Rescorla and others 1982; Seitz, Rosenbaum, and Apfel 1985), the Houston PCDC Program (Johnson and Walker 1987), the Rochester Nurse Home Visitation Program (Olds 1988; Olds and others 1986a, 1986b), the Montreal Home Visitation Study (Larson 1980), and the Gutelius Child Health Supervision Study (Gutelius and others 1972, 1977).

Seitz questions programs that focus on cognitive development of children, noting that raising IQ to normal levels does not guarantee school success several years later. Seitz also notes that educational programs with long-term effects involve parents and that family support programs lead to better parenting, better socioemotional development of children, and better life outcomes for parents. Based on these findings, Seitz proposes merging educational and family support models, as was done in the Gutelius and the Houston PCDC programs.

Social Competence and Juvenile Delinquency. In reviewing early childhood interventions as a preventive measure against juvenile delinquency, Zigler, Taussig, and Black (1992) study some of the same programs included in the reviews described above. They note that some early childhood intervention programs have lasting effects on social competence. Long-term evaluations are made in the Perry Preschool Project (Berrueta-Clement and others 1984, 1987), the Syracuse University Family Development Research Program (Lally, Mangione, and Honig 1988), the Yale Child Welfare Research Project (Provence and Naylor 1983; Seitz, Rosenbaum, and Apfel 1985), the Houston PCDC Program (Johnson and Walker 1987), the Rochester Nurse Home Visitation Program (Olds 1988), and the Gutelius Child Health Supervision Study (Gutelius and others 1972, 1977).

Positive effects on social competence from these programs include not engaging in delinquent behavior; fewer behavioral problems in children; better parental interaction with the children and more effective discipline; less aggressiveness and hostility, which are factors associated with later delinquency; and better surveillance by parents of their children's school performance, which contributes to better school adjustment for children.

All of the programs reviewed by Zigler, Taussig, and Black (1992) contain parental involvement, in most cases taking the form of parent education and support through home visits. The programs all sought to improve childrearing skills of parents, and the lasting benefits observed in children could be attributed to improved parenting. The programs also share continuity and comprehensiveness by targeting parents for change, which would continue over time and affect all areas of childrearing and a child's environment.

Finally, in reviewing prevention as offering cumulative protection from chronic delinquency, Yoshikawa (1994) recently studied twenty-two early education and family support intervention programs. Among the risk factors examined for chronic delinquency were a child's cognitive ability, early socioemotional development, school adjustment, parenting, family interaction, and socioeconomic status (SES).

Yoshikawa (1994) singles out some programs that show long-term reductions in antisocial behavior and affect multiple risk factors. The Perry Preschool Project (Berrueta-Clement and others 1984, 1987; Schweinhart and Weikart 1980; Schweinhart and others 1993) affected chronic delinquency, cognitive development, SES, and adult criminality. The Houston PCDC Program (Johnson and Walker 1987) affected parenting behavior, child cognitive development, and antisocial behavior in late childhood. The Syracuse University Family Development Research Program (Lally, Mangione, and Honig 1988) affected cognitive ability, early socioemotional competence, and chronic delinquency. The Yale Child Welfare Research Project (Seitz, Rosenbaum, and Apfel 1985) affected cognitive development, antisocial behavior in adolescence, and SES.

These four programs, which combined early childhood education with family support, were the most effective of the twenty-two reviewed. Yoshikawa (1994) notes that positive effects on a child's cognitive ability and on parenting preceded the long-term effects on delinquency; that is, the long-term effects were mediated by earlier effects on cognitive ability and parenting. Early childhood education programs (education given directly to a child) show principal effects on cognitive development and school achievement. Early family support programs (targeting parents and family) show principal effects on family variables such as parenting, maltreatment of children, attachment, and parents' educational attainment.

Overall, the results of the reviews discussed above indicate a number of beneficial outcomes for children and parents of early U.S. intervention projects targeting child development.

The Developing Countries' Experience

Most of the issues raised in U.S. research also apply to developing countries. However, obvious differences between the United States and these countries raise questions about generalizing U.S. findings to other sociocultural contexts (Woodhead 1985). Program variations and trends in developing countries are summarized below, and pertinent findings are reported.

Early childhood intervention lags behind in developing countries and shows great diversity in the services provided. Nevertheless, recent increases in available programs are notable, and the number of children in these programs is impressive. For example, childhood intervention programs in Brazil, Indonesia, and India serve millions of children. China provides preschool services to 16.3 million children, which is still a small percentage of its child population (Myers 1992).

Program Variations and Trends

As in industrialized countries, different types of intervention programs exist among developing countries. Some programs integrate health, nutrition, and early education such as the Integrated Child Development Services in India. Others are smaller-scale, experimental programs, involving mainly center-based enrichment or including home and community involvement. The quality of the different intervention programs varies considerably.

An important trend of intervention programs in developing countries is toward combining approaches that underlie different services for young children, women, and families. The Thai Nutrition Project (Kotchabhakdi and others 1987) is an example of an intervention program that integrated community-based primary health care, growth monitoring, supplementary food provision, and nutrition education with a psychosocial educational program. The education program sensitized mothers to the early development of sensation-perception in their infants, the value of early stimulation, and the importance of mother-child interaction. Other attempts to integrate services have sought to meet the intersecting needs of working women and children (Evans and Myers 1985).

In many developing countries, early childhood education programs follow the traditional Western pattern and are conceptualized in formal preschool terms. However, because preschools tend to be expensive, a limited number exist in developing countries, and they mainly serve urban, middle-class families who can afford to pay. Slowly, other models, such as the parent education and support model, are gaining favor and moving beyond urban centers. As new models are introduced, a growing number of reviews are emerging from developing countries.

Recent Reviews

Myers (1992) provides the most comprehensive review of intervention programs and their effects in several different countries. His findings on school adjustment and parent education are described below.

School Adjustment. Reviewing thirteen center-based educational interventions, Myers (1992) notes that six of them showed a difference in school promotion rates. For example, in Brazil only 9 percent of children receiving a nutrition and education intervention (The Preschool Feeding Program, PROAPE) repeated first grade, compared with 33 percent for a matched control group. Another study from Brazil showed a high rate (36 percent) of first-grade repetition for children who attended kindergarten, but it also showed a much higher rate (66 percent) for children in the control group.

Studies from Colombia showed higher gains from intervention among children in the most impoverished groups. In these groups, 60 percent of the intervention children reached the fourth grade, compared with only 30 percent of the children in the control group. The most impoverished groups in India and Argentina also benefited from intervention the most. In Argentina, 36 percent of the intervention children repeated the first grade, compared with 77 percent of the children in the comparison group. Also, in six of the nine studies from different countries with available information on school performance, children with early educational intervention performed better than children without.

Parent Education. Studies with a specific parent education component also had positive outcomes related to school. These studies are TEEP in Turkey (Kagitcibasi, Sunar, and Bekman 1988); Osorno (Parents and Children Project) in Chile (Richards 1985); and PROMESA in Colombia (Nimnicht and Posada 1986).

Myers (1992) also distinguishes home visiting and group approaches to parent education. The Israeli Home Instruction Program for Preschool Youngsters (HIPPY) (see Lombard 1981, this volume) and a Mexican national program of informal parent education organized at the community level are examples of the home visiting approach. Examples of group approaches to parent education are from Indonesia, China, Colombia, and Jamaica. Some of these examples and others are noted by Evans in this volume. Myers also gives several examples of child development services that are being integrated into existing community development programs.

Overall results from developing countries, although sparse, are encouraging because they show that early interventions can improve children's school performance, particularly for the most disadvantaged children. Early interventions appear to have positive effects despite unfavorable conditions in primary schools. Greater effects, particularly in the most impoverished areas, come from multifaceted programs that integrate nutrition and health with early education.

Summary of Findings

The above summary of intervention programs in the United States and developing countries suggests several general conclusions. These are noted below.

Multipurpose Programs Are More Effective. The more effective programs target both child education and parent education and support. Such multipurpose programs influence several factors, such as children's cognitive development, school adjustment, parenting, and family functioning. When promoted, these factors interact to mediate long-term, optimal development. As optimal development does not result from focusing only on children, the above interacting factors also create a contextual framework for parental involvement.

Parental Involvement is Crucial. To sustain children's growth and development, even in center-based programs, parents must be involved. Otherwise, when a program ends, children are left to rely on their own limited resources, and the immediate cognitive gains are not sustained (Kagitcibasi 1996). Optimal development requires parental involvement within a contextual framework. However, making such a framework operational raises questions of conceptualization and implementation, as noted below.

The Effectiveness of Home Visits Varies. In almost all cases, parent education takes the form of home visiting (an individual professional or paraprofessional visits a parent at home), and child education is defined as children receiving direct cognitive training at a center. Center-based and home-based approaches are compared on the basis of these particular conceptualizations and applications, and alternative types of parent education or various combinations of parent and child education typically are not considered.

Problems with home visiting could explain some of the findings reviewed by Farran (1990) that showed a low level of effectiveness on cognitive development. For example, regular home visiting may become an imposition and may undermine the authority of parents in their own home (Ball 1994). This negative effect could result if the goals of the home intervention program and family goals do not agree and if the home visitor is not well accepted. Clearly stated health goals shared by parents may be one reason that health outcomes are more pronounced than cognitive outcomes in home visiting (Wasik and others 1990).

Another problem with home visiting may be that home visitors can apply their own versions of the curriculum, or particularly in the case of paraprofessionals, they may not have a high level of expertise. Finally, home visiting involves working with single individuals; its effectiveness and cost-effectiveness may be limited without the facilitative effects of groups and other support systems.

Despite conceptual problems and possible limitations, home visits are effective in family support programs, as discussed above. Generally, home visits are more effective for family and parent support than for children's cognitive development, although there are exceptions. The model of a parent as teacher, if implemented solely through home visits, also may not produce optimal results because uneducated parents may be poor teachers (Eldering and Vedder 1993). This problem may be difficult to solve with a single home visitor, but it possibly could be helped through more effective feedback, which could be provided in group discussions.

Quality of Implementation Affects Outcomes. A more general implementation issue is how well a particular approach or program actually is applied in the field. Although obviously important, implementation often is less than adequate. As concluded from the reviews, generally programs are more effective with better implementation, including careful planning, intensive training and supervising of trainers, intensive application, availability of good materials, good rapport between parents and intervention implementers, and high level of participation from parents.

Conclusions regarding the effectiveness of a type of intervention (for example, child-focused in contrast to caregiver-focused) are based on program results. However, the effect of a program may have more to do with the quality of implementation than with the curriculum used (Zigler and Weiss 1985). Schweinhart (this volume) identifies and describes seven elements of quality for early childhood programs.

Variations in implementation may result in different outcomes for programs using the same content and approach. For example, HIPPY (Lombard 1981, this volume) achieved good results in Israel and Turkey; however, its effect with ethnic groups in the Netherlands was negligible (Eldering and Fedder 1993). The different outcomes resulted partly from implementation problems with ethnic minorities in the Netherlands, such as high attrition rates and language problems.

To apply the lessons from this overview of the effects of intervention programs in the United States and developing countries, TEEP is explained below. This Turkish intervention is an example of an early child development program with a broad focus. It is multifaceted, involves both education and family support, targets children and parents within the context of family and community, and addresses the relative effects of center- and home-based interventions. This example capsulizes the important elements of an intervention program targeting early child development and parent education.

Case Study: TEEP

The Turkish Early Enrichment Project comprises two studies spanning a period of 10 years (1982-92). The original study (Study I) was a 4-year intervention project in the low-income areas of Istanbul. The follow-up study (Study II) was carried out 6 years after completion of the original study and 7 years after completion of the intervention (Kagitcibasi, Sunar, and Bekman 1988; Kagitcibasi 1991, 1993, 1996; Bekman 1990, 1993). Study I was funded by the International Development Research Centre; Study II was funded by MEAwards Program of the Population Council.

Study I

Study I examined the relative effectiveness of early enrichment through home- and community-based parent education and center-based child education. In the first year of the study, extensive assessments were made of the cognitive, social, and emotional development of 280 children ages 3 and 5. The childrearing orientations, lifestyles, self-concepts, and world views of mothers also were studied along with the home environments. Baselines were established through direct testing of children, observations of children and mother-child interactions, and interviews with mothers.

Study Design

Two-thirds of the children attended childcare centers attached to factories where their mothers were employed as semiskilled or unskilled workers. One-half of the day-care centers were educational, and one-half were custodial. One-third of the children had nonworking mothers from homes in the same neighborhoods. These children were not attending a childcare center. Each context (educational day care, custodial day care, and home care) included 3- and 5-year-old children. Because children were not assigned randomly to the three contexts, this aspect of the study had a quasi-experimental design.

At the beginning of the second year, children from each context and their mothers were assigned randomly to experimental and control groups. In the second and third years of the project, the experimental group of mothers received project intervention (mother training). This aspect of the study used an experimental design. The overall study had a factorial design: two (mother training and no mother training) by two (ages 3 and 5) by three (educational, custodial, or home care).

In the fourth year, children and mothers were reassessed to establish pre- and postintervention differences between the experimental and control groups. Almost all of the first-year measures were repeated, except those rendered inappropriate by the increased ages of the children (7 and 9). Children's school achievement and attitudes toward school also were examined. During the 4 years of the project, the attrition rate was about 10 percent, lowering the number of total mother-child pairs to 255. Most attrition occurred in the first year of the intervention.

Study Intervention

The intervention introduced by TEEP was home- and community-based mother training. It had two components, cognitive training and mother support, which were designed to support the cognitive and socioemotional development of the child, respectively.

The Cognitive Training Program was HIPPY, developed by Lombard (1981, this volume). Mothers received training through a network of paraprofessional field workers alternating weeks at home or in group settings at a community center or the workplace. The mothers then worked on the cognitive materials with their children at home, assuming the role of a trainer with their children. Cognitive materials, in the form of weekly worksheets and study books, focused on preliteracy and prenumeracy skills and age-appropriate cognitive enrichment activities (including discrimination, generalization, concept formation, problem solving, verbal comprehension and expression, and word knowledge).

Most of the mothers had only a primary school education of 5 years or less. The trainers (group leaders) had at least a high school education and were trained by the research team. Mothers' aides, at the same low educational level and SES as the mothers, were trained by group leaders to help mothers mainly with home administration of the cognitive enrichment program.

The Mother Support Program was conducted in biweekly group discussion sessions. Topics ranged from health and nutrition to psychological needs of children, discipline, and communicating with the child. Sessions also focused on mothers' needs, expressing feelings, and communicating feelings to others. The goal was to support mothers and sensitize them to their children's development, empowering the mothers to cope with problems better. A special effort also was made to render the program culturally sensitive. For example, existing close family ties and "relatedness values" (Kagitcibasi 1990) were reinforced while introducing a new element, autonomy, to childrearing.

Techniques for group dynamics were used, often involving group decisionmaking about modifications to parenting behaviors. The contextual-interactional approach of the study capitalized on the effectiveness of community-based groups as a modified version of culturally familiar women's groups (Aswad 1974; Kiray 1981; Olson 1992).

Study Results

All TEEP results summarized in this chapter are statistically significant. More detailed analyses and results are available elsewhere (Kagitcibasi, Sunar, and Bekman 1988; Bekman 1990; Kagitcibasi 1991, 1993, 1996).

Fourth-year results of the project intervention (mother training) showed that intervention had positive effects on children's overall development and school achievement, as well as positive effects on mothers. On most of the cognitive measures [the Stanford-Binet Test, the Analytical Triad and Block Design of Wechsler Preschool and Primary Scale of Intelligence (WIPPSI), Piaget tasks, and achievement tests] children in the experimental group, with mothers participating in the training program, surpassed children in the control group. The former group also manifested better school adjustment and achievement than the latter. In socioemotional development, the children in the experimental group demonstrated less aggressiveness, more autonomy, and better emotional state than children in the control group (Kagitcibasi, Sunar, and Bekman 1988; Kagitcibasi 1991, 1993, 1996).

As for effects of the three contexts, children in educational day care surpassed children in custodial day-care and home-care groups on most cognitive measures and in school adjustment and achievement. Children attending educational day care whose mothers were trained consistently performed the best on virtually every measure. However, an interaction effect was not found, suggesting that the effects of mother training and educational day care were additive; there may have been a ceiling effect for children in the educational day-care group because their level of cognitive functioning was initially higher. Children cared for at home were more dependent and exhibited more emotional problems than day-care children. Overall, the results clearly showed the positive effects of mother training and educational day care through the third grade (for the older cohort).

Training also had notable effects on the mothers. In terms of orientation toward their children, trained mothers manifested greater satisfaction and better interaction with their children (more responsiveness, more supportiveness, and higher levels of verbalization) and higher educational aspirations and expectations for their children than untrained mothers. These orientations toward the children were assessed by interviewing the mothers and by observing mother-child interactions on the Hess and Shipman structured problem-solving task (Shipman and others 1977).

In terms of direct effects, trained mothers, compared with mothers in the control group, enjoyed a more equitable intrafamily status relative to their husbands in terms of having more interspousal communication, role sharing, and joint decisionmaking; and had a more positive outlook on life.

The fourth-year findings of TEEP indicated the beginning of a positive cycle, demonstrated by better school adjustment and achievement of children in the experimental group and by trained mothers' greater satisfaction with their children and higher educational aspirations and expectations for them. The general childrearing orientation and interaction style of trained mothers with their children also were more conducive to the children's overall development and success. Study II was done to assess whether this positive trend would continue.

Study II

For this follow-up study to test the long-term effects of the project intervention (mother training), 225 of the original 255 families were found, and 217 of them agreed to participate. Extensive interviews were conducted with mothers and children, who were now adolescents, and fathers were interviewed as well. Complete school records of the adolescents were obtained, and students were given the vocabulary subtest of the Wechsler's Intelligence Scale for Children-Revised (WISC-R), standardized in Turkey with Turkish word counts and urban low-SES norms (Savasir and Sahin 1988). Long-term effects were assessed for adolescents' cognitive development and school performance, academic orientation, socioemotional development and social integration, and perceptions of their mothers; parents' perceptions and academic orientation also were assessed.

Cognitive Development and School Performance

In Turkey where compulsory schooling is only for 5 years, attainment of education beyond primary school is a most important indicator of positive orientation toward education among adolescents in low-income areas. Because of economic pressures, unmotivated children or those who are unsuccessful in school tend to leave after primary school. For this crucial, objective indicator of educational attainment, a significant difference was found between adolescents in the experimental group and the control group; 86 percent of the former, compared with 67 percent of the latter, were still in school (x^2=9.57; p=0.002). This finding is probably the most important long-term effect of TEEP's early intervention.

For a second objective indicator, primary school academic performance, a significant difference was found between adolescents in the experimental group and the control group. Based on report card grades throughout 5 years, the trained children surpassed children in the control group on the Turkish language (t=3.08; p=0.001), mathematics (t=3.01; p=0.001), and overall academic average (t=2.82; p=0.002). Five years of better school performance must have contributed to the higher level of school attainment among adolescents in the experimental group. Differences between the two groups in school achievement beyond primary school are not significant. This finding is largely because of the self-selection factor in the control group; less successful students tend to drop out after the compulsory primary school, and better ones continue. A better primary school experience seems to pave the way toward higher educational achievement and more years of schooling.

Finally, as an indicator of cognitive performance, the WISC-R vocabulary scores also showed the superiority of adolescents in the experimental group over those in the control group (F=4.63; df=2, 216; p=0.03). This finding is important in view of research showing social class differences in vocabulary (Kagitcibasi and Savasir 1988; Bernstein 1974; Laosa 1984; Leseman 1993; Savasir, Sezgin, and Erol 1992). The finding shows that early enrichment, if successful, can have long-term effects, counteracting the adverse effects of low SES.

As for the long-term effects of context (educational day care, custodial day care, and home care), no significant difference in educational achievement was found among the three groups. Context did not relate to school grades, but children in the custodial group had more retentions in grade (failed one or more school years) than the other two groups (F=4.69; df=2, 216; p=0.0l). Class grades do not reflect retentions because the grade of the year failed is deleted. Context made a significant difference in the WISC-R vocabulary test (F=4.78; df=2, 216; p=0.009); children in the educational group scored the highest, followed by children in the custodial group. An interaction effect was obtained, showing that the project intervention (mother training) made a greater difference for children in the custodial day-care and home-care groups than for those in the more advantaged, educational day-care group; the latter group may have experienced a ceiling effect.

Several subjective indicators of development and school performance among adolescents were based on interviews and indicate positive, long-term effects of early intervention. Indicators for adolescents included their academic orientation and self-concept, social adjustment, retrospective perception of mothers, and current perception of families. Indicators for parents included their perceptions of the above adolescent characteristics, relationships with the family, and academic orientation regarding their children.

Academic Orientation
Adolescents in the experimental group, compared with those in the control group, were more pleased with their school success and thought that their teachers also were pleased with them. They felt that they could be the best student in the class if they studied hard. Their parents also had positive perceptions. Their fathers perceived them as more motivated to succeed in school, and their mothers perceived them as actually having greater school success. External pressure or negative reasons for going to school, such as having nothing better to do or following parents' wishes, were endorsed more by adolescents in the control group. Those in the experimental group, compared with the control group, felt that they were prepared for starting school, that preparation helped, and that it helped for a longer period. This difference shows the perceived importance of the project intervention (mother training) because two-thirds of adolescents in both the experimental and control groups had been in day care.

A negative effect of custodial day care was found on adolescent academic orientation. The custodial group adolescents perceived their parents and their teachers as less pleased with their school performance than did adolescents in the educational day-care and home-care groups. Compared with the day-care groups, children receiving home care were much less likely to think that they had been prepared well for school.

Socioemotional Development and Social Integration
Adolescents in the experimental group manifested more autonomy than those in the control group, which was shown by making their own decisions (t=1.73; p=0.045), and exhibited better social integration, which was shown by their ideas being accepted by their friends (t=2.06; p=0.02). Most of the adolescents in both groups have intact families, and trouble with the law is rare. The few (6 percent) who had such a problem all were from the control group. These findings indicate better social adjustment and greater autonomy for adolescents whose mothers had been trained.

The negative effects of custodial day care are again found. Adolescents in the custodial day-care group rated themselves as less intelligent than their classmates (F=3.68; df=2, 214; p=0.027) and had a near-significant tendency to exhibit less confidence in their ability to cope with difficult situations (F=2.4; df=2.214; p=0.09). Six of the eight adolescents who had been in trouble with the law were from this group; the other two received home care. Although the numbers are too small for statistical significance, the pattern is suggestive.

Retrospective Perceptions
The retrospective perception that adolescents had of their mothers indicates the accomplishments of the Mother Support Program. The adolescents whose mothers had

been trained remembered their mothers as more nurturant and more responsive than adolescents in the control group remembered theirs. Specifically, adolescents whose mothers had been trained perceived retrospectively that their mothers talked with them, consoled them, were interested in them more, and spanked them less than adolescents in the control group remembered. These childhood experiences show that trained mothers manifested a different style of parenting. This experience probably was the key difference between the environments of children in the experimental and control groups.

Parents' Perceptions and Academic Orientation

Results of the mother and father interviews further substantiate findings obtained from the adolescents. The results imply that changes in the mothers brought about changes in the family's emotional atmosphere and family relations. Parents from the experimental group reported better parent-child communication, better adjustment of the child in the family, less physical punishment, and closer, better general family relations. The intrafamily status of trained women relative to their husbands also was higher than that of nontrained women.

Parents in the experimental group, in contrast to the control group, showed higher educational expectations for their children, were more interested in what was going on in school, and provided more help with homework and more environmental stimulation. Families with trained mothers better supported children's role as students.

Summary

TEEP shows impressive short- and long-term effects of early enrichment through parent education on children, parents, and the family. Subjective and spontaneous reports of parents from TEEP and the current Mother-Child Education Program (MOCEP) confirm the study assessments. Sometimes mothers write letters to their group leaders after the program ends; a number of these letters are translated and printed in the Mother-Child Education Foundation (MOCEF) Newsletter #3, 1995. MOCEP and MOCEF are outgrowths of TEEP described later in this chapter.

Implications of TEEP Findings

The short- and long-term findings of TEEP show the relative effectiveness of early enrichment through home- and community-based parent education (mother training) and center-based child education. Both approaches were found effective in the fourth year. However, the follow-up study showed that more gains are sustained from mother training than from educational day care. Gains were sustained in school attainment, school achievement, academic orientation, socioemotional development, and social adjustment and integration. In the vocabulary measure, which indicated long-term main effects for both mother training and day-care context (educational day-care children surpassed custodial and home-care groups), children with trained mothers in custodial and home-care groups performed better than children with untrained mothers.

The difference between short- and long-term effects is important. Although a higher-quality educational day care might have produced a broader range of long-term effects, the educational day-care centers studied in TEEP were of sufficiently good quality to produce substantial short-term effects when compared with the other two contexts (custodial day care and home care). Also, expecting excellent quality in large-scale day care may not be realistic for developing countries; TEEP used the highest-quality educational day-care centers serving children of the working classes in Istanbul.

Long-term findings of TEEP also showed that far from being beneficial, custodial care can even be detrimental. This relative ineffectiveness of custodial care is cause for concern because, too often, day care for children of the poor, especially in developing countries, tends to be custodial (Bekman 1993).

Long-term findings of TEEP further show that early enrichment through parent education is a more viable model than center-based, direct child training. For sustained development, improving and supporting a child's environment, using an ecological or contextual approach, is better than only focusing on children because a supportive home environment gives a child necessary care and cognitive stimulation after the enrichment program ends. Immediate gains from an enrichment program cannot be sustained if the home environment is not improved because children are left to their own limited resources.

The policy implications of this finding on the relationship between home environment and sustained gains from intervention are clear. In impoverished areas of developing countries, where home environments do not provide children with adequate cognitive stimulation, parent education to improve these environments is necessary to sustain long-term developmental results. In socioeconomic areas where homes provide enriched environments for young children, center-based education can produce optimal results. A recent example from Sweden showed the long-term positive effects of early day care (Andersson 1992). This conclusion also is compatible with the results of successful programs in the United States and developing countries reviewed earlier that show long-term effects from center-based interventions that include some level of parental involvement. Indeed, Zigler and Styfco (1994) note that successful programs, even if they begin by focusing directly on children, evolve into programs affecting two and even three generations.

From Project to Program

Since the completion of TEEP, the similar MOCEP (Mother-Child Education Program) has been devised and applied in many contexts with many groups in Turkey. A new Cognitive Training Program has been developed for MOCEP, replacing HIPPY. The new program lasts 25 weeks, concentrating on the year before school entry. The program has discarded home visits and adopted a complete group orientation, with weekly rather than fortnightly group meetings, to conduct cognitive training and the Mother Support Program.

These adjustments made the program shorter and less costly but did not decrease quality. Now well-trained, more educated group leaders provide training rather than depending on less-educated mothers' aides to conduct training in home visits that alternated weekly with group meetings before. Also, the program is using fully the facilitating effects of group processes. Recent evaluation studies, one with mothers and two with children (Aycicegi 1993; Ercan 1993; Aksu-Koc and Kuscul 1994), show significant benefits from the program; a more comprehensive evaluation is under way.

MOCEP now is conducted in cooperation with the Turkish Ministry of Education. The United Nations Children's Fund and other local groups have cooperated. The ministry's adult education teachers are trained as group leaders and lead groups at adult education centers. The program has expanded tremendously, serving 10,320 mothers and children in twenty-three provinces throughout the country during the 1995-96 school year. From its inception until 1993, the program served 1,500 mothers and children, and from 1993 to the present, it has served a total of 18,490 mothers and children. This growth was made possible by the establishment of MOCEF in 1993, which operates the program in collaboration with the ministry, and by allocation of World Bank project funds to MOCEF through the ministry.

Absolute costs are minimal because adult education teachers are group leaders, which usually entails only upgrading and optimizing use of already existing personnel and facilities. MOCEF conducts training, provides materials, and ensures continued quality by closely supervising and regularly upgrading teachers and materials. Good implementation is considered top priority.

TEEP and the applications deriving from it have influenced educational policy in Turkey. Early childhood education formerly was conceived solely in center-based terms as preschools, and now a multipurpose, informal education model that includes parent education and early childhood education is accepted as a viable and more cost-effective alternative.

Essential Ingredients of Parent Education and Child Development Interventions

The parent education and child development program used in Turkey today (MOCEP) benefited greatly from the research and lessons of TEEP. The following seven essential ingredients of TEEP and MOCEP discussed below provide a basis for other successful parent education and child development programs:

- Whole Child Approach
- Contextual Approach
- Multiple Goals
- Empowerment
- Sharing Goals
- Optimal Timing
- Cost-effectiveness.

Whole Child Approach

TEEP and MOCEP targeted support to a child's overall development, including cognitive, language, socioemotional, and life skills development. This approach is crucial because human development is an integrated process, and attending to only one aspect of the process does not promote optimal development. The common emphasis put on cognitive development, therefore, remains limited because other aspects of child development are not supported. For example, children with low levels of self-concept and motivation will achieve at a level below their cognitive capacity. Also, cognitive and general psychosocial development are bound intricately with physical growth, nutrition, and health. A great deal of research findings substantiate this bond. The strong synergy and interdependence of different spheres of child development render ineffective any approach that is not holistic.

The importance of a whole child approach is generally agreed on, and no one questions its validity. The problem, however, is not with proving its validity, but with realizing it. At times the whole child approach receives only inadequate attention because it requires an interdisciplinary and multivariate approach in research and applications.

TEEP realized a whole child approach by attending to children's socioemotional development as well as cognitive and language development. TEEP also assessed physical development and health, but they were not included in the intervention because all children were at adequate levels. Current applications of MOCEP integrate health (including mothers' health and family planning), hygiene, and nutrition into the Mother Support Program in addition to cognitive, language, and socioemotional development.

Contextual Approach

Known also as an ecological approach (Bronfenbrenner 1974, 1979), the contextual approach targets a person in context, or in interaction with others. This approach is at the core of TEEP and MOCEP. The weight of the evidence reviewed in this chapter and the long-term findings of TEEP indicate that a contextual, holistic approach to child development interventions that involves parent education is more effective than an approach focused on the individual.

TEEP and MOCEP use the contextual approach on two levels. The first level is working on the mother and the mother-child interaction to promote overall child development, and this chapter has addressed the benefits of this level. The second level is working through the group context to support mothers.

The facilitating and supportive function of groups effectively promotes attitude and behavior change. In a sociocultural context characterized by close-knit human relations and women's support networks, an approach that is sensitive to culture favors community-based women's groups (Aswad 1974; Benedict 1974; Kiray 1981; Olson 1982). This approach is not unique to Turkey or to a non-Western context; it can be the case in Western societies as well. For example, Slaughter (1983) claims that group discussion is an intervention approach more culturally consonant than individual home visits for low-income black mothers in the United States. Capitalizing on groups as support mechanisms and agents of change makes sense in any culture of relatedness (Kagitcibasi 1990, 1996) with closely knit human bonds, which includes most developing countries.

Regularly meeting, small groups facilitate attitude and behavior change because individuals are active participants and they identify with the group, internalizing its norms. The pressure and responsibility they feel to carry out group decisions result in change that is difficult to achieve through lectures and other information dissemination techniques where recipients are passive. Furthermore, because members feel group support even when they are at home, they are empowered to resist possible opposition better than if they were alone carrying out their own individual decisions. The facilitating and supportive function of groups appears to underlie sustained group effects. Much social psychological research on group dynamics since Lewin's pioneering work (1951, 1958) gives scientific evidence for this function of groups.

Finally, group training is more cost effective than individual training (for example in home visits). In terms of investing time and personnel, the group setting is more economical than targeting individuals.

Multiple Goals

A program with multiple goals and targets that successfully achieves the goals and reaches its targets accomplishes more than a program with one goal and one target can accomplish with the same investment. The former program is not only more cost effective, but also more likely to have greater overall outcomes because of interaction and mutual reinforcement of the different goals and targets. Growth from interaction and mutual reinforcement can be expected in a contextual approach with a systemic perspective. For example, change in one element (target of intervention) of the family system (such as the mother) leads to changes in other elements of the family system (such as the father and children).

All the evidence reviewed in this chapter shows that programs targeting children, parents, and the family have greater effects than those focusing solely on children. All three models described earlier, the parent therapy model, the parent training model, and the parent-child interaction model (Marfo and Kysela 1985), can be pursued in the same intervention. Similarly, the cognitively oriented (childhood) educational model and the family support model of intervention (Seitz 1990; Yoshikawa 1994) can be integrated successfully.

TEEP is an example of an integrated program, and its short- and long-term positive effects indicate the viability of a multipurpose approach. Deriving from TEEP, the expanding MOCEP is a multipurpose, informal education program, combining adult education and early child development. Its multiple goals for the mother include education and support in parenting, family planning, and reproductive health; development of communication skills; and building a sense of well-being, efficacy, coping skills, and empowerment. Multiple goals for the children include cognitive enrichment (school readiness), more optimal psychosocial development, and better health and nutrition.

Empowerment

Another essential ingredient of a good parent education program is empowerment rather than compensation for deficiency. Subscribing to an empowerment rather than a deficiency model does not imply that existing conditions are optimal for child development. Optimal conditions would need no intervention. The intervention of an empowerment model builds on existing strengths to change the conditions and promote optimal development. Empowerment strengthens what is adaptive in order to change what is maladaptive. TEEP used active group participation and decisionmaking to capitalize on the existing capacity and knowledge of mothers.

As a specific example, TEEP and MOCEP changed the conceptualization of a mother's role through empowerment. The commonly held definition of parenting among lower-SES groups involves loving and caring for children but not preparing them for school; this definition contrasts with middle-class views of parenting, which include preparing children for school (Kagitcibasi 1996). TEEP introduced the latter, more comprehensive definition, which was shown by a great deal of research to be more favorable for a child's school readiness (Coll 1990; Goodnow 1988; LeVine and White 1986; Slaughter 1988). In fact, parents assume the role of teacher in cognitively oriented, parent-focused interventions. Mothers in TEEP were empowered to take this self-enhancing role despite their low levels of formal education. The same approach is used in current applications of MOCEP.

Sharing Goals

An intervention program that shares the goals of parents will be more successful than one that does not take family goals into consideration. For example, although lower-SES and less-educated parents do not see themselves as contributors to a child's school readiness, they are interested in the schooling of their children as well as in their health and overall well-being. A program whose goal is to enhance children's school readiness as well as their overall development can reach parents without much difficulty if the goal is made very clear. Because parents share the goal of the intervention program, the program has greater likelihood of success than one seen by parents as an outside imposition. A program with shared goals also can reach parents to accomplish other goals, such as building positive attitudes and behavior toward family planning.

When goals are shared, parents can become partners instead of passive recipients. Schorr (1991) notes that successful programs emphasize the importance of relationships with recipients in a flexible structure with a coherent, integrated broad spectrum of services that are adapted to the needs of the people they serve.

Optimal Timing

Another essential ingredient of a good parent education program is optimal timing. Important questions for conceptualization and implementation of an intervention are how early it should start and what its duration should be. In general, it is assumed that the earlier an intervention starts and the longer it lasts, the better it will be. However, this generalization may not apply to all types of interventions with different goals and targets. For example, a later preschool intervention that also covers primary school years may be more effective than an early preschool intervention (Farran 1990), and later intervention may produce more optimal results than early (infant) intervention (Yoshikawa 1994). When health and nutrition goals are important, especially with young primiparous mothers of low education, intervening during pregnancy is required; however, a later starting date would be more reasonable for school preparation.

The right timing involves not only how early the intervention should start, but also when the target is most receptive to intervention. For example Brazelton (1982) talks about touchpoints, or times when parents are most receptive to new information, such as during pregnancy and just after birth. For a program with educational goals, the time before school may be a touchpoint.

MOCEP uses the year before school entry as the period of intervention. The initial TEEP intervention lasted for 2 years before school; however, afterward it was condensed to a 1-year program and is now applied during the year before school entry. Because a 1-year program is less demanding of mothers' time and commitment, more mothers can be reached. Also the year just before school is more of a touchpoint than 2 years before. The condensed and more intensive version of MOCEP appears to be as effective as the longer version.

Finally, shorter programs are more economical than longer ones, especially if they accomplish the same goals in a shorter period. A cost-effective program achieves the purpose of the intervention, and this requires optimal timing and duration of the intervention as well as shared goals.

Cost-effectiveness

Cost-effectiveness is a final essential ingredient of a good parent education program as seen in TEEP and MOCEP. Indeed, cost-effectiveness is an important consideration for any early child development intervention, as noted by van der Gaag and Barnett in this volume.

A number of factors already discussed contribute to a program's cost-effectiveness: multiple goals (for example, children's cognitive development, parental self-enhancement and empowerment, family planning, and family functioning); multiple targets (children, parents, and families); group rather than individual (home visiting) approaches to educating parents; and timely, optimal duration. All of these factors make TEEP and MOCEP more cost-effective because a single investment has multiple effects.

Other factors that make TEEP and MOCEP economical include using existing personnel (teachers) and facilities. In general, informal home- or community-based programs that employ paraprofessionals, volunteers, and parents tend to be less costly than formal, center-based preschool programs that employ professionals. Informal programs are more cost effective and usually involve a broader provision of services (such as health, nutrition, and education) than costly formal programs, which focus mainly on education.

Cost-effectiveness is a relative, not an absolute, concept. For example, an inexpensive program can be expensive in absolute costs if it does not produce results, making a more expensive program with long-range benefits more cost effective. Although the cost-effectiveness of TEEP has not been analyzed, the program exemplifies a multipurpose, informal education model with multiple targets and sustained benefits, and it appears to be a good investment. As has already been demonstrated, TEEP does have great potential for expansion. Myers (1992: 121) notes that "parent education for early childhood development is the most feasible low-cost approach to programming on a large scale."

Evaluation Issues and Planning Elements That Require Attention

The essential ingredients of parent education and child development interventions identified above apply to the implementation of interventions as well as the planning and evaluation of interventions. Experience with TEEP and MOCEP suggests several issues and elements that deserve particular attention when evaluating existing programs and designing new interventions. These issues and elements are addressed below. Related issues pertaining to quality are addressed by Schweinhart in this volume.

Evaluation Issues

Evaluation of early child development programs raises several conceptual and methodological issues. These pertain to a child's overall development, the child in context, short- vs. long-term effects, evaluating process as well as outcome, and evaluation measures.

The Whole Child in Context. Two issues in evaluating early childhood intervention programs, already discussed in this chapter, are conceptualizing and measuring child development only in cognitive terms and focusing on a child out of context (Kagitcibasi 1996). Exclusively evaluating IQ gains diverts attention from other possible developmental benefits of intervention programs; cognitive development is only one aspect of overall child development, and the different spheres of development are interdependent. Intervention, and evaluation, therefore require a whole child approach. Also, an intervention should not focus on children out of context but should support a child's immediate social environment. Evaluation, therefore, must focus not only on the child, but on the relationship between a child and its context as well as the context itself (parents, family).

Short- vs. Long-Term Effects. A third issue in evaluating intervention research and programs is the timing of the evaluation. Because human development is a continuous process, knowing when to measure an effect is difficult. Although short-term effects typically are measured, they do not establish sustainability. Also, long-term effects can be stronger than short-term ones, as seen in the Yale Child Welfare Research Project (Seitz and Provence 1990) and TEEP. Although difficult, long-term effects should be evaluated whenever possible.

In summarizing these three important issues in properly evaluating an intervention program or model, the long-term impact on more than one target (child, parent, family) must be studied in more than one sphere of functioning (health, cognitive development, socioemotional development, school adjustment, school performance, school attainment, parenting, parental self-concept and world view, family interaction). If reliable long-term gains are found in several spheres, the approach and the program can be candidates for serious consideration, replication, expansion, and possibly adoption in other similar contexts. TEEP has fared well in short- and long-term evaluations comparing center- and home/community-based interventions.

Process Evaluation. In addition to its outcomes, a program may be evaluated by its process. Process evaluation focuses on actual implementation of the program. As noted earlier, the quality of implementation is important for the eventual outcome of a program. If implemented improperly, even a good program will fail.

Evaluation Measures. The conceptualization and methodology of program evaluations are dictated by program goals. Several indicators for desired outcomes must be established along with specific assessment criteria. For example, TEEP used psychometric tests, Piaget tasks, and achievement tests for cognitive development criteria. School-related criteria in long-term evaluation included objective measures of school attainment, school achievement, and adjustment as well as subjective measures of attitudes toward education.

Measures with single criterion are methodologically weak because they are vulnerable to statistical artifacts such as ceiling effects and regression toward the mean in repeated testing. Therefore, several criteria are best, and *multifaceted assessment* is necessary. *Objective outcome measures* should be used as much as possible to avoid the vulnerability that self-report measures have to subjectivity and social desirability. However, subjective measures can be useful; they add a richness, reflecting real subjective experience, that is lacking in objective outcome measures. Still, as less robust measures, they should supplement more robust objective indicators rather than be used alone. Also, all evaluations should use *culturally sensitive measures*. In evaluating programs in developing countries, measures imported from the West must be used carefully. Culturally sensitive measures are an important methodological issue in cross-cultural assessment of all kinds, not just evaluation research. A general principle is to use a measurement that makes sense in the context where it is applied.

Planning Elements That Require Attention

Several important elements generally have not been included adequately in planning or refining parent education and early child development interventions. By giving closer attention to untapped resources (such as the media), well-defined goals, standards of quality, characteristics of specific contexts, and economic dimensions, the success of these interventions can be enhanced.

Untapped Resources (Media). Valuable resources remain untapped or underused even though their potential importance is accepted. The mass media (television, radio, and the printed press) is an example of an untapped resource whose effective use for information dissemination and communication can have far-reaching consequences. Using the media to strengthen demand and awareness for early childcare and development has already been highlighted by Evans in this volume as a key programming strategy.

Communication through the media can target caregivers, families, and children. However, because exposure to the media is voluntary and depends on the inherent attractiveness of the medium or message, there are no captive audiences; effectiveness is contingent on self-initiated exposure. To be effective, the information communicated must be made interesting rather than didactic.

The Sesame Street program is a prime example of effective use of the media. It has been shown in more than 100 countries. A wide-scale study of its effects in Turkey (Sahin 1989) showed a gain in cognitive development of about 1 year among 5-year-old children as a result of regular exposure to the Turkish Sesame Street program.

Effective use of the media also can be highly beneficial to parent education. This use requires good planning; for example, media appeal can enhance an education program that includes discussion of media material in community groups. Myers (1992) provides several examples of successful programs that use the media, including the printed press, for parent education in developing countries.

Well-defined Goals. Another element that has not figured adequately into the planning of parent education is well-defined goals. Program goals should include a statement of desired outcomes and criteria for assessing these outcomes. Without such well-defined goals, evaluating the worth of a program or approach to child development is impossible. Furthermore, goals should be realistic and achievable, and the time allotted for achieving them should be specified.

Standards of Quality. The debate continues on standards of quality. The two main contrasting views are the relativistic and universalistic perspectives. As shown earlier, cultural context needs to be taken into consideration when setting goals and targets, and programs should be culturally and ecologically sensitive. If the targeted skills and orientations are not functional or acceptable in a cultural context, they should not be imposed from the outside. However, the limits within which cultural norms apply and where universal standards start is an unresolved issue (Kagitcibasi 1996).

An example of the limits of cultural relativism in the face of changing environmental demands is the social change occurring in every country that is undergoing an unprecedented movement of people from traditional rural areas to urban environments. Urban living conditions, in particular schooling, require certain common orientations and cognitive skills that call for universal standards. Yet, universal standards should not be imposed from outside. The standards of quality must be developed jointly by educators and the parents and families who are partners in the education process, taking into account the requirements of their changing life-styles. These standards also should be applied to preparing children for schools and preparing schools for children (Myers 1992). For further discussion of the elements of quality, see the chapter by Schweinhart in this volume.

Characteristics of Specific Contexts. All planning for parent education must include the characteristics of specific contexts. Major differences in contexts should be taken into consideration particularly when transferring programs and materials from one context to another. This attention is especially important when adapting programs from an industrial country to the context of a developing country. With recent advances in applications in some developing countries, it may be profitable for these countries to develop networks among themselves and to learn from each other's experiences rather than depending entirely on input from industrial countries with less similar cultural contexts.

Economic Dimensions of Programming. Finally, economic dimensions of programming often are not incorporated adequately into the planning of parent education. Cost-effectiveness is an essential ingredient of a successful program and is crucial for turning projects into large-scale programs. The economic aspects of programs cannot be ignored, particularly in developing countries. Although calculating cost-effectiveness exactly is not easy, the costs of many projects and programs can be analyzed to inform policies. Economics must be integrated into program plans and applications if programs are to be expanded (see also van der Gaag and Barnett, this volume).

Conclusion

The best investments in early child development and parent education appear to be programs with multiple outcomes (cognitive and socioemotional development; better school adjustment, performance, and attainment; better social adjustment; better parenting; increased women's status; and better spousal relations and family interactions) and multiple beneficiaries (children, parents, and families). The short- and long-term results of TEEP include all of these outcomes. Particularly in developing countries, such multipurpose approaches to parent education and early child enrichment promise to contribute to the societies' human potential.

Long-term results of TEEP show that investing in parent education results in sustained gains in children's attainment that pave the way for eventual, significant improvement in the development of human capital. A parent education program that integrates a contextual approach with multiple goals and multiple targets, empowerment, shared goals, proper timing, and cost-effectiveness can benefit parents and children in mutual interaction. This interaction sets off a dynamic positive cycle that can be self-sustaining over time, rendering such an approach worthy of investment. Programs like TEEP and MOCEP should be supported widely to reach a large number of families because they promote the development of human capital in socioeconomic contexts where it is needed most.

References

Aksu-Koc, A., and H. O. Kuscul. 1994. Turkish Middle and Working Class Homes as Preliteracy Environments and the Effects of Home Enrichment on Literacy Skills. Paper presented at the AERA Conference, New Orleans, April 4-8, 1994.

Andersson, B. E. 1992. Effects of Day-care on Cognitive and Socioemotional Competence of 13-Year-old Swedish Schoolchildren. *Child Development* 63:20-36.

Andrews, S. R., J. B. Blumenthal, D. L. Johnson, A. J. Kahn, C. J. Ferguson, T. M. Lasater, P. E. Malone, and D. B. Wallace. 1982. The Skills of Mothering: A Study of Parent-Child Development Centers. *Monographs of the Society for Research in Child Development* 47(6). Serial No. 198. Chicago: University of Chicago Press.

Aswad, B. 1974. Visiting Patterns among Women of the Elite in a Small Turkish City. *Anthropological Quarterly* 47:9-27.

Aycicegi, A. 1993. *The Effects of the Mother Training Program.* Master's thesis, Bogazici University, Istanbul.

Ball, C. S. 1994. Start Right: The Importance of Early Learning. The Royal Society for the Encouragement of Arts, Manufacture and Commerce (RSA) Report. London.

Bekman, S. 1990. Alternative to the Available: Home Based vs. Center Based Programs. *Early Childhood Development and Care* 58:109-19.

———. 1993. The Preschool Education System in Turkey Revisited. *OMEP International Journal of Early Childhood* 25:13-19.

Benedict, P. 1974. The Kabul Gunu: Structured Visiting in an Anatolian Provincial Town. *Anthropological Quarterly* 47:28-47.

Bernstein, B. 1974. *Class, Codes, and Control: Theoretical Studies toward a Sociology of Language.* Rev. ed. New York: Shocken.

Berrueta-Clement, J. R., L. L. Schweinhart, W. Barnett, A. Epstein, and D. Weikart. 1984. *Changed Lives: The Effects of the Perry Preschool Programme on Youths through Age 19.* Ypsilanti, Mich.: High/Scope Press.

Berrueta-Clement, J. R., L. L. Schweinhart, W. S. Barnett, and D. P. Weikart. 1987. The Effects of Early Educational Intervention on Crime and Delinquency in Adolescence and Early Adulthood. In J. D. Burchard and S. N. Burchard, eds., *Primary Prevention of Psycho-pathology.* Vol. 10. *Prevention of Delinquent Behaviour.* Newbury Park, Calif.: Sage.

Brazelton, T. Berry. 1982. Early Intervention: What Does It Mean? In H. E. Fitzgerald, ed., *Theory and Research in Behavioural Pediatrics.* New York: Plenum.

Bronfenbrenner, U. 1974. Is Early Intervention Effective? *Columbia Teachers College Record* 76: 279-303.

———. 1979. *The Ecology of Human Development: Experiments by Nature and Design.* Cambridge: Harvard University Press.

Campbell, D. T., and A. Erlebacher. 1970. How Regression Artifacts in Quasi-experimental Evaluations Can Mistakenly Make Compensatory Education Look Harmful. In J. Hellmuth, ed., *Compensatory Education: A National Debate.* Vol. 3. New York: Brunner/Mazel.

Cicirelli, V. G., J. W. Evans, and J. S. Schiller. 1969. *The Impact of Head Start: An Evaluation of the Effects of Head Start on Children's Cognitive and Affective Development.* Washington, D.C.: Westinghouse Learning Corporation, Ohio University.

Coll, C. T. G. 1990. Developmental Outcome of Minority Infants: A Process-oriented Look into Our Beginnings. *Child Development* 61:270-89.

Eldering, L., and P. Vedder. 1993. Culture-Sensitive Home Intervention: The Dutch Hippy Experiment. In L. Eldering and P. Leseman, ed., *Early Intervention and Culture.* Paris: United Nations Educational, Scientific, and Cultural Organization.

Epstein, A., and D. Weikart. 1979. *The Ypsilanti-Carnegie Infant Education Project.* Monographs of the High/Scope Educational/Research Foundation. No. 6. Ypsilanti, Mich.: High/Scope Press.

Ercan, S. 1993. *The Short-term Effects of the Home Intervention Program on the Cognitive Development of Children.* Master's thesis, Bogazici University, Istanbul.

Evans, J. L., and R. G. Myers. 1985. *Improving Program Actions to Meet the Intersecting Needs of Women and Children in Developing Countries: A Policy and Program Review.* The Consultative Group on Early Childhood Care and Development. Ypsilanti, Mich.: High/Scope Educational Research Foundation.

Farran, D. C. 1990. Effects of Intervention with Disadvantaged and Disabled Children: A Decade Review. In S. J. Meisels and J. P. Shonkoff, eds., *Handbook of Early Childhood Intervention.* Cambridge: Cambridge University Press.

Field, T., S. Widmayer, R. Greenberg, and S. Stoller. 1982. Effects of Parent Training on Teenage Mothers and Their Infants. *Pediatrics* 69:703-07.

Garber, H. L. 1988. *The Milwaukee Project: Preventing Mental Retardation in Children at Risk.* Washington, D.C.: American Association on Mental Retardation.

Garber, H., and R. Heber. 1983. Modification of Predicted Cognitive Development in High-risk Children through Early Intervention. In M. K. Oetterman and R. J. Sternberg, eds., *How Much Can Intelligence Be Increased?* Norwood, N.J.: Ablex.

Goodnow, J. J. 1988. Parents' Ideas, Actions, and Feeling: Models and Methods from Developmental and Social Psychology. *Child Development* 59:286-320.

Gordon, I. J., B. J. Guinagh, and R. E. Jester. 1977. The Florida Parent Education Infant and Toddler Programs. In M. C. Day and R. K. Parker, eds., *The Preschool in Action.* 2nd ed. Boston: Allyn & Bacon.

Gray, S., B. Ramsey, and R. Klaus. 1983. The Early Training Project 1962-1980. In the Consortium for Longitudinal Studies, ed., *As the Twig Is Bent.* Hillsdale, N.J.: Lawrence Erlbaum Associates.

Gray, S., and K. Ruttle. 1980. The Family-Oriented Home Visiting Program: A Longitudinal Study. *Genetic Psychology Monographs* 102:299-316.

Gutelius, M. F., A. D. Kirsch, S. MacDonald, M. R. Brooks, and T. McErlean. 1977. Controlled Study of Child Health Supervision: Behavioral Results. *Pediatrics* 60:294-304.

Gutelius, M. F., A. D. Kirsch, S. MacDonald, M. R. Brooks, T. McErlean, and C. Newcomb. 1972. Promising Results from a Cognitive Stimulation Program in Infancy: A Preliminary Report. *Clinical Pediatrics* 11:585-93.

Halpern, R. 1990. Community Based Early Intervention. In S. J. Meisels and J. P. Shonkoff, eds., *Handbook of Early Childhood Intervention.* Cambridge: Cambridge University Press.

Harrell, R. 1983. *The Effects of the Head Start Program on Children's Cognitive Development: Preliminary Report of the Head Start Evaluation, Synthesis and Utilization Project.* Washington, D.C.: U.S. Department of Health and Human Services.

Hauser-Cram, P. 1983. *A Question of Balance: Relationships between Parents and Teachers.* Doctoral diss., Harvard Graduate School of Education.

Jester, R. E., and B. J. Guinagh. 1983. The Gordon Parent Education Infant and Toddler Program. In the Consortium for Longitudinal Studies, ed., *As the Twig Is Bent.* Hillsdale, N.J.: Lawrence Erlbaum and Associates.

Johnson, D. L., and T. Walker. 1987. Primary Prevention of Behavior Problems in Mexican-American Children. *American Journal of Community Psychology* 15:375-85.

Kagitcibasi, C. 1990. Family and Socialization in Cross-cultural Perspective: A Model of Change. In J. Berman, ed., *Cross-cultural Perspectives: Nebraska Symposium on Motivation, 1989.* Lincoln: Nebraska University Press.

———. 1991. *The Early Enrichment Project in Turkey.* UNESCO-UNICEF-WFP Notes, Comments...No. 193. Paris: United Nations Educational, Scientific, and Cultural Organization.

———. 1993. A Model of Multipurpose Non-formal Education: The Case of the Turkish Early Enrichment Project. In L. Eldering and P. Leseman, eds., *Early Intervention and Culture.* The Hague, Netherlands: United Nations Educational, Scientific, and Cultural Organization.

———. 1996. *Family and Human Development Across Cultures: A View from the Other Side.* Hillsdale, N.J.: Lawrence Erlbaum Associates.

Kagitcibasi, C., and I. Savasir. 1988. Human Abilities in the Eastern Mediterranean. In S. H. Irvine and J. W. Berry, eds., *Human Abilities in Cultural Context.* Cambridge: Cambridge University Press.

Kagitcibasi, C., D. Sunar, and S. Bekman. 1988. *Comprehensive Preschool Education Project: Final Report.* Ottawa: International Development Research Centre.

Kiray, M. B. 1981. The Women of Small Town. In N. Abadan-Unat, ed., *Women in Turkish Society.* Leiden: Brill.

Klaus, R. A., and S. W. Gray. 1968. The Early Training Project for Disadvantaged Children. *Monographs of the Society for Research in Child Development* 33(4). Serial No. 120.

Kotchabhakdi, N. J., P. Winichagoon, S. Smitasiri, S. Dhanamitta, and A. Valya-Sevi. 1987. The Integration of Psychosocial Components in Nutrition Education in Northeastern Thai Villages. *Asia Pacific Journal of Public Health* 2:16-25.

Lally, R. J., P. L. Mangione, and A. S.Honig. 1988. The Syracuse University Family Development Research Program: Long-range Impact on an Early Intervention with Low-income Children and their Families. In D. Powell, ed., *Parent Education as Early Childhood Intervention: Emerging Directions in Theory, Research and Practice.* Norwood, N.J.: Ablex.

Laosa, L. M. 1984. Ethnic, Socioeconomic, and Home Language Influences upon Early Performance on Measures of Abilities. *Journal of Educational Psychology* 76:1178-98.

Larson, C. 1980. Efficacy of Prenatal and Postpartum Home Visits on Child Health and Development. *Pediatrics* 66:191-97.

Lazar, I., and R. Darlington. 1982. Lasting Effects of Early Education: A Report from the Consortium for Longitudinal Studies. *Monographs of the Society for Research in Child Development* 47(2-3). Serial No. 195.

Leseman, P. 1993. How Parents Provide Young Children with Access to Literacy. In L. Eldering and P. Leseman, eds., *Early Intervention and Culture.* The Hague, Netherlands: United Nations Educational, Scientific, and Cultural Organization.

Levenstein, P. 1970. Cognitive Growth in Preschoolers through Verbal Interaction with Mothers. *American Journal of Orthopsychiatry* 40:436-42.

Levenstein, P., J. O'Hara, and J. Madden. 1983. The Mother-Child Home Program of the Verbal Interaction Project. In the Consortium for Longitudinal Studies, ed., *As the Twig Is Bent.* Hillsdale, N.J.: Lawrence Erlbaum and Associates.

LeVine, R. A., and M. I. White. 1986. *Human Conditions: The Cultural Basis of Educational Development.* London: Routledge & Kegan Paul.

Lewin, K. 1951. *Field Theory in Social Science.* New York: Harper.

———. 1958. Group Decision and Social Change. In E. E. Maccoby, T. M. Newcomb, and E. L. Hartley, eds., *Readings in Social Psychology.* New York: Holt, Rinehart & Winston.

Lombard, A. 1981. *Success Begins at Home.* Lexington, Mass.: Heath.

Maciuika, L., and H. Weiss. 1987. Issues and Trends in Parent Education. Cambridge: Harvard Graduate School of Education, Harvard Family Research Project.

Marfo, K., and G. M. Kysela. 1985. Early Intervention with Mentally Handicapped Children: A Critical Appraisal of Applied Research. *Journal of Pediatric Psychology* 10:305-24.

McKey, R. H., L. Condelli, H. Ganson, B. J. Barret, C. McConkey, and M. C. Plantz. 1985. The Impact of Head Start on Children, Families and Communities. Final Report of the Head Start Evaluation, Synthesis and Utilization Project. Washington, D.C.: U.S. Department of Health and Human Services.

Myers, R. 1992. *The Twelve Who Survive: Strengthening Programs of Early Childhood Development in the Third World.* London: Routledge.

Nimnicht, G., and P. E. Posada. 1986. The Intellectual Development of Children in Project Promesa. A Report Prepared for the Bernard van Leer Foundation. Research and Evaluation Reports, No. 1, October. Medellín, Colombia: Centro Internacional de Educación y Desarrollo Humano (CINDE).

Olds, D. L. 1988. The Prenatal/Early Infancy Project. In E. L. Cowen, R. P. Lorion, and J. Ramos-McKay, eds., *Fourteen Ounces of Prevention: A Handbook for Practitioners.* Washington, D.C.: American Psychological Association.

Olds, D. L., C. R. Henderson, R. Chamberlain, and R. Tatelbaum. 1986a. Preventing Child Abuse and Neglect: A Randomized Trial of Nurse Home Visitation. *Pediatrics* 78:65-78.

Olds, D. L., C. R. Henderson, Jr., R. Tatelbaum, and R. Chamberlain. 1986b. Improving the Delivery of Prenatal Care and Outcomes of Pregnancy: A Randomized Trial of Nurse Home Visitation. *Pediatrics* 77:16-28.

Olds, D. L., C. R. Henderson, Jr., R. Tatelbaum, and R. Chamberlain. 1988. Improving the Life-course Development of Socially Disadvantaged Mothers: A Randomized Trial of Nurse Home Visitation. *American Journal of Public Health* 78:1436-45.

Olson, E. 1982. Duofocal Family Structure and an Alternative Model of Husband-Wife Relationship. In C. Kagitcibasi, ed., *Sex Roles, Family and Community in Turkey.* Bloomington: Indiana University Press.

Provence, S., and A. Naylor. 1983. *Working with Disadvantaged Parents and their Children: Scientific and Practice Issues.* New Haven: Yale University Press.

Ramey, C. T., D. Bryant, J. Sparling, and B. Wasik. 1985. Project CARE: A Comparison of Two Early Intervention Strategies to Prevent Retarded Development. *Topics in Early Childhood Special Education* 5:12-52.

Ramey, C. T., K. O. Yeates, and E. T. Short. 1984. The Plasticity of Intellectual Development: Insights from Preventive Intervention. *Child Development* 55:1913-25.

Rescorla, L., S. Provence, and A. Naylor. 1982. The Yale Child Welfare Research Program: Description and Results. In E. Zigler and E. Gordon, eds., *Daycare: Scientific and Social Policy Issues.* Boston: Auburn House.

Richards, H. 1985. *The Evaluation of Cultural Action.* London: The Macmillan Press Ltd.

Rodriguez, G. G. 1983. Final Report: Project CAN PREVENT. San Antonio, Tex.: Avance.

Rodriguez, G. G., and C. P. Cortez. 1988. The Evaluation Experience of the Avance Parent-Child Education Program. In H. B. Weiss and F. H. Jacobs, eds., *Evaluating Family Programs.* New York: Aldine de Gruyter.

Royce, J. M., R. B. Darlington, and H. W. Murray. 1983. Pooled Analysis: Findings across Studies. In the Consortium for Longitudinal Studies, ed., *As the Twig Is Bent.* Hillsdale, N.J.: Lawrence Erlbaum and Associates.

Sahin, N. 1989. Televizyondan Ogrenme (Learning from Television). In *Turkiye' de cocugun durumu* (The Situation of the Child in Turkey). Ankara: UNICEF (United Nations Children's Fund) and DPT.

Savasir, I., and N. Sahin. 1988. *Wechsler çocuk zeka ölçeði* (WISC-R) (Wechsler Intelligence Scale for Children). Ankara: Milli Eðditim Basýmevi.

Savasir, I., N. Sezgin, and N. Erol. 1992. 0-6 Yaþ çocuklarý için geliþim tarama envanteri geliþtirilmesi (Devising a Developmental Screening Inventory for 0-to 6-Year Old Children). *Türk Psikiyatri Dergisi* 3:33-38.

Schorr, L. B. 1991. Effective Programs for Children Growing Up in Concentrated Poverty. In A. C. Huston, ed., *Children in Poverty: Child Development and Public Policy.* Cambridge: Cambridge University Press.

Schweinhart, L. J., H. V. Barnes, D. P. Weikart, W. S. Barnett, and A. S. Epstein. 1993. *Significant Benefits: The High/Scope Perry Preschool Study Through Age 27.* Ypsilanti, Mich.: High/Scope Press.

Schweinhart, L. J., and D. P. Weikart. 1980. *Young Children Growup.* Monograph No. 7. Ypsilanti, Mich.: High/Scope Press.

Seitz, V. 1990. Intervention Programs for Impoverished Children: A Comparison of Educational and Family Support Models. *Annals of Child Development* 7:73-103.

Seitz, V., and S. Provence. 1990. Caregiver-focused Models of Early Intervention. In S. J. Meisels and J. P. Shonkoff, eds., *Handbook of Early Childhood Intervention.* Cambridge: Cambridge University Press.

Seitz, V., L. K. Rosenbaum, and N. H. Apfel. 1985. Effects of Family Support Intervention: A Ten-year Follow Up. *Child Development* 56:376-91.

Shipman, V. C., J. Barone, A. Beaton, W. Emmerich, and W. Ward. 1977. *Disadvantaged Children and their First School Experiences: Structure and Development of Cognitive Competencies and Styles prior to School Entry.* Princeton, N.J.: Educational Testing Service.

Slater, M. 1986. Modification of Mother-Child Interaction Processes in Families with Children At-risk for Mental Retardation. *American Journal of Mental Deficiency* 91:257-67.

Slaughter, D. 1983. Early Intervention and its Effects on Maternal and Child Development. *Monographs of the Society for Research in Child Development* 48(4). Serial No. 202.

———. 1988. Black Children, Schooling, and Educational Interventions. In D. T. Slaughter, ed., *Black Children and Poverty: A Developmental Perspective.* San Francisco: Jossey-Bass.

Smilansky, M. 1979. Priorities in Education: Preschool Evidence and Conclusions. World Bank Staff Working Paper 323. Washington, D.C.: World Bank.

Smith, M. S., and J. S. Bissell. 1970. Report Analysis: The Impact of Head Start. *Harvard Educational Review* 40:51-104.

Travers, J., M. J. Nauta, N. Irwin, B. Goodson, J. Singer, and C. Barclay. 1982. *The Effects of a Social Program: Final Report of the Child and Family Resource Program's Infant-Toddler Component.* Cambridge, Mass.: Abt Associates, Inc.

Wasik, B. H., C. T. Ramey, D. M. Bryant, and J. J. Sparling. 1990. A Longitudinal Study of Two Early Intervention Strategies: Project CARE. *Child Development* 61:1682-96.

Weiss, H. B. 1988. Family Support and Education Programs: Working through Ecological Theories of Human Development. In H. B. Weiss and F. H. Jacobs, eds., *Evaluating Family Programs.* New York: Aldine de Gruyter.

Weiss, H. B., and F. H. Jacobs. 1988. Family Support and Education Programs–Challenges and Opportunities. In H. B. Weiss and F. H. Jacobs, eds., *Evaluating Family Programs.* New York: Aldine de Gruyter.

White, S. H. 1970. The National Impact Study of Head Start. In J. Hellmuth, ed., *Disadvantaged Child.* Vol. 3. New York: Brunner/Mazel.

Woodhead, M. 1985. Pre-school Education Has Long Term Effects: But Can They Be Generalized? *Oxford Review of Education* 11(2):133-55.

———. 1988. When Psychology Informs Public Policy. *American Psychologist* 43:443-54.

Yoshikawa, H. 1994. Prevention as Cumulative Protection: Effects of Early Family Support and Education on Chronic Delinquency and its Risks. *Psychological Bulletin* 115:28-54.

Zigler, E., and W. Berman. 1983. Discerning the Future of Early Childhood Intervention. *American Psychologist* 38:894-906.

Zigler, E., and S. Muenchow. 1992. *Head Start: The Inside Story of America's Most Successful Educational Experiment.* New York: Basic Books.

Zigler, E., and S. J. Styfco. 1994. Head Start: Criticism in a Constructive Context. *American Psychologist* 49:127-32.

Zigler, E., C. Taussig, and K. Black. 1992. Early Childhood Intervention: A Promising Preventative for Juvenile Delinquency. *American Psychologist* 47(8):997-1006.

Zigler, E., and J. Valentine, eds. 1979. *Project Head Start: A Legacy of the War on Poverty.* New York: Free Press.

Zigler, E., and H. Weiss. 1985. Family Support Systems: An Ecological Approach to Child Development. In R. Rapaport, ed., *Children, Youth, and Families: The Action-Research Relationship.* Cambridge: Cambridge University Press.

1997 Elsevier Science B.V.
Early Child Development: Investing in our Children's Future
M.E. Young, editor.

Two Home-Based Programs for Early Child Education

Avima Lombard

In their early years, children undergo rapid physical growth, acquire language and cognitive skills, develop social behaviors, and evolve a concept of self. Through experience and guidance in every aspect of daily life at home and in school, they acquire the essential skills for functioning independently in new settings.

The value of early education programs in helping children develop these skills has been demonstrated repeatedly as noted in the preceding chapters. The various program models that have been developed and studied indicate that high-quality, center-based interventions can significantly help children develop and function successfully in formal school settings (Bronfenbrenner 1974). Studies also show conclusively that involving parents in early education programs enhances the effects of these programs, especially their long-term outcomes (Gray and Halpern 1989; Clark-Stewart and Apfel 1979; Lombard 1992b).

This chapter highlights the importance of parental involvement in early education by describing two successful programs in which parent education is a major component. Both of these programs were developed at The National Council of Jewish Women (NCJW) Research Institute for Innovation in Education, School of Education, The Hebrew University of Jerusalem, Israel. The Home Instruction Program for Preschool Youngsters (HIPPY) targets educationally disadvantaged mothers and preschool children; the Home Activities for Toddlers and Their Families (HATAF) program targets families with children 10-36 months old. Success with HIPPY led to development of HATAF and adaptation of HIPPY in many other countries (see Evans and Kagitcibasi, this volume). A brief review of the expectations, objectives, and planning issues related to home-based programs precedes the HIPPY and HATAF case descriptions in this chapter.

Home-Based Education: Expectations and Objectives

Intervention programs for home-based early education have the following characteristics. They take place in the family home, are initiated by an external agency, have clear objectives, involve regular contact with one or both parents, and provide parents with directions for engaging their child in educational activities.

Expectations

Certain expectations drive the planning and development of home-based programs. A key premise is that although preschool education is important for young children, it addresses only a small part of a child's early educational environment. Home learning is the basis for all other experiences and increases a child's potential success in school (Lombard 1991). To be effective, the existence and quality of parent teaching in the home must relate to a child's preparatory needs for school. In this regard, studies show that the quality of parent teaching reflects a parent's education level. Children of more highly educated parents are generally better prepared for school than are children of less educated parents, possibly because higher educated parents are more aware of a child's preparatory needs for school.

Another expectation for home-based programs is that because children and parents interact constantly, affecting each other in a dynamic relationship, changing the input from either participant may effect changes in both the dynamics and results of this relationship. Using the home for educational purposes capitalizes on the role of parents as educators, makes it easy for mothers to participate, and enables parents to interact with their children in a nonthreatening and noncompetitive setting (Lombard 1996). Studies show that home-based programs for young children in population groups at higher risk and with multiple needs are especially beneficial (Gomby and others 1993; Schlossman 1983).

It is also recognized that the learning environment in the home differs substantively from the learning environment in a preschool classroom. On entering the formal education system, a preschool child is expected to be both ready for learning and ready for school. Home-based programs can foster this readiness. Studies suggest that readiness for learning represents a match between the cognitive dispositions of a child and the material to be taught (Watson 1994) and that all children will have certain beliefs, expectations, and assumptions that must be taken into account to ensure successful learning (Ramey and Haskins 1981). School readiness relates to the ability of a child to function within a school and to meet its myriad social, physical, and intellectual demands.

Expectations regarding this preparation and the role of formal education differ between schools and parents (Lightfoot 1978). Schools generally view parents as responsible for preparing children for entry into school, encouraging children throughout school, and supporting the school and teachers' expectations for their children. Parents expect schools and teachers to give children the skills and knowledge needed that parents cannot provide. Parents' often overly high expectations may lead to parent-school conflict, especially when children do not succeed within the formal school system. Home-based programs can thwart the probability of this type of conflict by involving parents early in their child's education, thereby making them more like equal partners in the child's education, and helping the child to succeed later in school.

Objectives

Three main objectives for home-based early child education are (a) bridging the gap between home and school, (b) preventing school failure, and (c) reducing dropout rates. To bridge the gap between home and school, teachers can initiate activities to augment their classroom teaching. They may suggest home activities to supplement a child's classroom learning, invite parents to meetings to discuss subjects covered in the classroom and to learn about possible related home activities, and recommend that the school provide home tutors for children needing additional help.

Home-based early education programs can be especially effective for preventing school failure and reducing dropout rates. The target for these programs is usually preschool children (Zigler, Taussig, and Black 1992). The aim is to encourage development of the children's cognitive and mental abilities, a goal that has become a critical component of home-based early education, especially for disadvantaged children and families. Incorporation of this component is based on the recognition that parents of most children who fail in school have a poor educational background and lack the skills or information needed to promote their child's intellectual growth. Parents' sense of failure over their own education, and the feelings of inadequacy and shame that often result, make them reluctant to become involved in this aspect of their child's development, expecting the schools to fulfill this function. Yet it is in the home through interacting with parents that a child acquires the experiences and information necessary for intellectual growth (Harmon and Brim 1980; Ramey and Haskins 1981).

Planning Home-Based Programs

In planning home-based programs for early education, eight questions must be addressed:

1. What are the characteristics of the populations to be served and how will they be targeted? Related questions are: Is home visiting suitable for all targeted families? Can one program meet the needs of all the families, given their differences in education, culture, family status, and other aspects? Will the program augment, replace, or fill a gap in available preschool services? Will participation be compulsory or voluntary?

2. What will be the focus of the program? Can factors relating to school readiness and school success, other than cognitive skills, be identified?

3. Under what administrative auspices will the program operate? Will it be a "stand-alone" program, part of the services offered by a health department or school district, or affiliated with a national model?

4. What will be the duration and intensity of the program (that is, the age at which children will enter and complete the program, the frequency of home visits, and the level of parents' expectations of the program)?

5. What will be the relationship between the planned programs and other community services?

6. How will staff be selected, trained, and supervised? Will the staff include paraprofessionals and professionally trained personnel experienced in the culture and language of the families targeted?

7. How will the program be monitored and evaluated to maintain quality control and meet accountability requirements?

8. What budgets are required for program development and operation?

Planning for home-based early education must focus on the primary participants: the parents and children. Program materials should be appropriate for the ages targeted, promote the program objectives, and meet the requirements of adult education. Identification of parents' attitudes and expectations as well as other factors influencing and reinforcing parents' participation in the program is important (Lombard 1991).

Two Case Models: HIPPY and HATAF

The design and implementation of HIPPY and HATAF incorporated the planning objectives and considerations noted above. A brief description of each case model is given below. These two descriptions are followed by a summary of three aspects common to both HIPPY and HATAF, which are important for home-based early education.

Home Instruction Program for Preschool Youngsters (HIPPY)

HIPPY was designed in 1969 as an experiment to examine the effectiveness of home-based educational activities for educationally disadvantaged mothers and their preschool children. An underlying assumption was that home instruction can improve children's ability to learn. This case description summarizes HIPPY's target population, program focus, funding support, duration, intensity, staffing, and activities.

Population. The initial target population was the children of recent immigrants to Israel from Asian and African countries. This population had a relatively high dropout rate from school, which suggested that the children had difficulty learning and that their home environment did not provide the experiences needed to succeed in school. The parents' educational levels were low, as was their sense of adequacy in performing home teaching roles. Families were generally large and most of the mothers did not work outside of the home. Literacy levels were low, although almost every family had at least one literate member.

Focus. HIPPY focuses on the development of cognitive skills in preschool children through home-based experiences that stimulate acquisition of the knowledge, skills, and attitudes expected by preschool teachers. The program also emphasizes stimulation of parents' sense of adequacy and control regarding their children's early school careers.

Funding Support. HIPPY was initially a field experiment funded through a special grant from abroad. All aspects of program operation, including service delivery and training, were developed at the NCJW Research Institute. Later, the Israeli Ministry of Education assumed operational and fiscal responsibility for the program; the institute retains responsibility for quality control.

Duration. HIPPY is a 3-year program which children begin at age 3 and complete at age 6. More than 90 percent of Israeli children attend preschool beginning at age 3; formal schooling begins at age 6, and free and compulsory kindergarten is required beginning at age 5. HIPPY thus overlaps in the third year with kindergarten. In this way, the program reinforces parents' awareness of the importance of their role as educators even after their children have entered the formal school system.

Intensity. Parents receive instruction through both home visits and group meetings. In both settings parents are provided with special packets of activities to do with their children. They are expected to devote about 20 minutes daily for 5 days each week to these activities. Parents' interaction with their child is reviewed in the home setting and individualized instruction is given as needed. In the group meetings the parents share their impressions and experiences and develop a sense of community involvement in education. The meetings include a half-hour enrichment period, led by a professional coordinator, to enhance the parents' knowledge and understanding in fields related to their roles as parents (for example, child development, education, health, hygiene, nutrition, psychology).

Staffing. HIPPY is a community-based program that utilizes community personnel as much as possible. A professional program coordinator who meets HIPPY's requirements is selected by the community and attends a week-long pretraining period. After this training, the coordinator selects paraprofessional home visitors from the target mothers. These home visitors attend a very short pretraining and weekly, 4-hour inservice training sessions. In the weekly sessions, they report on the week's work, prepare for the next week, and discuss issues concerning their work with the families.

Home visitors see each parent weekly, alternating between home visits and group meetings. They instruct parents, but normally have no direct contact with the children. The program coordinators are trained and supervised by a representative from the central HIPPY office. The coordinators meet monthly to discuss their work, review activities to be distributed to the families, and plan special training for home visitors. Both home visitors and professional coordinators maintain written records of their work. These records are monitored by the central staff at the university, where statistical data on the families and program are entered into a data base.

Training at all levels involves role play, an excellent way of working with educationally disadvantaged children and adults. The role play emphasizes action rather than talk, is concrete and easy, and has an informal, game-like tempo. Mothers and home visitors alternate in playing the role of mother or child, allowing problems and misunderstandings to be handled naturally. Home teaching is enacted, with the trainer playing the role of parent and the parent playing the role of child. This nonthreatening way to learn new behaviors and materials enables all participants to identify with the child as learner and enhances the parents' sensitivity to their child.

The position of home visitor is valued. It provides employment in a relatively high status position (teacher), allows flexible working hours, and offers personal advancement through special training and continuing education. HIPPY encourages home visitors to seek other employment after 3 or 4 years in the program to prevent job fatigue and to enable others in the community to become home visitors. Coordinators are responsible for preparing home visitors for departing the program. They may include them in job-training courses, contact other community agencies that have job openings, and help explore various job options.

Activities. HIPPY activities are guided by a desire to create an educational program for young children that can be implemented successfully at home by parents with low education levels. The written instructional activities create situations in which parents can interact successfully on educational activities with their child. Five criteria, which reflect planning decisions on what is important, what is possible, and what is expected to work, guide the selection of HIPPY activities. The criteria are as follows.

1. The activity is appropriate for the developmental ages of the participating children. Because developmental differences among children are likely to be considerable, the activities selected for HIPPY are appropriate for children within a 6-month chronological age range. The components of each activity are designed in step-wise progression so that it can be adjusted to each child's developmental level. Slow developers can learn at their own pace, and more advanced children can attain a sense of mastery.

2. The activity will contribute to a child's potential school success. HIPPY activities focus on three broad cognitive areas: language, perceptual and sensory discrimination, and problem-solving. Because these areas are considered primary to a child's ability to learn, the activities emphasize each cognitive area as much as possible.

3. The activity is attractive to children. Activities are not valued by children if they do not enjoy them or want to do them, and activities not liked by children could promote parent-child conflict and loss of interest in HIPPY. Recognizing that children will enjoy some series of activities more than others, HIPPY makes every attempt to ensure that the vast majority of activities are attractive and fun for all participating children.

4. The activity can be accomplished at home, using little or no special equipment. To promote parents' willingness and ability to participate actively in the home education of their children, HIPPY emphasizes that "you can do it." This message is reinforced throughout all materials. Activity and story books are simple and inexpensive. The activities accommodate the limited space in most homes and utilize furniture, eating utensils, and kitchenware available in even the poorest of homes.

5. The activity "makes sense" to the parent. The connection between each activity and the skills expected by school teachers is made clear to the parents to encourage them to approach each activity seriously. For example, although scribbling is known to be an excellent precursor of writing, it is not accepted by most target families as a serious undertaking. Thus, HIPPY emphasizes a variety of more directive activities to develop a child's control over paper and writing tools, such as pencils, crayons, or markers. In this way, HIPPY elicits the involvement of parents and educates them on how their children use these tools, making parents more receptive to different ways of improving their child's writing skills, including scribbling (Lombard 1992a).

Home Activities for Toddlers and Their Families (HATAF)

The HATAF program was developed at the NCJW Research Institute in 1973. Adopting the successful HIPPY model, this new program targeted children 10-36 months old. HATAF is described below in terms of the same topics used for HIPPY.

Population. HATAF targets parents who do not feel comfortable and knowledgeable in creating enriching interactions for their toddlers. Often these parents have low educational levels and their own parents did not engage them in early stimulation activities.

Focus. In contrast to HIPPY, which is targeted to children 3-6 years old, HATAF focuses on toddlers 10 months to 3 years old. Like HIPPY, however, HATAF focuses on empowering parents to assume an active role in educating their children. By changing parents' behaviors and attitudes, it is expected that HATAF will positively affect children's physical, emotional, and intellectual development. The primary objective for HATAF is to produce changes in parents' awareness and skills relating to the following five areas:

1. Understanding a child's developmental stages in the first 3 years of life. Through HATAF, parents are given extensive information on children's growth and development, including the stages of development and factors that affect a child's passage from one stage to the next. HATAF emphasizes the importance of providing children with opportunities for exploration and experimentation and demonstrates the significant role adults can play in a child's development.

2. Recognizing the importance of reading, speaking, and playing with children. Because language learning takes place in verbal exchanges between adults and children, HATAF guides parents in using stories, pictures, and language that will encourage children to talk and learn basic language concepts and uses.

3. Using natural learning settings in the home. HATAF encourages parents to consider every aspect of their toddler's life as a teaching and learning situation. HATAF activities derive from daily routines and occurrences, providing opportunities for parents to acquire basic skills while "teaching on the fly."

4. Using a variety of reinforcement techniques appropriately and effectively. Because parents often misuse reinforcements in their interactions with children, HATAF encourages parents to use immediate positive reinforcement in ways that are meaningful to the child and appropriate to the situation.

5. Adopting new techniques for playing with young children. HATAF teaches parents how to select and adapt toys that are appropriate to their child's interest level and ability and that encourage a child's exploration and discovery. To encourage creativity, HATAF also teaches parents how to draw on children's natural inclination to play imaginary games, encouraging the parents to add materials and converse with their children in a way that encourages self-expression.

Funding Support. Like HIPPY, HATAF was funded initially by a grant from abroad. All aspects of program operation, including service delivery and training, were based on the HIPPY model developed at the NCJW Research Institute. Later, the Israeli Ministry of Education assumed operational and fiscal responsibility for the program; the institute retains responsibility for quality control.

Duration. Families join HATAF for 2 years when their child is about 10 months old. It is expected that during these important developmental years, HATAF can produce lasting changes in parents' attitudes and skills, promote children's acquisition of basic skills and self-concept, and provide a strong base for all subsequent development.

Intensity. Like HIPPY, HATAF provides instruction to parents through home visits and group meetings. Also like HIPPY, this instruction is provided by paraprofessional home visitors selected from the community and guided by a professional coordinator. In contrast to HIPPY, home visitors interact directly with toddlers, instructing parents by modeling behavior and activities.

Home visits are weekly during the first year and twice monthly during the second year. Parent discussion groups occur monthly during the first year and twice monthly during the second year. These group meetings are devoted to topics of interest to the parents, such as child development, sibling rivalry, and children's sleeping and eating problems. The professional coordinator leads these discussions and parents are encouraged to share ideas on the issues addressed.

In addition to these monthly group meetings, HATAF convenes the parents and children about every 2 months for afternoon workshops. At these workshops, parents and children move among a variety of activities and parents receive guidance and encouragement from the home visitors and coordinator as they engage their child in each activity.

Staffing. HATAF home visitors are expected to model desired behaviors and attitudes. They are selected not only for belonging to the larger target group, but for displaying appropriate parenting skills and a willingness to learn more about children and parents. They are selected from among the more mature mothers in the neighborhood, rather than from the general target population of young mothers.

HATAF home visitors attend a 1-week pretraining program. Thereafter they receive weekly training from the professional coordinator at staff meetings and periodic training throughout the year at special inservice sessions for all home visitors in a region. Weekly training is focused on modeling the weekly activity to be taught; other sessions address general issues pertaining to child development and parent-child relationships.

Both home visitors and professional coordinators maintain written records of their work. These records are monitored by the central staff at the university, where statistical data on the families and program are entered into a data base.

Like HIPPY, HATAF home visitors are expected to work no more than 3-4 years before obtaining new employment. The coordinator is responsible for helping each home visitor prepare for this move.

Activities. HATAF activities relate to basic developmental areas: gross and fine motor development, language, eye-hand coordination, creativity, and social and emotional development. They are age-appropriate, suitable for implementation at home, and utilize materials easily found at home. Story books and a few basic toys are provided as integral parts of the program. Each activity is accompanied by a guide sheet for parents that emphasizes the primary objective and message for the week. The guide sheet is given to the parents to include in a looseleaf HATAF notebook.

Three Important Aspects

HIPPY and HATAF demonstrate three important aspects of home-based early education programs: community base, cultural sensitivity, and cost-effectiveness.

Community Base

Both HIPPY and HATAF are community-based programs. All funding is provided directly to interested local community agencies, which enter into agreements to operate the programs in coordination with the NCJW Research Institute. The institute provides guidelines, but the programs are operated by the community agencies which, in consultation with institute staff, select target populations and program staff. Local staff are directly involved in locating and enrolling families, determining and collecting participation fees, providing information on the programs, and interpreting community needs to institute staff. As home-based programs, HIPPY and HATAF importantly serve as "windows" to the families in a community, enabling local staff to connect families with other community services.

Cultural Sensitivity

Israeli families represent a variety of cultures and languages. To respond to this cultural diversity, HIPPY and HATAF are structured so that all program components can be understood easily and adapted to local needs and interests. For example, because the programs are intended to promote parental involvement in education and enhance cognitive and language growth in children, parents are encouraged to use their home language in interacting with their children. Hebrew is the language used in most Israeli schools and thus HIPPY and HATAF materials are written in Hebrew.

Special needs are met as required, however. For example, special simplified versions of the materials in Hebrew were prepared for use by newly arrived immigrants from Ethiopia until they are able to acquire greater language and literacy skills in Hebrew. During this transition, the home visitors for this population, who are Ethiopian as well, serve as interpreters while engaging the participants in the planned activities. Also, to meet the needs of Israeli Arab schools, in which Arabic is used, the materials are written and presented in Arabic. HIPPY materials also are being used in many other countries and have been translated into English, Spanish, Dutch, Turkish, German, and Papamiento.

Cost-Effectiveness

The costs of operating HIPPY and HATAF include (a) salaries for professional coordinators and paraprofessional home visitors, (b) production or purchase of written materials for the parents and home visitors, and (c) associated operating expenses such as rent, office services, travel, and fee reductions. Costs vary among the sites and budgets are determined locally. In Israel, the average annual cost for participating in HIPPY or HATAF per family is US$400.

Families are expected to pay an annual fee to participate in the programs. The amount of this fee is determined locally and is intended to give families a sense of pride in participating and to help meet operating expenses.

Most of the cost of operating the programs in Israel is borne by the Division for Educational Welfare, Ministry of Education and Culture, supplemented by small grants from foundations. Various and different sources provide the funding for programs in other countries, with government support provided in most cases.

HIPPY is an effective and successful program, as noted by Evans and Kagitcibasi in this volume. In both HIPPY and HATAF, the intermediary change agent for a child is the primary caregiving parent of the child. Parents transfer knowledge and skills to children, producing immediate and possibly short-term effects. Increased parental interest in gaining more knowledge through courses or other ways results in long-term, favorable effects on the assistance parents give their children. Both HIPPY and HATAF thus stimulate circular positive effects that ultimately benefit the participating children.

Through their involvement and education, parents receive practical and social support, enabling them to be more effective as parents than others who may feel stressed and alienated. By improving family functioning, HIPPY and HATAF help create a supportive home environment that enables the child to relate well to family and peers, succeed in school, and avoid delinquent activities or school dropout.

In entering into HIPPY agreements with communities outside of Israel, NCJW Research Institute requires both a continuing and summative evaluation of the program operation. Data on the effectiveness of HIPPY are consistent across HIPPY sites throughout the world. The findings indicate that participating mothers undergo substantial growth in their self-concept, community involvement, and willingness to be involved in their children's and their own continuing education. The children participating in HIPPY are better prepared for school (Gumpel 1996), feel better as students over the years, and are less likely to drop out of school.

Studies conducted over the years also indicate that parents participating in HATAF undergo significant changes in their attitudes and expectations and in certain areas of interaction with their children. Parents do less "testing" of their children and, instead, provide expanded language descriptions and encourage interactions with their children (Lombard 1989).

Implications for Future Planning

Increasingly, research studies emphasize the importance of the early years in a child's development (Begley 1996). During these years, children's education and stimulation are provided by their parents, most of whom are unaware of the importance of their role in this regard. Home-based educational programs, such as HIPPY and HATAF, which directly involve parents, are one way of improving learning in the home and enabling children to succeed in school. Home-based programs can be offered alone, in conjunction with school or center-based programs, or as a component of a range of coordinated community services.

HIPPY and HATAF demonstrate well the importance of integrating services for families and children. One concept deserving further exploration is family support centers, as described by Mayfield (1993). Designed to address both adult and child needs, these centers provide adults with information and activities related to social networks, child development, and community resources and services. Combining home-based programs such as HIPPY and HATAF with such center-based programs offers exciting possibilities for achieving well-integrated and coordinated services that meet the needs of parents *and* children in a community setting.

References

Begley, Sharon. 1996. Your Child's Brain. *Newsweek International*, February 10, 41-44.

Bronfenbrenner, U. 1974. Is Early Intervention Effective? *Day Care and Early Education* 2(2):14-18, 44.

Clark-Stewart, K. A., and N. Apfel. 1979. Evaluating Parental Effects on Child Development. In L. S. Shulman, ed., *Review of Research in Education.* Itasca, Il.: F. E. Peacock.

Gomby, Deanna S., Carol S. Larsen, and Eugene M. Lewit. 1993. Home Visiting: Analysis and Recommendations. In Richard E. Behrman, ed., *Future of Children*, Vol. 3, No. 3. Los Altos, Calif.: Center for the Future of Children, The David and Lucille Packard Foundation.

Gray, E., and R. Halpern. 1989. *Early Parenting Intervention to Parent Child Abuse: A Meta-Analysis of Preventative Early Parenting Inventions*. Final Report. Grant #90-CA-1333. Washington, D.C.: National Center on Child Abuse and Neglect, U.S. Department of Health and Human Services.

Gumpel, T. 1996. A Measure of Teacher Assessment of Readiness for School. Unpublished research report.

Harmon, D., and O. G. Brim, Jr. 1980. *Learning to be Parents: Principles, Programs and Methods*. Beverly Hills, Calif.: Sage.

Lightfoot, S. L. 1978. *Worlds Apart*. New York: Basic Books.

Lombard, A. D. 1989. Mothers of Very Young Children: A Study of HATAF. Unpublished research report. Jerusalem: Hebrew University.

———. 1991. Home Instruction, for Whom, When and Why? Unpublished paper presented at Utrecht University, Netherlands. November.

———. 1992a. *A Handbook for HIPPY Coordinators*. Jerusalem: Hebrew University, School of Education, NCJW Research Institute.

———. 1992b. Involving Parents in Early Childhood Education. Unpublished paper presented at conference on Education in Israel, Jerusalem.

———. 1996. Parents and Preschool Education: Lowering the Risk of Failure [in Spanish]. *Reflejos IV*. Jerusalem: Hebrew University, Department of Spanish and Latinamerican Studies.

Mayfield, M. I. 1993. Family Support Programs: Support for Urban Families in a Multi-Cultural Setting. *International Journal of Early Childhood* 2:45-50.

Ramey, C. T., and R. Haskins. 1981. The Modification of Intelligence through Early Experience. Paper presented at the biennial meeting of the Society for Research in Child Development, March 15-18, San Francisco.

Schlossman, Steven L. 1983. The Formative Era in Parent Education: Overview and Interpretation. In R. Haskins and D. Adams, eds., *Parent Education and Public Policy*. Norwood, N.J.: Ablex.

Watson, R. 1994. Rethinking Readiness for Learning. In D. Olson, ed., *Handbook of Education and Human Development: New Models of Learning, Teaching and Schooling*. London: Blackwell.

Zigler, Edward, Clara Taussig, and Kathryn Black. 1992. Early Childhood Intervention: A Promising Preventative for Juvenile Delinquency. *American Psychologist* 47(8): 997-1006.

III. Investing in Early Child Development: Economic and Policy Considerations

Early Child Development: Investing in our Children's Future
M.E. Young, editor.

Early Child Development: An Economic Perspective

Jacques van der Gaag

Early child development (ECD) is a powerful investment in the future, both socially *and* economically. Stimulating children's development and helping them reach their full potential are beneficial not only to children and their families, but also to societies and the entire global community. Well-developed children become successful, productive adults who are better able to contribute to a society's economy and to instigate a cycle of positive effects as they become parents, and grandparents, of the generations that follow.

The preceding chapters in this volume have well stated the short- and long-term benefits of improved nutrition, health, and education for children and families participating in ECD programs. In describing these benefits, the authors have emphasized the interrelationship and synergistic effects of nutrition, health, and cognitive stimulation. They also have documented the substantial negative effects for these children and their families of not intervening early in life against poor health, malnutrition, and unstimulating environments. These effects are synergistic as well and, if allowed to continue, can undermine entire societies and countries; these are not steady-state situations and can proceed in a downward negative spiral across generations.

Positive action can take different forms, as indicated by the various conceptual frameworks presented in this volume. Many options for promoting early child development are available and have been utilized by different countries throughout the world. With sufficient will, this knowledge, which already exists, can be examined closely and exploited to good advantage.

The will to take action often involves having the means to take action. The purposes of this chapter are to substantiate that ECD programs are a good investment *economically* and to suggest a broad general framework for addressing the economics of early child development.

Early Child Development: Benefits and Choices

Two immediate questions for policymakers and government administrators are: Why worry about the economics of early child development? Why talk about ECD as "an investment"? The answer is simple: The success and inventiveness of researchers and the

---

This chapter was developed from the keynote address, "Investing in the Future," presented at the conference.

lessons learned from their studies of early child development have resulted in many effective ECD strategies and programs that have been shown to benefit children. Interventions in nutrition, health care, preschool and primary education, and related areas (for example, water and sanitation) have all been shown in various settings, using different delivery mechanisms, to improve children's health, nutrition status, growth, and cognitive and behavioral development.

Some of these interventions focus on a single area (for example, education or health), whereas others are combined as complementary programs (for example, nutrition *and* education) or serve as alternative approaches (for example, home-based or center-based preschool education). To select a strategy and the programs that implement the strategy requires consideration of two key questions: Given limited resources, how can government maximize the number of children who will benefit from a program? How can government utilize the lessons learned to form coherent public policies for young children?

Some choices are easy; some strategies and programs work, others do not. Other choices are constrained; some programs are effective at certain ages, others are not. Researchers, for example, continue to accumulate evidence of "windows of opportunity" for the development of children's abilities; when a window is closed, interventions in the area of interest may not succeed or be effective. Figure 1 summarizes the known windows of opportunity for five abilities. These windows are the critical periods in a child's development when the capability for physical, emotional, social, and cognitive (verbal and spatial) functioning is established. The figure shows that these five capabilities are established between the prenatal period and 6 years of age.

Other choices are more difficult; some interventions yield greater benefit when combined horizontally as integrated programs for a specific age group, others are more effective when organized vertically for a range of ages. Additional questions to ask are: Should all programs be available universally, or should some programs be targeted to children at high risk? Are programs always more effective in formal settings with trained caregivers, or can programs in informal settings without trained caregivers be equally or

Figure 1. Windows of Opportunity

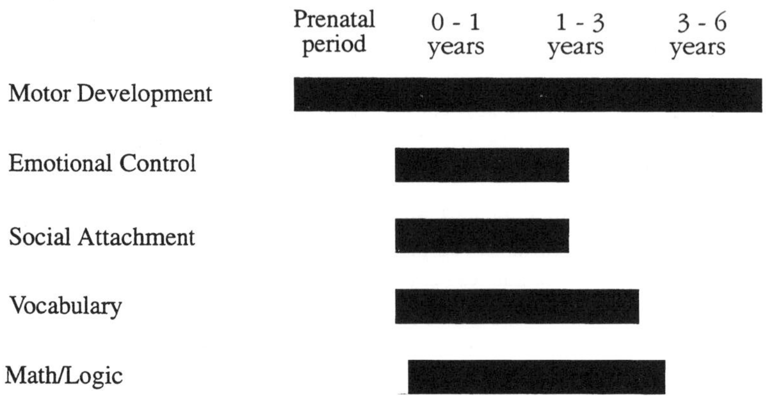

even more effective? These additional questions are especially difficult to resolve for interventions with multiple objectives, as is often the case with ECD programs.

Yet, even if an intervention's objective is seemingly simple, such as achieving good nutrition, the choices can be complex. For example, can good nutrition be provided best by assuring adequate food distribution, or by providing food stamps or making food-for-work programs available? Are school feeding programs preferable, or would mothers' education programs, which are not directly linked to food, be more effective in promoting good nutrition?

All of these questions, which guide the selection of strategies and programs, need to be addressed. The choice of a particular strategy or program will reflect the amount of resources available and the objectives to be achieved.

As a first step toward addressing these questions, the effectiveness of existing strategies and programs must be evaluated rigorously for different groups and settings. Subsequently, an intervention, or set of interventions, that is optimal for a given situation must be selected from among the options available. A useful tool for conducting this rational examination of ECD programs is benefit-cost analysis.

Benefit-Cost Analysis

Policymakers and government administrators will utilize economic criteria for forming coherent public policies regarding children and making decisions on ECD strategies and programs. To ensure that these policies and decisions are "optimal," the criteria need to be expressed in terms of benefits and costs.

Applying economic criteria to programs that benefit a child's health, nutrition, and development may appear unnecessary but can be illuminating and serve to document potential returns on investment, thereby encouraging public and private action. Cost-benefit analysis has been used, for example, to document economic returns on investment for education, leading to major national and global initiatives in this field. An example of the type of analysis that would be useful for ECD programs is given below for education.

> In this example, a young girl grows up healthy, well nourished, and without damage to her cognitive and behavioral development. She stays at home until age 12 and then starts working. She may work with her parents in the fields, with a family member in the household, or with others in a local store. The girl has not attended school and cannot read, write, or perform basic mathematical calculations. During her first year of work, her productivity is low but she learns from experience. Her productivity (and her income) increases during her early years of work but, lacking education, she soon reaches her maximum productivity level. She retires at age 55.

Figure 2 shows the pattern of this woman's productivity over her lifetime. This productivity pattern is called her "age-earnings profile."

> Now consider the same young girl again in a different scenario. This time she attends school from age 6 to age 12. When she enters the work force at age 12, she can read sufficiently well to comprehend instructions and labels and can operate a cash register. Her productivity, with schooling, is higher initially than it would be without schooling

and she will maintain this higher productivity *for the rest of her work life*. Again, she retires at age 55.

Figure 3 shows this woman's productivity, or age-earnings profile, with schooling in comparison with her profile without schooling. By comparing the increase in her lifetime productivity (*P* on figure 3) to the cost of her education (*I*), the economic returns of education can be calculated, as is done for any other investment.

In fact, the returns to schooling are very high (table 1). The literature on the benefit-cost of education shows that 1 extra year of primary education increases a person's future

Figure 2. Age-earnings Profile without Schooling

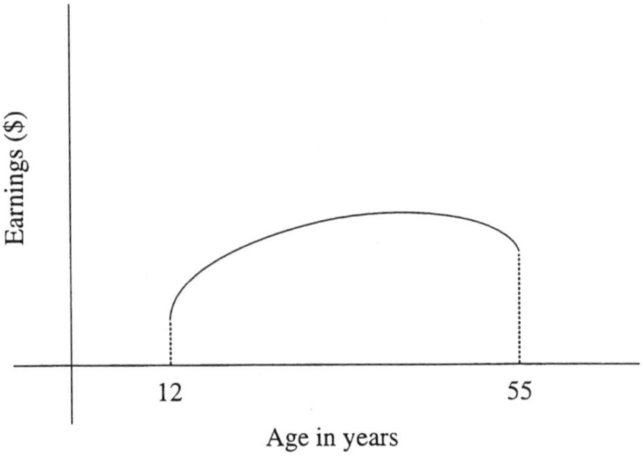

Figure 3. Age-earnings Profile with and without Schooling

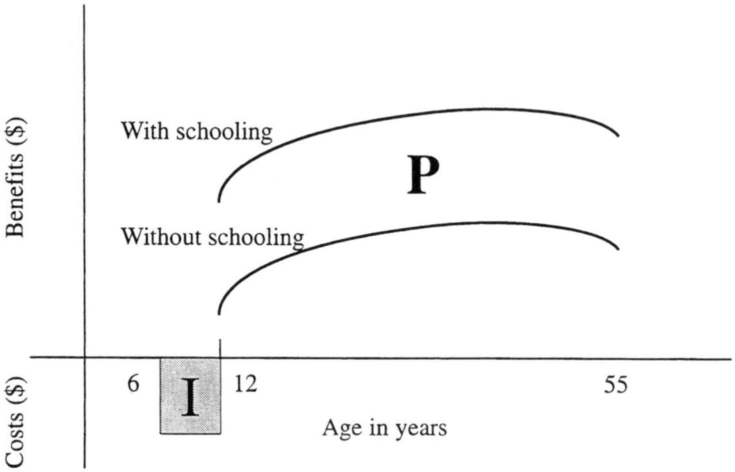

Table 1. Economic Returns to Investments (Percent Increase in Future Productivity) of 1 Extra Year of Primary Education

Country	Percent increase	Country	Percent increase
Argentina	10.0	Nigeria	30.0
Bolivia	9.8	Pakistan	20.0
Brazil	9.7	Philippines	18.3
Cyprus	15.4	Spain	31.6
Ethiopia	35.0	Yemen	10.0
India	19.8	Zimbabwe	16.6

Source: Psacharopoulos 1994.

productivity (that is, hourly wage rate) by 10 to 30 percent (Psacharopoulos 1994). These high economic returns are among the main reasons why the global development community is urging "Education for All." Economic analysis has shown that education is the surest way out of poverty because education has a very high rate of economic return.

Social Indicators and Productivity

In the first example described above, the young girl lacks schooling but is healthy, well nourished, and cognitively and behaviorally well developed. She is ready to learn. If she is able to enter school, the benefits to her and her family are high. Unfortunately, the situation for most children in many developing countries is much grimmer and programs are needed to break the cycle of poverty and its associated effects.

The Developing World: Grim Statistics

Despite tremendous progress made during the past 3 decades, the struggle for survival continues for young children in low-income countries and in poor, remote areas of middle-income countries. In twenty-five of forty low-income countries, the infant mortality rate (IMR) still exceeds 100. International efforts are needed to complete this unfinished agenda of increasing child survival and lowering the IMR in all low-income countries. The knowledge is available to accomplish this.

But mere survival is not enough. Many children who survive today often suffer from malnutrition as a result of insufficient dietary intake of protein or essential micronutrients. The damage from malnutrition is often irreversible, as noted by Martorell in this volume.

Also, despite major advances in extending education to children in all parts of the world, the rates of enrollment in primary school in some countries are less than 60 percent and even lower for girls. Many of those who enroll repeat grades or drop out before they graduate, remaining functionally illiterate and unable to function fully and productively within their communities and society. Table 2 shows typical levels of social indicators pertaining to children in low-income countries and poor regions of middle-income countries.

How do all of these statistics relate to early child development? The answer: They indicate the severity of the health, nutritional, and educational needs of young children in

Table 2. Typical Levels of Social Indicators in Low-income Countries and Poor Regions of Middle-income Countries

Indicator	Value
Infant mortality rate	150 deaths per 1,000 live births
Child mortality	50 deaths per 1,000 children
Malnutrition	50% of all children
Enrollment in primary school	60% of children in the appropriate age group for primary school
Average late enrollment in primary school	2 years
School dropout rate	30% of all schoolchildren
Grade repetition rate	30% of all schoolchildren

many countries throughout the world. Perhaps the best way of illustrating the severity of this situation is to consider a hypothetical cohort of 100 children from a low-income country. In this country, with the social indicators shown in table 2, more than half of the 100 children in the cohort will never have a chance to reach their full potential. Some will die, although most will survive. Of those who survive, many will become subsistence farmers, inhabitants of shanty towns, and illiterate and ill-prepared parents.

Sound public policies need to be designed for the children that survive to protect them from malnutrition and disease and to provide the health care, early childcare, and education that will enable them to reach their full potential. Without appropriate intervention, the vicious cycle of poverty that entraps them will continue and will be passed on to the next generation and generations thereafter.

Breaking the Cycle

ECD policies and programs can break this cycle and help these children achieve a fulfilling and productive life. Adopting the schema used in figure 3 to explain a young girl's loss of productivity potential without schooling, figure 4 depicts the loss of the entire cohort's productivity potential. Losing part of this cohort to malnutrition and disease reduces the potential for the entire cohort. Failing to enroll part of the cohort in school at ages 6-8 results in additional loss to the cohort [age 6 is used arbitrarily in the figures to signify the age when children enter primary school]. Allowing children to drop out and others to complete school, and yet remain functionally illiterate, further reduces the cohort's full potential.

Any efforts to mitigate the loss of future productivity shown in figure 4 will increase the overall cohort's chance of success, adding children to the number who will survive well as productive adults. For each child that is added back, an entire family benefits, and so does the community and overall society.

Intervention: A Comprehensive Approach

The knowledge exists for breaking the terrible cycle of poverty. Consider a cohort of newborns. As much as 60 percent may be at risk in some countries, and yet their primary

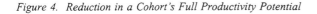

Figure 4. Reduction in a Cohort's Full Productivity Potential

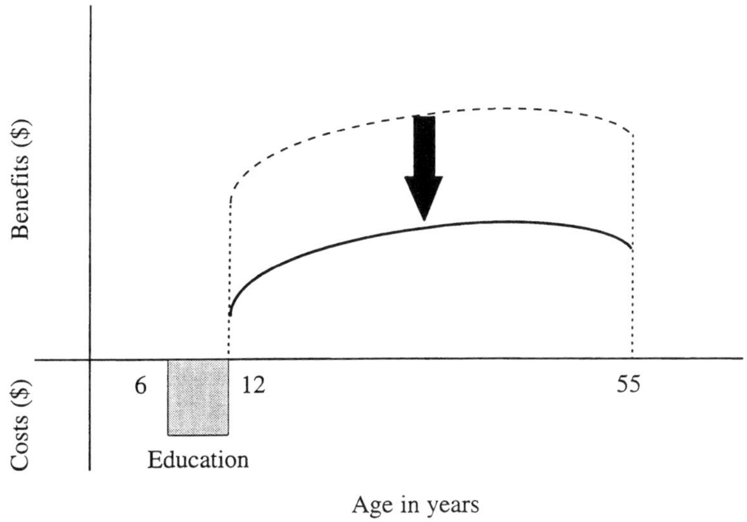

needs are known: shelter, food, health care, stimulation. Programs are available to assure their survival, reduce malnutrition and illness, and foster development. If these programs are implemented broadly, with a focus on infants at high risk, the cohort can proceed healthy, well nourished, and active into the next stage of life.

The needs of the young children at ages 1-3 also are known, and programs are available to assure that these needs are met. By implementing these programs broadly, favorable outcomes can be obtained and the children can enter their preschool years with vigor. Figure 5 summarizes the needs and areas of intervention for children at these three stages: 0-1 years, 1-3 years, and 3-6 years.

As indicated by figure 5, the needs and interventions for one age group are related to those for the other age groups. Because they are related, intervention strategies and programs need to be comprehensive and integrated horizontally as well as vertically. The aim at each stage of life is to decrease the likelihood of irreparable damage and to increase the likelihood of successful transition to the next stage.

Arguably, programs for even earlier stages (prenatal care, mothers' health care, safe birthing practices) and later stages (high-quality secondary school education) should be included as part of an integrated, comprehensive approach. The first step, however, is to offer children ages 0-8 a solid foundation on which to build. This age range accommodates the different ages around the world when children enter primary school.

ECD programs can provide the foundation needed. Returning to the cohort of 100 children whose productivity potential was reduced (see figure 4), figure 6 depicts the gains to be made in this cohort's potential by investing in ECD programs for children aged 0-8. As figure 6 suggests, the costs of this investment in the early years yield a substantial return on investment, in regained productivity, for the *entire cohort across the lifespan*.

Figure 5. Needs and Interventions for Young Children

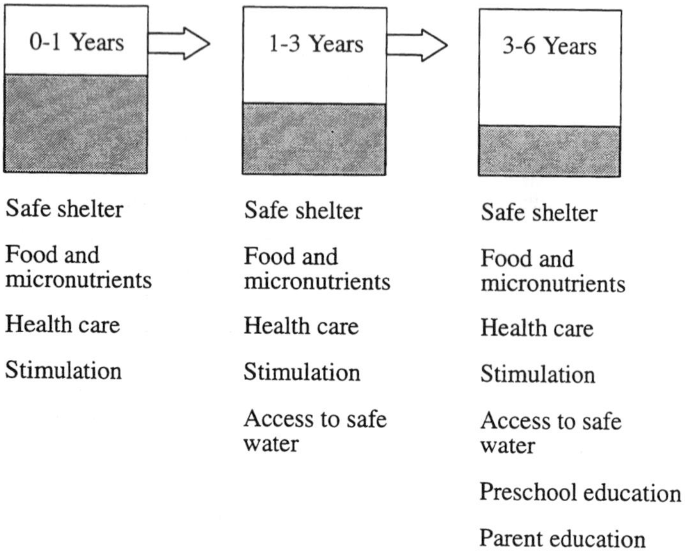

Figure 6. Regaining the Lost Productivity Potential

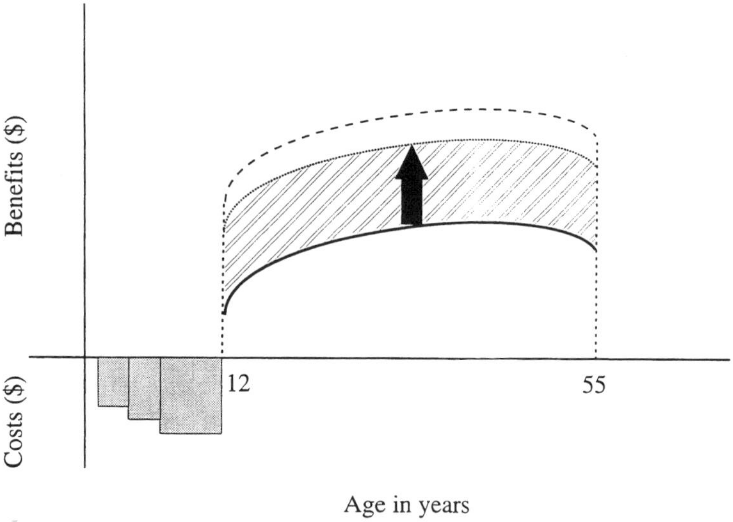

Conclusion

Productivity potential is a useful concept for understanding the benefits of ECD programs. Already applied to education, this concept enables policymakers to estimate the overall effect of a policy and helps administrators select the most cost-effective and appropriate interventions from among the many strategies already proven to be effective.

An increase in productivity potential, however, is an important but not the only benefit of ECD programs. Children who participate in these programs are likely to become more responsible citizens and better parents. They also will influence their siblings as they become better role models. ECD programs enable older siblings to pursue their own developmental directions in school and work by releasing them from the responsibility of providing daily childcare for their younger brothers and sisters.

Parent involvement is a key aspect of many ECD programs. By their participation in these programs, parents acquire knowledge about good nutrition, health risks and healthy behaviors, learning and cognition, parent-child interactions and family relationships, and other subjects related to early childcare and development. Their new knowledge and awareness benefit not only them but also the entire family. With improved self-esteem, these parents also may become more active in community activities. While their young children are attending an ECD program, parents, and particularly mothers, have more time for these activities and other productive endeavors.

All of these benefits must be counted in any analysis of ECD programs although they may be difficult to quantify economically. A rigorous effort is needed to delineate both the benefits and costs of available ECD strategies and programs. A framework for addressing the broad range of considerations that will be required in such benefit-cost analyses is suggested by Barnett in the next chapter.

By applying benefit-cost analysis to early child development, researchers can rationally document anticipated future returns of investment from ECD strategies and programs. Such documentation can be expected to stimulate design and implementation of ECD policies and programs that will address concerns about the well-being of the world's children.

References

Psacharopoulos, George. 1994. Returns to Investment in Education: A Global Update. *World Development* 22(9):1325-43.

Early Child Development: Investing in our Children's Future
M.E. Young, editor.

Costs and Financing of Early Child Development Programs

W. Steven Barnett

How much do highly effective early child development (ECD) programs cost? How should ECD programs be financed? These are simple questions, but they do not have simple answers.

The selection of ECD programs and of options regarding cost and financing must be based on expected economic benefits of the programs as well as local cultural, political, and economic constraints. These local variables are complex, and no single best solution exists for every situation. The costs and benefits of the same ECD program will vary among places and times and with different political, social, and economic conditions.

In the preceding chapter, van der Gaag addresses the benefits and choices related to ECD and introduces the concept of benefit-cost analysis. Relating this concept to social indicators and productivity, he calls for a comprehensive approach to interventions for early childhood and for research that will define the benefits and costs of such investments. Many of the benefits have been documented in the research literature on early child development, as summarized in the chapters throughout this volume. The *economic* benefits, however, have not been assessed systematically nor have the economic costs of these programs been examined. A combined benefit-cost analysis would help governments decide on specific program strategies that meet their society's needs and characteristics.

This chapter provides a general approach for obtaining information on the costs and benefits of ECD programs and a framework for guiding decisions regarding the cost and financing of these programs. The chapter opens with a discussion of alternative ECD arrangements, highlighting the advantages of integrating childcare with other ECD services. The sections that follow describe steps for assessing cost and initiating a cost analysis, major determinants of cost, cost variations between formal and informal programs, indicators for evaluating program benefits, and public and private approaches to financing. Emphasizing the need for research, several approaches are recommended, including the resource cost model and experimental or quasi-experimental studies utilizing a randomized or regression-continuity design.

Alternative ECD Arrangements

ECD programs are investments in the well-being and development of children. A major goal of these programs in developing countries, and in many industrialized countries as well, is to improve the development of children living in poverty. Considerable evidence indicates that poverty affects child development and that detrimental effects on child development increase as the depth and persistence of poverty increase. Moreover, the detrimental effects of poverty during early childhood are cumulative and long lasting.

Because the benefits from even modest ECD interventions can be substantial and permanent for poor children in developing countries (Grantham-McGregor and others 1994; McKay and others 1978; Pollitt and others 1993), government policy regarding ECD programs can influence national economic progress as well as children's well-being and development. Governments may finance or provide ECD programs by investing nationally in child development that focuses on poor children or by investing nationally in systems of health care, nutritional support, early childcare and education, and child financial support (for example, child allowances) that serve all families.

ECD programs encompass a wide range of interventions and focus on all domains of development, physical, social, emotional, and cognitive. As described earlier in this volume, ECD services include early childcare and education, nutritional supplementation, health care, and parent education. Many ECD services can affect multiple domains. However, programs that address different domains of development or provide different services tend to be administered by different government agencies. Inevitably, this makes coordination difficult, and each agency tends to focus only on the services and benefits relevant to the agency's specific mission.

Research, evaluation, and planning of ECD programs must avoid the fragmented views that tend to be held by government agencies and must include consideration of all the potential benefits from ECD programs. For example, theory and research suggest that early education, nutrition, and health interact with and complement each other and that the effects of this interaction increase with the severity of poverty in which a child lives (Selowsky 1981; Grantham-McGregor and others 1994). Also, interactions and complementarities indicate significant economic advantages to designing programs that deliver multiple services.

ECD services can be delivered using a variety of strategies and in various settings, primarily a child's home, another home, or some type of center. Table 1 classifies alternative arrangements for delivering ECD services. These arrangements are described in greater detail in the preceding chapters. Important differences among the approaches include the setting; a child's relationship to service providers; the professional status and training of providers; the formal or informal nature of the ECD arrangement; and the inclusion or lack of childcare among the services provided. (Paraprofessionals may be included in all settings. These persons may be day-care home mothers or employees of home visiting programs, childcare centers, preschool programs, or other ECD organizations who receive training but do not have the formal qualifications of teachers, nurses, or other professionals.) All of the differences in setting, service, and caregivers affect cost and also may affect benefits.

Integrating Childcare with Other ECD Services

One of the most important program distinctions is whether or not a program delivers services in conjunction with childcare. This distinction overlaps substantially with the distinction between home visiting and center-based programs, but is not exactly the same. For example, childcare can be provided in and around homes, and home visitors can work in family childcare homes and with other in-home caregivers.

Table 1. Alternative ECD Arrangements

Setting	Service	Caregiver status
Own home	Home visits	Professional, paraprofessional
	Childcare and education	Parent, sibling, other kin, untrained neighbor, nanny, babysitter
Another Home	Part-time, full-day, part-day childcare, education, and other services	Kin, untrained neighbor, paraprofessional
Centers	Part-time, full-day, part-day childcare, education, and other services	Professional, paraprofessional, untrained

Determining whether a program delivers services in conjunction with childcare is critical because providing childcare with ECD services may save on costs and generate added benefits. Integrating childcare with other services is relevant to policies for improving the lives of women and children, particularly as changes in family structure lead to the feminization of poverty (Evans 1994). The importance of nonparental childcare varies across and within countries, but with the need for childcare growing rapidly worldwide, nonparental childcare is a vital consideration in developing, planning, and evaluating ECD services (Leslie and Paolisso 1989).

Childcare is central to interactions among maternal employment and earnings, intrafamily resource allocation, fertility (number, timing, and spacing of births), and early education and development of children. Improvement in the quality of children's lives that enhances their development may be the most obvious and direct effect on children of providing free or subsidized high-quality childcare. Without such interventions, poor children will likely be in poor-quality environments that endanger their development; poor-quality childcare, which may be the only alternative available, has negative effects (Lamb and Sternberg 1990). At least one study shows that children cared for by preteen siblings in a developing country had lower weight for height, even after adjusting for social and economic differences (Engle 1991).

Although evidence of the effects of length-of-day or service mode is sparse, high-quality, full-day programs should produce more effects than part-day programs or programs that deliver services even less frequently (for example, in weekly home visits). Both quantity and quality affect efficacy. Cross-study comparisons suggest that centers are more effective than home visitors in improving child development (Barnett 1995; Boocock 1995). One exception is the parent education program studied by Kagitcibasi, which suggests that parent education in conjunction with home visiting or home visiting and childcare improves child development (see both Kagitcibasi and Lombard, this volume).

The indirect effects of childcare also may be quite substantial. Unfortunately, research on the effects of partially or fully subsidized high-quality childcare on maternal employment and productivity is lacking. Clearly, such programs would add to family income, contributing to improved child development. Studies show that maternal earnings increase the percentage of total family resources devoted to children's needs (Blumberg 1988; Engle, forthcoming). By adding to family income and increasing the share of family funds devoted to children's needs, partially or fully subsidized ECD programs could have a more than proportionate effect on child development and well-being (Pollack 1985).

In addition to increasing family income, childcare subsidies indirectly affect maternal fertility, which as it declines also increases a child's well-being by spreading funds among fewer children. Although the net effects of subsidies on fertility are unclear, subsidies increase maternal employment and decrease the frequency and extent of time out of the labor force. Experimental research is greatly needed on the effects of childcare on all aspects of maternal behavior. Interestingly, one home visiting program has affected fertility among low-income women in the United States, suggesting useful combinations of home visiting and childcare (Olds and Kitzman 1993).

Cost and Cost Analysis

Examining the cost of ECD programs involves several considerations. These include understanding the impact of the cost for developing countries, obtaining informative cost data, and adopting an appropriate methodology for estimating program costs. Each of these considerations is explored below.

Impact of Cost for Developing Countries

Cost affects the feasibility and desirability of ECD programs everywhere, but it especially limits widespread provision of ECD services in developing countries. In comparison with industrial economies, developing countries have lower incomes and a much larger percentage of their population in preschool years. The World Bank (1993) defines low-income countries as those with per capita gross national product below $635 in 1991 (all dollar amounts in this chapter are U.S. dollars). Many ECD model programs in high-income countries cost 5-10 times this amount, and some are even more expensive (Barnett 1993; Barnett and Escobar 1990). Although operating such models in developing countries at lower costs may be possible because of lower labor costs, the total costs still may be prohibitively high.

Even among developing countries, what they can afford varies tremendously. Their per capita incomes vary by more than an order of magnitude, and the percentage of the population under age 5 varies from 10 to 20 percent. Poorer countries tend to have higher percentages of young children, making the percentage of the population to be served by ECD programs highest where the ability to pay for services is lowest.

Government-sponsored ECD programs of some developing countries, such as professionally staffed nursery schools and childcare centers, are far out of reach for other, lower-income developing countries (Lira 1994). Even in the countries where they were developed as the primary ECD approach, the relatively high cost of such formal programs may prohibit their expansion to more than a small percentage of young children. Each country must carefully develop and implement ECD programs that are sufficiently low cost to be feasible on a large scale.

Need for Cost Data

In general, greater attention must be paid to obtaining cost data on ECD programs and to developing low-cost, highly effective model programs. These efforts require increased focus on cost analysis during ECD program research and evaluation. Researchers of ECD programs in developing countries rarely report program costs. Little information is available on the costs of alternative ECD approaches (see Lira 1994 for an exception), and virtually none of the cost information is accompanied by evidence of program effectiveness. Data are needed on income and wages, average and marginal costs, and number of children served.

Income and Wages
In providing cost data on ECD programs and models, information on local and national per capita income and average wages should be presented to put the cost data in perspective. Obviously, obtaining this information is difficult from communities where much of the work and many workers are not in the monetary sector of the economy or where underemployment is extensive. Nevertheless, in many circumstances the information can be obtained and would provide a rough way of indexing costs, enabling analysts and administrators in developing countries to assess the economic feasibility of alternative programs transferred to their own situation.

Average and Marginal Costs
Most often cost analysis involves average or marginal costs for each child rather than total costs of a program. Average cost for each child, sometimes referred to as unit cost or cost per child, is total cost divided by the number of children served. Marginal cost is the additional cost required to serve another child.

When national ECD efforts are relatively modest, marginal cost can be substantially lower than average cost because significant fixed costs can be divided among a larger number of children. Even with a single, small program marginal cost can be lower than average cost. For example, the costs of serving an additional child in each crèche or family day-care home might be lower than the average cost if a child were added without increasing the number of staff or the amount of space. Of course, whether such changes in adult-child ratios or square feet for each child are desirable depends on how both benefits and costs are affected.

Alternatively, if ECD programs are implemented first in the most densely populated or easily accessible areas with the greatest infrastructure, the marginal cost of expansion to more remote urban and rural areas may be higher than current average cost. For example, the costs of one informal ECD program in the Federal District of Mexico were an estimated $30 for each child, while the costs of extending the program to other areas of Mexico were an estimated $76 to $145 for each child (Lira 1994).

Number of Children Served
Focusing on average or marginal costs requires measuring another important variable, the number of children served. To obtain estimates of accurate costs for each child, accurate estimates are required of the number of children served. The number of children served must be estimated accurately whether the cost calculations are rough estimates for a nation,

which are based on government expenditures and community contributions, or highly precise estimates for a pilot program, which are based on detailed observations.

Accurately estimating the number of children served is difficult for at least two reasons. First, programs and agencies have incentives to exaggerate the number of children served. For example, programs may receive funding on a per-child basis, and agencies may have goals for numbers of children served that they are expected to achieve by specific dates. Second, absences and turnover make the number of children served somewhat ambiguous. Program administrators must carefully specify what counts as a child served and how the number of children served is to be computed. Average daily attendance, which must be converted to full-time equivalents when some children attend part-day and others full-day, is the most relevant concept in estimating average and marginal costs for each child. A survey indicating that roughly 300,000 children were served by an informal ECD program that officially was reported to serve nearly 900,000 children (Lira 1994) illustrates the importance of these issues.

Other important measures for number of children served include the number of children ever served during a year; the number of children who attend for a full year; the average number of days that a child attends and the average number of absences; and the annual turnover rate. Also useful would be knowing whether children and families who leave a program are simply moving from one program to another and continuing to receive services or whether they cease to receive services when they leave. Another important question to consider is whether a minimum amount of participation is required for a program to be minimally effective. In an extreme case, a program could be filled to capacity every day without any child or family receiving enough service to significantly affect child development.

Estimating Program Costs: The Resource Cost Model

Estimating program costs is more than an exercise in accounting. A standard method of cost analysis is the ingredients, or resource cost, model (Levin 1983, Chambers and Parrish 1994). This method begins by identifying required resources and listing quantities necessary to produce a program. After identifying the resources required, the various costs associated with these resources must be measured and the organizations paying for the costs must be determined.

Identifying Required Resources

Table 2 illustrates the type of resources that should be included for several different elements of a possible ECD system. Identifying required resources must be followed by specifying amounts of each resource needed to serve a certain number of children and expected costs of each resource. With this information, any government or other agency can estimate the cost of a model or approach to ECD in specific circumstances.

The resource cost model should be quite detailed about identifying the ingredients that affect cost most; usually these ingredients will be the direct service staff, supplies, equipment, and facilities. Such details are especially critical when communicating with an international audience because homogeneity of the qualities for ingredients cannot be assumed, particularly qualifications of the direct service staff. For example, specifying that

Table 2. Resource Cost Model Outline for National ECD System

Elements of national administration for early childhood investment	*Elements of childcare center*
	Recurrent Costs
Director	
Deputy director for training and curriculum development	Personnel
	Director
Deputy director for health and nutrition	Curriculum specialist or trainer
Deputy director for evaluation	Teachers
Deputy director for planning and budgeting	Assistant teachers
Regional assistant directors	Parent volunteers
Program inspectors or monitors	Secretary
Technical support staff	Health care professional (part-time)
Clerical support staff	
Consultants	Nonpersonnel
Office supplies and equipment	Office supplies
Communications	Classroom supplies
Publication of training and curriculum materials	Food or nutritional supplements for children's meals
Transportation	Medicines or vaccines
Utilities and facilities	Telephone
	Postage
Elements of a family childcare home	Utilities
	Insurance
Mother's time and effort	Advertising
Training and planning materials for mother	
Educational materials and supplies	Capital Costs
Toys	Classroom equipment
Food or nutritional supplements	Playground equipment
Additional wear and tear on home or home improvements needed	Office equipment
	Building and land

one teacher and one assistant teacher are required for every thirty children ages 3-5 years is not detailed enough. The training and qualifications of these caregivers also must be specified. Similarly, requiring one classroom for every thirty children is insufficient detail; the size of the classroom and its equipment and supplies also must be specified.

Measuring Resource Costs

Once all of the ingredients in the resource cost model have been identified, the cost of each ingredient must be measured. This cost, which economists refer to as the opportunity cost, is assessed as the value of a resource in its best alternative use. In a relatively well-functioning market, the price of an ingredient purchased from the market economy provides a reasonable estimate of its opportunity cost. However, this equation will not always be the case.

For example, the market wage is too high when hired staff would otherwise be unemployed or underemployed. Also, when wage and benefit levels are set administratively, the paid wages and compensation may be too high or too low, such as when part of the compensation is access to privileges, goods and services, or opportunities that are not recognized formally as fringe benefits. Sometimes, program staff would not otherwise participate in the monetary economy, and no alternative wages are comparable. Some programs may even require substantial donations of time, effort, and materials from participating families. Again, even the travel time required to reach a day-care center is a cost that should not be neglected in planning and comparing alternatives.

When no ready market values exist for ingredients and making any inference from markets is difficult, sensitivity analysis can be useful. In a sensitivity analysis, the cost analyst proposes a range of reasonable low, medium, and high cost estimates for an ingredient and examines the effect on overall program cost.

In some cases the cost of an ingredient may have little effect on overall cost and can be considered irrelevant. In other cases, the effect on overall cost may be so great that the ECD program only makes sense if the ingredient's cost is assumed to be low. In this case, the program should only be implemented when there is reasonable certainty that the ingredient is low-cost. For example, ECD programs should only use parents on a rotating basis as unpaid caregiver assistants when the cost of the parents' time plus the costs of organizing and managing parent volunteers is lower than the costs of paid teacher assistants or when added benefits from using parents outweigh the added costs.

In addition to showing what ingredients or resources are required and their costs, a cost analysis model must show all costs, direct and indirect, initial as well as ongoing. Costs include those of administering, supporting, and starting up a program as well as the costs of providing the service. Capital costs, annual operating costs, and costs that are not paid for by the government or program sponsor also must be included in the model.

For example, developing a national system of day-care centers and family day-care homes might require creating a national administration like the one outlined in table 2. Other requirements might include regional administrative units; a preservice and inservice training system for teachers and caregivers; developing curriculum and publishing curriculum materials; constructing and equipping new facilities; services from local health care providers that are accessible to childcare providers; and a research and development agency to facilitate program and policy improvement. Resource cost models may be developed for each of the different types of requirements and for each of the basic types of service delivery organizations.

Direct Costs. Because most costs result from direct services, the resources necessary to administer and support a program (infrastructure resources) must be separated from the resources necessary to provide services at a local or community level (direct service resources). In most ECD programs, resources necessary for delivering direct services, such as education, at the local level are distinguished as recurrent and capital costs by how long the cost is relevant (Tsang 1994). Recurrent costs are the ongoing operating costs of goods and services consumed in the current year. Capital costs are the costs of equipment, buildings, land, and anything else that lasts for more than a year. In most instances, for example, the costs of preservice and inservice training for administrators, teachers, and others are properly considered capital costs.

As shown in table 2, personnel costs are recurrent and usually account for the majority of program costs. They may be subdivided into administrative and support services, paid direct services, and parents and other volunteers. Further breakdown of personnel costs by type of activity may be useful if separate staff members have responsibility for nutrition, health, and educational or childcare activities. In developing countries where labor costs are relatively low and programs seek to improve nutrition, food can be a substantial part of direct costs, and close attention must be paid to the efficient purchase, preparation, and distribution of food and special supplements.

Examining the distribution of direct costs across categories increases understanding of program operation and of resource allocation to various types of activities. For example, evaluators frequently wish to know what percentage of costs goes to direct service staff, to facilities that provide direct services, to transportation, to administrators, and to support staff at all levels. No firm rules exist for how much should be allocated to each type of activity, but insight regarding the efficiency of allocations may be gained by looking at variations in the percentages over time and among programs and by making comparisons to other types of education and human service programs.

Generally, programs that are more efficient allocate a relatively large percentage of resources to direct services and provide services at low, average total costs. Of course, care must be exercised when making comparisons or imposing rules on resource allocations, such as ruling that no more than 10 percent of cost goes to administration. Misallocation of resources may result from failing to recognize important differences among programs, and quality may be inadvertently sacrificed in efforts to contain costs.

If programs cut administrative costs (which might include supervision, training, and evaluation) too much, quality may fall. Some programs may have hidden service costs (such as donated facilities or large quantities of unpaid labor) that result in inaccurate comparisons when comparing only government budgets. As another example, although the percentage of administrative costs might be relatively high for a program of family childcare homes that provides significant amounts of ongoing training to caregivers who are paid by parents, when compared with a program that uses preschool teachers with university degrees to provide services, the family home childcare program may be more efficient administratively and overall.

Indirect Costs. ECD programs also must consider indirect costs, although these may be more difficult to identify than direct costs. For example, in many countries, private sources contribute a substantial portion of the resources for primary education (Tsang 1994) and preprimary education, which is particularly supported by families of the participating children. Private costs may be direct (such as when fees are paid to cover the costs of resources employed by the program) or indirect (such as when costs imposed by participation are not resources provided by the program).

All too often indirect costs imposed on parents and children who participate in ECD programs are ignored. The most important of these indirect costs for parents tends to be travel cost, the cost of getting children to and from a program that is far from home or work. Location and hours of operation are highly important considerations in minimizing indirect costs to families as is the recognition that families may need care and education for several children of different ages. Access to the program by mass transit and colocation of infant, preschool, and school-age programs near homes might significantly lower indirect costs.

Other indirect costs result from withdrawing children from some other productive activity. In many cases, preschool children are not sufficiently productive in work at home or in the market to make this cost significant. However, older preschool children sometimes provide useful services for their families and others; they may be providing childcare for their younger siblings (although this might be considered costly rather than valuable from the perspective of society as a whole). ECD programs should take into account all direct and indirect costs to parents and children.

Initial Costs. Planning and budgeting for an ECD system also must include preparation for unusually high initial costs. One-time start-up costs and capital costs usually require large initial expenditures. Administrative, monitoring, and training costs may be relatively high at first because of the extra effort required to launch a new enterprise and figure out how to make it work. Once the enterprise is launched, knowledge and skills can become institutionalized and passed on at relatively low cost. Some investments in human capital, however, will continue to be necessary because of staff turnover and because skills and knowledge eventually need to be updated. Still, investments in staff development will be highest in the first several years.

The cost for new facilities can pose an initial financing problem for governments or other organizations that may already have high debt levels or high borrowing costs. Strategies for dealing with this problem include developing new facilities slowly, relying on communities to develop the facilities, and making use of existing community and family resources. Existing resources include religious organizations' buildings, businesses, markets, courtyards and other community spaces, and homes. Clearly, ECD programs can lower costs by using existing facilities that serve other purposes. Lack of specialized facilities should not hinder an ECD program from beginning.

Determining Public and Private Contributions

Along with identifying all costs, a cost analysis must distinguish between public and private costs (who pays) (Tsang 1994). In many cases, the government's share covers only part of the program's cost, and looking only at government costs can be misleading. Community contributions may be needed and indicate the value a community places on a program. In some circumstances an ECD program is feasible *only* if others share the costs with government. However, a program may still fail if the government requires more cost sharing than parents or communities can afford or more than is justified by perceptions of private benefits, which may be less than social benefits. When replicating a model developed elsewhere, recognizing the extent to which international organizations, businesses, community organizations, or families contributed to costs is critical. If these contributions are not replicated, government may have to pay more.

Major Determinants of Cost

Table 1 shows alternative arrangements for delivering ECD program services. These arrangements can be collapsed into three basic models: home visitor programs, family childcare homes, and center-based programs. The models differ in cost primarily because of differences in nine program characteristics that influence cost and are easily mandated or regulated. These nine program characteristics are described below: age at start, frequency, duration, ratio of children to staff, staff qualifications, supervision and administration, health and nutrition components, parental involvement, and community and family context.

Age at Start

This factor is the most obvious influence on cost because it determines how many children must be served and for how long. Generally, providing ECD services at an early age is relatively ineffective if the services are discontinued before school entry. For a given program configuration, serving children for 2 years beginning at age 3 costs twice as much as serving them for 1 year at age 4. Because of higher staff-child ratios necessary for infants and toddlers, childcare in centers from birth to age 3 may cost even more than twice as much as serving children from ages 3-6.

The relative cost advantage of home visitor programs over the other two models and of family childcare homes over center-based care is considerably higher at the youngest ages than for children ages 3-5. Because of changes in relative cost, changing the mode of delivering ECD services from one age to another may make the program more cost-effective. Of course, no matter how services are provided, costs rise when the age at which ECD service begins is lowered.

Frequency

Frequency refers to the number of days each week or month that services are delivered. A home visitor program might entail meeting with children and their parents once a week or once a month. Children might attend a preschool program at a center or participate in a playgroup in their neighborhood for 2 or 3 days a week or every day. Many preschool education programs operate only 8 or 9 months of the year, but childcare programs tend to operate all 12 months. Also, some variations in scheduling may occur when mothers work outside the home only during certain seasons.

Duration

Duration is the length of each session in which children and parents participate. Home visits typically last between 1 and 2 hours. Center-based programs commonly last for one-half day (2-2.5 hours), a whole school day (4-6 hours), or a whole work day (8-10 hours). Childcare programs sometimes provide services on a drop-in or as-needed basis, and the amount of care each child receives varies according to the parent's work schedule.

Ratio of Children to Staff

Another determinant is the number of children for each staff member. In a home visitor program this ratio is called caseload. Caseload is determined by the duration and frequency of home visits and the time required for travel, preparation of lessons and other activities, office work, and any other activities the home visitor must conduct. Increasing caseload is one way to decrease cost, but it may reduce quality and eventually does reduce either the duration or frequency of home visits.

In a home- or center-based program, the number of children in the home or center and the number of staff determine the ratio. Sometimes specifying ratios for various types of staff is useful. For example, ratios may be specified for teachers alone; teachers and their paid assistants; and teachers, paid assistants, and volunteers (including parents). When all

similarities also exist across rural contexts. For example, most women face seasonal increases in intensity and hours of their work. In urban sectors, women are classified as formal or informal sector workers. Within the formal sector, a distinction can be made between women who have relatively well-paying jobs with fringe and social benefits and women who do not.

Family structure varies within all sectors across communities and families. ECD programs should take into account the presence or absence of fathers (influenced by male migration for work, which may be seasonal); the availability of extended family to care for children; and the extent that older children are the caregivers (especially during school years). Finally, ethnic and religious diversity may require programmatic diversity and affect cost (Yeoh and Huang 1995).

Costs of Formal and Informal Programs

Another important area for ECD intervention research is the relative merits of formal and informal programs. Formal programs provide ECD services in a center or school and are staffed by professional teachers and teacher assistants. They have relatively high costs. In many developing countries, formal programs may be too expensive for large-scale use. If they are used, they may consume such a large percentage of the public funds for ECD investment that only a small percentage of the population receives service, resulting in inefficient and inequitable allocation of ECD resources.

Informal programs operate in one of three ways. First, they may train community volunteers or others to educate parents, which improves parental efforts to foster the development of their own children. Second, informal programs may train staff to make home visits (typically weekly) and work directly with children. Third, they may train community women to care for children in their homes or in community facilities, often improving services already offered by women in such settings.

Informal programs have much lower costs than formal programs, and some evidence indicates that they can produce benefits equivalent to those of formal programs (Myers 1992). Many alternative models of ECD services might be developed and tested in the vast middle ground that exists between current formal and informal models.

Apparent Cost Advantages of Informal Programs

For both formal and informal models and those that lie between, application of the nine important program characteristics described earlier would be useful. In principle, informal ECD programs seem to have cost advantages. For example, from the perspective of government funding, which excludes parental costs, the cost comparison is most favorable toward informal programs. However, few data are available on parent and community costs for either type of program. Although cross-program and cross-country generalizations are risky because information is lacking on contributions of local conditions, customs, and cultures to program success, the magnitude of the differences between costs of formal and informal programs is so large that general comparisons seem useful despite their limitations.

Costs for formal, center-based programs for young children tend to be measured in thousands of dollars. For example, Lira (1994) reports unit costs of $3,611 in 1994 for full-day programs and $1,959 for half-day programs in Argentina. The World Bank (1992) shows a unit cost of $1,406 in 1991 for full-day programs in Mexico.

Costs for informal programs tend to be an order of magnitude lower. For example, The cost to the government of an informal Colombian program of government-sponsored family day-care homes, called Hogares Comunitarios de Bienestar (HCB), was reported in 1991 to be as low as $130 each year, but the full social cost is more than twice that, $298 (Lira 1994). Estimated costs for other informal programs, such as home visitor and family home childcare models, are about $100 per child (World Bank 1992). Several programs, such as the Integrated Child Development Services in India, PROAPE (Programa de Alimentaçao de Pre-escolar) in Brazil, PRONOEI (Programa No Formal de Educación Inicial) in Peru, and Initial Education Project in Mexico, have estimated costs between $25 and $50 per child (Myers 1992; World Bank 1992).

Difficulties in Estimating Costs

Caution should be exercised when comparing formal and informal ECD programs based on the cost estimates given above. For example, cost estimates for informal education programs other than HCB also may include only government or cash costs, and costs to the community may be relatively difficult to estimate.

Previous reviews of cost estimates for early intervention programs indicate that costs are underestimated (see Barnett and Escobar 1990 for a review of problems encountered in the U.S. literature), and recent studies cited by Lira (1994) suggest that underestimation can be quite serious. Some costs actually may be omitted, and the number of children served may be overestimated, possibly a widespread problem for informal programs that are not subject to standard auditing and accountability procedures. In some cases, informal models may have been implemented first, in the least expensive circumstances, and expansion requires higher costs.

A conservative lower boundary for cost estimates of informal ECD models might be $100 per child (at least in Latin America), and some informal models may cost several times this amount. The true figure could be lower, but a range of estimates should be used in sensitivity analyses for low-cost models to ensure that projects will be feasible or efficient even if costs are higher than expected. Even with costs higher than expected, informal programs are low cost compared with formal programs. Unfortunately, comparison of benefits is unclear among high-cost formal programs, somewhat lower-cost programs and very-low-cost informal programs.

Evaluating Program Benefits

Few evaluations of ECD programs have been conducted in developing countries, and most that have been conducted have serious methodological limitations. The strongest information on ECD programs in developing countries comes from the few studies using true experimental designs and longitudinal follow-up (McKay and others 1978; Powell and Grantham-McGregor 1989). Long-term follow-up of experimental studies of interventions for low-income populations in the United States remains an important source of additional information (Barnett 1995). However, these studies focus on higher-cost models.

Studies of low-cost, informal ECD programs in developing countries generally use weak, quasi-experimental designs, small samples, short follow-ups, and rudimentary (or no) statistical analyses (Myers 1992). Small samples limit statistical power to detect effects, which can be especially serious if effects vary with child and family characteristics and social context as predicted by the ecological theory of human development (Bronfenbrenner 1989). Short follow-ups leave unanswered questions about the persistence of effects and later consequences.

Selection Bias

The single greatest threat to the validity of these studies of high- and low-cost ECD models probably comes from selection bias (Campbell 1991; Moffit 1991). Without random assignment, participation in ECD programs (that is, selection by families of one ECD program over another) is influenced by family characteristics that also influence child growth and development. For example, families that are more intensely concerned about child development and education are more likely to enroll their children in ECD programs. Families with higher status, higher incomes, and better political connections (even within a generally poor community) are more likely to succeed in enrolling their children in programs that are in limited supply.

Such initial differences between program and no-program groups or between groups attending different programs tend to bias estimates of program effects. Because the bias results from self-selection, it is called selection bias. More generally, several selection processes may bias results. For example, selection bias also can result when programs select participants and when nonrandom attrition occurs. When measured after intervention, preexisting differences that lead to selection (for example, maternal influence on family decisionmaking or parental concern for child development and education) may themselves be mistaken for program effects.

Incorporating Pretest Measures. At the very least, measures of child development and family characteristics likely to affect child development (parental education, attitudes, behavior, and family economic resources) should be measured before and after program participation. Although incorporating these control variables into statistical analyses does not guarantee unbiased estimation of program effects, and true experiments are preferred (especially when control variables are measured imperfectly), pretest measures at least allow researchers to check for some initial selection differences and attempt to control for them (Campbell 1991; Hausman and Wise 1985; Heckman and Robb 1985; Mullahy and Manning 1995).

Advantages of Experimental Research

Experimental studies are the primary means for assuring that research findings are valid and replicable. Two possibilities for ECD programs are "true" experiments utilizing random assignment of participants and quasi experiments utilizing the regression-discontinuity design.

True Experiments with Random Assignment

Although common arguments claim that true experiments are difficult to conduct, they have been conducted successfully and are used commonly in other fields, such as health care research. Most people feel that program assignment by lottery is fair. When services cannot be provided to all the families who would benefit, experiments have the added advantage of distributing services more equitably than would occur without the experiments. Random assignment does not need to be made by individual child or family, but can be performed by city blocks, neighborhoods, villages, or other units; analyses should take this factor into account because independence within sampling units cannot be assumed.

Common arguments against true experiments also claim that attrition introduces the same problem as selection anyway. However, attrition can be kept low enough so that it has little influence on estimated effects, and the combination of selective participation and attrition only complicates statistical analyses. Experiments provide superior estimates of program effects, and they are relatively easy for public officials and the general public to understand. Using true experiments to compare two alternative ECD programs is beneficial because both programs are expected to have positive effects and only their relative cost-effectiveness is in question.

Quasi Experiments with Regression-Continuity Design

True experiments may be unnecessary or inappropriate, for example, when improvement is highly improbable without intervention, or when dire consequences are imminent for specific children, *and* the intervention is certain to have no negative consequences. In such cases, a strong alternative is the regression-discontinuity design, which admits children to the ECD program by intensity of their needs or severity of their conditions.

Using the regression-discontinuity design, if ECD services can be provided at no cost to 500 children in an area, children could be ranked according to degree of poverty or degree of malnutrition (for example, by weight for height), and the poorest or most malnourished 500 children could be accepted. The next 500 who rank higher on income or nutrition would be the comparison group. Health and nutrition programs that treat individuals in the poorest condition first parallel this design.

Because the rules used for assignment and cutoff between treatment and comparison groups are known, the effects of the ECD program can be estimated without selection bias. Compared with random assignment, the design's disadvantages include requiring a much larger sample size to yield the same statistical power, which is more costly, and the potential for having an interaction between the level of need (the selection criterion) and effects of the intervention, which creates doubt about producing unbiased results (Cook and Campbell 1979).

Potential Indicators of Benefit

The wide range of goals for ECD programs and the interaction among outcomes make specifying a concise list of benefit indicators difficult. Some indicators can be identified from previous research findings. Others have not been observed but are suggested by theory or empirical research, which indicates that they are consequences of effects that have been observed. Benefits produced by the interaction of program elements will be especially complex. For example, programs that facilitate child development as well as maternal employment and productivity also may affect fertility patterns. As noted earlier, few studies reliably estimate the effects of free or subsidized childcare (as part of an ECD program) on maternal employment and earnings, but such effects clearly are to be expected (Gustafsson and Stafford 1992; Joshi and Davies 1992; Maume 1991).

Table 3 provides a comprehensive list of potential benefit indicators. In practice, the most important will be simple indicators of child health and development; child injury and maltreatment; school success and progress (age of entry, school completion or dropout rates, educational attainment, grade repetition, and test scores); parental employment and earnings; and family size and structure.

Table 3. Measurable Benefit Indicators from ECD Programs

Maternal reports on child health and medical services	Achievement test scores
Maternal reports on child behavior	Disability and developmental delay
Maternal reports on child development	Involvement in crime and delinquency
Maternal reports on child injuries	Home literacy environment
Clinic records on health, services, and immunizations	Parental literacy
Hospitalization rates	Family health practices
Height and weight	Maternal report on stress
Anemia	Mother-child interaction
Condition of teeth	Child-mother interaction
Neonatal and infant mortality rates	Maternal health and nutritional status
Birthweight and gestation period	Maternal employment
Nutritional status	Maternal earnings
Grade level for age	Maternal role in family decisionmaking
Grade repetition	Family food budget and allocation
Age at school entry	Fertility rates
Dropout rate	Number, timing, and spacing of subsequent births
	Unwanted pregnancy and abortion

Financing

ECD programs can be financed through public and private arrangements and by international organizations.

Combining Public and Private Resources

Relying on a combination of public and private resources has important advantages. Public funds can support services directly with no charge to parents, can support subsidies that allow programs to lower prices, or can support subsidies that parents use to purchase services. Funding and services can be provided at any government level or combination of levels. Funds can be raised from taxes (payroll, income, sales, value-added, and property taxes) on individuals or businesses. Private funds include parents' payments and donations of labor and goods, employer contributions, and contributions from other community organizations including religious organizations, political parties, and charitable and service organizations.

To distribute the burden of funding ECD programs, most countries depend on funds from several levels of government (public) and from private sources. In the United States, local community agencies (mostly nongovernmental, but in some cases local school districts) operate federally funded Head Start programs. The federal government funds 80 percent of the Head Start program contingent on a 20 percent match from the community. The 20 percent community match is provided by many sources, but much comes from parents who donate time as volunteers in the program. These parents may acquire training and education that allows them to enter paid positions; about one-third of Head Start's teachers first encountered the program as parents. Facilities are another common donation from community organizations.

In Sweden, local governments provide ECD services with funds from the national government (49 percent), local government (41 percent), and parents (10 percent), who pay fees on a sliding scale that increases with income (Gustafsson and Stafford 1995). In Singapore, parents bear most of the cost although the government subsidizes monthly fees at government childcare centers for women who work outside the home and provides funds to help start childcare centers.

Politicians should decide which taxes or combination of taxes should be used, taking into consideration the feasibility and economic effects of alternative taxes in specific circumstances. Several important considerations can be specified. For example, some taxes may be favored because they are less conspicuous. Also, governments may favor using a wide range of taxes to support new programs so that no single tax is much affected and the increase will arouse less resistance from specific interest groups. Alternatively, taxes may be tied explicitly to program benefits to show to the public the connection between payment and benefits. For example, ECD programs that are part of a social security system tied to employment typically are financed by payroll taxes.

Gaining Business Participation

Businesses cannot be expected to lead financing for ECD programs, but they can be an important part of an overall approach to improve ECD services. They can be encouraged to provide ECD services or funds just as they are encouraged to provide health care benefits, through special tax incentives such as exempting ECD employee benefits from taxation. Also, businesses may be encouraged to adopt preventive interventions and improve the quality of health care because of potential savings from reduced medical expenses.

One key to gaining successful business participation would be specifying a well-defined set of reforms that businesses could adopt easily. For example, a study of health and health care among employees and their dependents (8,000 including 900 children under age 5) at a privately owned mine in Peru showed high morbidity rates despite an annual expenditure of $1.7 million for welfare and medical care (Foreit and others 1991). Infant mortality was 120 per 1,000 live births. The study showed a lack of well-baby care, low vaccination rates (less than 5 percent of children under age 5 were fully vaccinated), high incidence of care for diarrhea and respiratory infections, overmedication, and use of inappropriate medications. Children under age 5 accounted for 50 percent of all clinic use.

By hiring an additional physician and nurse to provide well-baby and maternal care (at an annual cost of about $10 for each employee) and by following World Health

Organization guidelines for treatment, the company was able to obtain substantial savings in pharmaceutical expenditures within the first 2 years. These savings were projected to exceed costs after several years. In addition, vaccination coverage exceeded 75 percent for children under age 5; 90 percent were enrolled in growth monitoring, and malnutrition rehabilitation was provided as necessary. Government can facilitate these types of improvements on a large scale by distributing a plan for businesses to follow that includes guidelines for well-baby and maternity care, treatment, and malnutrition rehabilitation.

Forms of Government and International Support

Government and international support for ECD programs can take a variety of forms short of full funding. For example, government can support local initiatives on either the supply or demand side of the market by:

- Matching funds for an organization or matching payments for each child served
- Matching government payments to private maternity savings associations or individual maternity and childcare accounts
- Paying more for programs that meet public or private standards of quality
- Paying child allowances to mothers
- Improving credit access for small businesses and cooperatives
- Offering technical assistance and training for ECD service providers
- Providing childcare homes and other informal programs with nutritional supplements, oral rehydration therapy (ORT), and other resources, including credit for renovations
- Passing legislation that requires employers to provide parental leave, childcare, and other ECD services
- Passing legislation that regulates ECD program quality
- Passing legislation that secures women's rights to land, other property, and income
- Sponsoring public information campaigns and parent education on water purification, food preparation, immunizations, breastfeeding, ORT, and injury prevention
- Sponsoring public information campaigns and parent education on the importance of quality adult-child interactions for infants and young children in childcare settings and at home
- Passing regulations for employers to facilitate women's efforts to breastfeed infants

- Coordinating public transportation schedules and routes with parents' needs for childcare

- Coordinating hours of school-age childcare and hours of childcare for younger children.

Some of these examples may be relatively ineffective or have negative consequences. For example, mandated, paid parental leave and ECD service benefits raise the cost of employees to business and government. This increased cost could result in (a) employment discrimination against women, if they are perceived as more likely than others to use such benefits; (b) decreased employment of low-skilled workers, especially in government agencies with fixed budgets and in the presence of a minimum wage; and (c) a decline in cash wages (Barnett and Musgrave 1991).

Innovative Efforts

Several developing countries show promising examples of innovative government efforts. In Colombia, the government improves family childcare homes by providing food supplies (food accounts for an estimated 40 percent of the cost) and credit for renovating the homes (Young 1996). In Brazil, as an incentive to participate in training, caregivers receive free milk and priority for services at health care clinics for children in their care (Thomas 1984).

In Bolivia, an interactive radio program, *Jugando en el PIDI*, teaches children under age 6 who attend child development centers and improves child-teacher interactions (Young 1996). This effort suggests the possibility of using radio to broadcast daily programs of activities (for example, stories, songs, and games) for parents and their children and for informal programs, such as family childcare homes and courtyard or neighborhood cooperatives. Such broadcasts may improve the curriculum of informal programs, especially if accompanied by training from a network of supervisors or trainers who work with caregivers and prepare them for using the radio sessions. Television and video could be used similarly (at least for centers) where television sets are widely available. Evans and Kagitcibasi (this volume) highlight the media as a potent, virtually untapped resource for a national strategy on early child development.

Local Effects and Alternative Approaches

Advantages and disadvantages of alternative approaches to government support for ECD programs will vary depending on local conditions. For example, a number of industrial and developing countries have legislation that ties ECD benefits, such as maternity leave and childcare, to employment in the formal sector of the economy. Such a policy may be effective when labor markets are tight and a large percentage of women with children work in the formal labor market. This policy may be particularly effective if most women work in the public sector where government can readily prevent discrimination against those who take time off during the first year of their child's life. However, in labor-surplus situations such policies may decrease employment of women and significantly lower their earnings.

Moreover in countries with legislation that ties ECD benefits to employment in the formal economy, when large percentages of the population are not in the formal economy, distribution of ECD services can be extremely inequitable and may be inefficient (for example, those with the greatest need receive nothing). Problems are exacerbated if government provides, or requires that others provide, ECD programs using expensive formal models whose cost may exceed wages paid to a typical worker in many communities.

Informal programs may have important advantages in addition to low cost. These include a high degree of parental involvement, comprehensive attention to all of a child's needs, sensitivity to each child's real needs, cultural appropriateness, and improved productive capacity of parents and communities.

However, because informal programs rely to a large extent on community and parent resources, they may have difficulty achieving the desired level of quality in some, or even many, communities. For example, low levels of education on the part of parents may make acquiring the knowledge and skills necessary for child development or parent education difficult. Lack of education may create difficulties in transmitting knowledge and abilities to older preschool children that would help them to succeed in school. In some cases, the nutritional, health care, and other physical resources contributed by a community also may be low quality. Quality becomes an especially serious problem when communities experience unusual stress from economic or political crises that reduce available resources to an even lower level. Similar difficulties have been noted when primary schools are highly dependent on community resources, as with harambee schools in Kenya (Bray 1994).

Systems to provide ECD programs also vary greatly from country to country, depending on social and economic conditions and prevailing attitudes and beliefs about the appropriate roles of government and the family, about women and their participation in the labor force, and about childrearing and education. The ethnic and religious diversity of a population also affects ECD systems; the more diverse a country is, the greater the need for a system that responds to different demands from groups and individuals.

Some countries emphasize full-day childcare programs that enable mothers to work, while other countries emphasize part-day programs and family subsidies that enable mothers (and in some cases fathers) to stay home with children. Such policies may vary by the ages of children. For example, Sweden provides an extensive public childcare system, but also offers parents paid leave for the first year of a child's life. Some countries offer universal public ECD programs; other countries provide free public programs only to low-income families. Some countries provide ECD services directly through the government; others offer parents subsidies to help purchase private services.

Conclusion

Analyzing the costs and benefits of ECD programs through rigorous, systematic benefit-cost analysis will provide a framework for addressing how much should be invested in early child development and at what unit cost in specific circumstances. Governments, international agencies, and other organizations have limited resources. To make informed decisions, they must understand the tradeoffs of alternative national investments, including early child development, and of alternative ECD programs for improving the growth and development of young children.

The Need for Research

As investments, ECD programs must be judged by their payoffs in economic and human terms, recognizing that placing a monetary value on important ECD outcomes is not always possible. Research on economic returns of ECD investments might help reverse the tendency of many governments to underestimate the value of ECD programs (particularly for the poorest children) in relation to other expenditures. Research also would provide more definitive information about the critical elements of program delivery, such as which services or combination of services should begin at what ages and how they should be staffed, located, and financially supported.

Understanding the Benefits of ECD

Knowledge has been accumulating in recent years on the benefits of ECD programs in industrialized and developing countries. The preceding chapters in this volume summarize current knowledge on the health, nutrition, and cognitive benefits of these programs. A great deal of information, however, is still unknown. To enhance understanding of these benefits, either an experimental approach using randomized trials or a strong quasi-experimental design should be used for estimating costs and benefits. Low-income countries cannot risk their resources on ECD interventions without solid evidence of high returns.

Although sound estimates of ECD program costs are relatively easy and inexpensive to produce, they generally are not available, even for nutritional interventions that show relatively strong evidence of effectiveness. Sound estimates of benefits are more difficult to produce, but should be pursued to identify especially effective programs and thereby avoid costly, large-scale investments in inefficient programs or failure to invest in beneficial programs because of the lack of convincing evidence. In weighing the costs and benefits of alternative research strategies, it is important to remember that randomized trials produce the largest statistical power for a given sample size and, as a result, are relatively low in cost.

Weighing Costs and Benefits

Special research attention needs to given to analyzing the costs and benefits of informal programs, which are more likely to be utilized in developing countries. Comprehensive systems of services, including childcare, may be especially promising. To facilitate benefit-cost analysis, the resource cost model can be used to great advantage.

Informal Programs

For ECD programs to be feasible worldwide, options must be affordable for low-income countries with a large percentage of their population under age 5. Future research, therefore, on ECD programs should target promising informal models that claim to have low costs and should estimate their costs and benefits in contrast to more expensive formal models. For example, government costs may be kept low by investments to improve the quality of existing plaza or courtyard nurseries and family day-care homes. A research program should be developed to illuminate the tradeoffs between cost and quality faced by informal ECD programs. Informal programs are engaged in the difficult task of trying to transfer human capital and other resources to young children at low cost in environments where these resources are scarce.

Comprehensive Systems that Include Childcare
The complementary interactions among health, nutrition, education, and childcare needs of mothers imply that an efficient approach to investing in ECD will consist of a comprehensive, coherent system of services that provides continuity in services from the beginning of childcare through primary school. A single program that provides all these services may or may not be the most efficient approach. Specialization may offer advantages, and cross-program coordination will be necessary. To date the most neglected benefit from ECD appears to be childcare benefits for mothers. The potential is great for large economic benefits from joint, low-cost childcare and ECD programs, but no studies provide sound estimates.

An ECD system can consist of multiple programs involving policymakers and researchers who take a systemic view to planning, developing, and evaluating the programs and coordinating with schools, employers, and mass transit. However, the components of an efficient ECD system will vary from one country to another and even within countries in accordance with parent and child needs, resources, and costs. Nevertheless, researchers should be able to provide information about desirable alternatives for ECD programs and systems in various types of communities.

Resource Cost Model
To ensure that analysis results are useful to as many countries as possible, cost studies should utilize a resource cost model approach and should index costs to local wage rates or per capita income. In estimating unit cost, more attention must be given to accurately measuring the number of units of service provided. Estimating the number of children who enter a program in a year or the number of places provided is not enough. Research must accurately estimate the number of children who are served for a specific period of time, as well as turnover and absentee rates for children, to enable estimation of the number of child-days of service and the number of children receiving a minimally adequate amount of service.

Benefit studies should not rely on existing data sets that have been designed for other purposes, such as public school records. Such data tend to be collected for annual cross-sections (for example, all children in third grade) rather than for cohorts, making change over time difficult to track accurately. Moreover when data are used for accountability purposes, administrators, local authorities, and others may seek to manipulate the results. Data from school achievement tests have these serious problems. Data on school progress, such as school entry, dropout, and educational attainment rates may have less serious problems, but even these data should not be accepted without investigation. Long-term benefits will vary by socioeconomic status and within local contexts, such as the affordability of an adequate diet, employment situation, and quantity and quality of health and educational services.

Scaling Up Programs

As evidence accumulates on the costs and benefits of model programs or exemplary programs that have only been implemented in limited areas, more research on going to scale will be necessary. A small-scale program can lose many of its benefits when expanded into a large-scale government program, but research is unclear on the reason this occurs. One reason may be that governments underestimate costs and expand programs with much less funding for each child served than the model used. Some programs may expand easily into national efforts, and others may not. Strategies for building infrastructure, including administration and training, may facilitate successful expansion. Limiting program expansion to a manageable annual rate of growth may be advantageous. A study of these issues could reveal much about realizing the tremendous potential of investing in ECD programs.

References

Barnett, W. S. 1993. Benefit-cost Analysis of Preschool Education. *American Journal of Orthopsychiatry* 63(4):500-08.

———. 1995. Long-term Effects of Early Childhood Programs on Cognitive and School Outcomes. *The Future of Children* 5(3):25-50.

Barnett, W. S., and C. M. Escobar. 1990. Economic Costs and Benefits of Early Intervention. In S. Meisels and J. Shonkoff, eds., *Handbook of Early Intervention.* Cambridge: Cambridge University Press.

Barnett, W. S., and G. L. Musgrave. 1991. *The Economic Impact of Mandated Family Leave on Small Businesses and Their Employees.* Washington, D.C.: National Federation of Independent Business Foundation.

Blumberg, R. L. 1988. Income under Female versus Male Control. *Journal of Family Issues* 9:51-84.

Boocock, S. S. 1995. Early Childhood Programs in Other Nations: Goals and Outcomes. *The Future of Children* 5(3):94-115.

Bray, M. 1994. Community Financing of Education. In T. Husen and T. Postlethwaite, eds., *International Encyclopedia of Education.* 3rd ed. Oxford: Pergamon.

Bronfenbrenner, Urie. 1989. Ecological Systems Theory. *Annals of Child Development* 6:187-249.

Campbell, D. T. 1991. Quasi-experimental Research Designs in Compensatory Education. In E. M. Scott, ed., *Evaluating Intervention Strategies for Children and Youth at Risk.* Proceedings of an OECD Conference. Washington, D.C.: U.S. Government Printing Office.

Chambers, Jay, and Thomas Parrish. 1994. Modeling Resource Costs. In W. S. Barnett and H. Walberg, eds., *Cost Analyses for Education Decisions: Methods and Examples.* Vol. 4. *Advances in Educational Productivity.* Greenwich, Conn.: JAI Press.

Cook, T. D., and D. T. Campbell. 1979. *Quasi-experimentation: Design and Analysis Issues for Field Settings.* Boston: Houghton Mifflin.

Engle, P. L. 1991. Maternal Work and Child-care Strategies in Peri-urban Guatemala: Nutritional Effects. *Child Development* 62:954-65.

———. n.d. Influences of Mother's and Father's Income on Children's Nutritional Status in Guatemala. *Social Science and Medicine.* Forthcoming.

Evans, Judith. 1994. Early Childhood Interventions. In T. Husen and T. Postlethwaite, eds., *International Encyclopedia of Education.* 3rd ed. Oxford: Pergamon.

Fogel, R. W. 1995. The Contribution of Improved Nutrition to the Decline in Mortality Rates in Europe and America. In J. L. Simon, ed., *The State of Humanity.* Cambridge, Mass.: Blackwell.

Foreit, Karen, Delia Haustein, Max Winterhalter, and Ernesto La Mata, E. 1991. Costs and Benefits of Implementing Child Survival Services at a Private Mining Company in Peru. *American Journal of Public Health,* 81(8):1055-57.

Grantham-McGregor, Sally, Christine Powell, Susan Walker, Susan Chang, and Patricia Fletcher. 1994. The Long-term Follow-up of Severely Malnourished Children who Participated in an Intervention Program. *Child Development* 65:428-39.

Gustafsson, Siv, and Frank Stafford. 1992. Child Care Subsidies and Labor Supply in Sweden. *Journal of Human Resources,* 27(1):204-30.

———. 1995. Links Between Early Childhood Programs and Maternal Employment in Three Countries. *The Future of Children* 5(3):161-74.
Harkavy, Oscar, and J. T. Bond. 1992. Program Operations: Time Allocation and Cost Analysis. In M. Larner, R. Halpern, and O. Harkavy, eds., *Fair Start for Children: Lessons Learned from Seven Demonstration Projects.* New Haven: Yale University Press.
Hausman, Jerry, and David Wise. 1985. *Social Experimentation.* Chicago: University of Chicago Press.
Heckman, J. J., and Richard Robb. 1985. Alternative Methods for Evaluating the Impact of Interventions: An Overview. *Journal of Econometrics* 30:239-67.
Hill, Kenneth. 1995. The Decline of Childhood Mortality. In J. L. Simon, ed. *The State of Humanity.* Cambridge, Mass.: Blackwell.
Joshi, Heather, and Hugh Davies. 1992. Day Care in Europe and Mothers' Forgone Earnings. *International Labor Review, 132*(6):561-79.
Lamb, M. E., and Sternberg, K. J. 1990. Do We Really Know How Day Care Affects Children? *Journal of Applied Developmental Psychology* 11:351-79.
Leslie, J., and M. Paolisso, eds. 1989. *Women, Work, and Welfare in the Third World.* Boulder, Co.: American Association for the Advancement of Science and Westview Press.
Levin, H. M. 1983. *Cost-effectiveness: A Primer.* Beverly Hills, Calif.: Sage.
Lira, M. I. 1994. Costas de Los Programas de Educación Pre-escular no Convencionales en America Latina Revision de Estudios. Santiago, Chile: Centro de Estudios de Desarrollo y Estimulación Psicosocial.
Maume, David J. 1991. Child-care Expenditures and Women's Employment Turnover. *Social Forces* 70(2):495-508.
McKay, Harrison, Leonardo Sinisterra, Arlene McKay, Hernando Gomez, and Pascuala Lloreda. 1978. Improving Cognitive Ability in Chronically Deprived Children. *Science* 200:270-78.
Moffit, Robert. 1991. Program Evaluation with Nonexperimental Data. *Evaluation Review* 15(3):291-314.
Mullahy, John, and Willard Manning. 1995. Statistical Issues in Cost-effectiveness Analyses. In Frank Sloan, ed., *Valuing Health Care.* Cambridge: Cambridge University Press.
Myers, Robert. 1992. Early Childhood Development Programs in Latin America: Toward Definition of an Investment Strategy (A View from LATHR No. 32). Washington, D.C.: World Bank.
Olds, David, and Harriet Kitzman. 1993. Review of Research on Home Visiting for Pregnant Women and Parents of Young Children. *The Future of Children* 3(3):53-92.
Poleman, T. T. 1995. Recent Trends in Food Availability and Nutritional Well-being. In J. L. Simon, ed., *The State of Humanity.* Cambridge, Mass.: Blackwell.
Pollack, R. A. 1985. A Transaction Cost Approach to Families and Households. *Journal of Economic Literature* 23(2):581-608.
Pollitt, Ernesto, K. S. Gorman, P. L. Engle, R. Martorell, and J. Rivera. 1993. Early Supplementary Feeding and Cognition: Effects over Two Decades. *Monographs of the Society for Research in Child Development* 58(6), Serial No. 235.
Powell, C., and Sally Grantham-McGregor. 1989. Home Visiting of Varying Frequency and Child Development. *Pediatrics* 84:157-64.
Selowsky, Marcello. 1981. Nutrition, Health, and Education: The Economic Significance of Complementarities at an Early Age. *Journal of Economic Development* 9:331-46.
Thomas, Margaret. 1984. *Investment Appraisal of Supportive Measures to Working Women in Developing Countries* (Proceedings of a working group). London: Commonwealth Secretariat and World Health Organization.
Tsang, Mun. 1994. Private and Public Costs of Schooling in Developing Nations. In T. Husen and T. Postlethwaite, eds., *International Encyclopedia of Education.* 3rd ed. Oxford: Pergamon.
World Bank. 1992. Staff Appraisal Report, Mexico Initial Education Project (Report No. 10821-ME). Washington, D.C.: World Bank.
———. 1993. *World Development Report: Investing in Health.* New York: Oxford University Press.
Yeoh, B. S. A., and S. Huang. 1995. Child Care in Singapore: Negotiating Choices and Constraints in a Multicultural Society. *Women's Studies International Forum* 18(4):445-61.
Young, M. E. 1996. *Early Child Development: Investing in the Future.* Washington, D.C.: World Bank.

Policy Issues and Implications of Early Child Development

Mary Eming Young

Policies link research to action. Policymakers can transform research findings and recommendations into demonstration and intervention programs. The transfer of knowledge that makes this possible, however, is not easy and does not occur passively. Expected results must be articulated, goals must be identified, benefits and costs must be weighed, and sufficient reason to act must be communicated. Even so, policies will be prescribed by persons acting in their own and, perhaps, others' interests.

Many players participate in formulating and enacting social, economic, and political policies at local or national levels. They may be well informed of the knowledge base for pertinent issues, they may have particular contributions to make, or they may expect to benefit from the policy at hand. All of these players are important stakeholders who will come together or separate depending on the policy messages that are developed and promulgated. Even a well-constructed policy could fail if it is not founded on sound research and supported by key stakeholders.

Early child development is a field in need of effective national policies and international cooperation. A great many local, and a number of national, efforts have already proven that early child development (ECD) programs can be a wise investment. The preceding chapters convey research and intervention findings which show that properly designed and implemented programs in all parts of the world can have multidimensional benefits. ECD programs enhance school readiness, increase the efficiency of primary school investments and human capital formation, foster valued social behavior, reduce social welfare costs, stimulate community development, and help mothers become income earners.

There are many varieties of ECD programs from which to choose; some will be more appropriate and beneficial than others in some settings. The authors in this volume suggest several frameworks for choosing among, or combining, the options available. Quality and effectiveness are paramount concerns, and criteria are offered for assessing these outcomes. Frameworks also are provided for evaluating and comparing the benefits and costs of ECD programs.

It is now time to act: to communicate the importance and promise of early child development to all social and economic sectors, to encourage policymakers to respond to

---

This chapter was developed from a panel discussion on policy implications, held at the conference. The panel was chaired by Armeane M. Choksi and included Sir George A. O. Alleyne, David de Ferranti, William Foege, James Kunder, and Avima Lombard.

this information, and to enlist the support of all stakeholders at local and national levels. To help stimulate the transition from research to action, this chapter summarizes current understanding of the overall need for and benefits of early child development programs, and it suggests major policy issues for discussion in national and international arenas.

Early Child Development: Common Themes

Engaging governments and public citizens in a discussion of the benefits of investing in early child development is probably the most effective means for increasing the number and scale of ECD interventions worldwide. Common themes for this discussion, presented in the preceding chapters, include:

- Many of the world's children live in a continuing state of poverty, which has ramifications for them, their families and communities, and their countries. Poverty is often passed on from generation to generation; ECD programs offer one important way of intervening in and breaking this vicious cycle.

- The poverty experienced by many of these disadvantaged children is magnified by the effects of undernutrition and malnutrition, disease, and environmental toxins and results in compromised development; ECD programs can successfully address the nutritional, health, and educational aspects of young children's development.

- Nutrition, health, and education are interactive and have synergistic effects; consequently, quality ECD programs that include all these areas, utilizing a comprehensive, whole-child approach, will be maximally effective.

- Readiness and preparedness for primary school are major factors contributing to successful learning and work experiences; the most effective ECD programs are likely to be those that offer coordinated interventions for children from birth to 8 years of age.

- The time frame, or "window of opportunity," for developing many capacities (for example, emotional, social, verbal, spatial) is 0-8 years old, with some authors indicating that 0-3 years is the critical period; ECD programs that include interventions designed for the 0-3 age group offer special promise for enhancing the potential of disadvantaged children.

- Parents usually are children's primary caregivers and first teachers; enhancing parenting skills is a critical component of ECD interventions.

- Children live in and respond to a complex and varied environment; ECD programs that are supported and sustained as part of a broad network of community services are likely to be more effective.

- Disadvantaged children are found in all parts of the world, including both developing and developed countries; ECD programs are appropriate for any region, but they must be tailored to "fit" the social, cultural, political, and economic context in which they are offered.

- Early child development is an important responsibility not only for parents and extended families, but also for communities, societies, and nations; a national and international commitment to high-quality ECD programs is needed, with participation of both the public and private sectors and at the highest policy levels.

- A variety of ECD strategies and approaches have been proven to be effective in different locales and settings. Now is the time to assess the benefits and costs of these programs systematically and to identify especially effective programs that could be scaled up from local to national levels.

- Investment in quality, effective ECD programs can result in manyfold returns to that investment in both the short and long term and for both individuals and societies.

Policy Implications

ECD programs face some of the same difficulties as health care interventions or programs for the aged: Obtaining the scientific information to demonstrate the importance of intervention is relatively easy, but initiating or changing policies to implement or enhance interventions is much more difficult. Science is always ahead of other disciplines—politics, law, theology, and sociology. As noted in the common themes above, researchers have demonstrated the importance and effectiveness of early child development. Some of the major policy implications of these findings are described below.

Appreciating Differing Views of Children

Two key issues are: How does a society view its children? What is children's value in society? Views of children and their importance vary considerably within and among societies and cultures. Each country expresses its views of children differently as indicated, for example, by the amount of money spent on children's health, or the opportunities given for education. Because these views vary and because children have different needs in different settings and countries, the importance and effectiveness (including cost-effectiveness) of ECD programs will be judged differently.

Differences in the views, importance, and needs of children and in the perception of effectiveness influence a society's discussions and decisions on policies related to children. As a result, these discussions and decisions will differ, sometimes significantly, among countries. One policy will not "fit" all countries or even all settings within one country. Regardless of the settings, however, children should remain at the center of any policy discussions and decisions affecting them.

Also, placing children at the center of a country's larger socioeconomic plans and development efforts has salutary effects because of the implied focus on a longer time horizon (15 years or longer). Economic development over time by definition involves children, and communities can be mobilized by centering their efforts around children.

Developing Shared Definitions and Goals

For policy discussions, a specific, clear, and readily understandable definition of early child development must be generated for each country and, ideally, across countries. Components of this definition are suggested throughout this volume. They include parental involvement and a synergism among health, nutrition, and stimulation/education programs.

Definition(s) of early child development will reflect national, and international, views of children. For example, although "play," which is what children do, may be appropriate to include in an operational definition of early child development, many societies might not support this notion. Child's play is viewed differently in different societies, and many societies would not view play as how children learn. Yet, in this volume, the authors encourage ECD programs that focus on the whole child, which would include play and all its aspects—art, music, and other forms of expression; and affective outcomes (trusting relationships, loving relationships, creativity).

Formulation of shared goals for early child development will depend on achieving a common understanding of what early child development is. These goals must accommodate regional and local differences and, at the same time, support basic principles of early child development. Defining, publicizing, and applying overall goals for early child development can be useful processes for engaging and mobilizing all partners, including donors and the public, to expend resources for ECD programs.

Shared definitions and goals are critically important. ECD strategies and programs will have to be culturally sensitive and appropriate to local situations, but if there is clamor rather than a symphony of voices when talking about early child development, the chances of developing coherent national and international policies are reduced significantly. As noted by one panelist, "If we have an idea of where we want to go, we're likely to get there. If we don't have an idea where we want to go, we'll never get there."

While developing definitions and goals, the momentum of intervention must be maintained. Action is needed now, and many ECD programs are already under way. Continuing to develop and apply ECD programs based on the knowledge that already exists will be important even while seeking shared definitions and goals for early child development.

Fostering an Integrated Approach

For governments and policymakers, two sets of priorities for early child development must be communicated: tending to the most urgent (survival) needs first, while also making a strong commitment to meeting developmental needs. The importance of balancing these two sets of priorities must be noted. These two needs, which have short- and long-term effects, must be met simultaneously.

Survival and development are simultaneous processes. Can anyone say which is more important to a child's well-being: good health; adequate nutrition; or the ability to reason, express one's self, and form close relationships with family and community members? If any of these elements is missing, the whole child is not being served and the world forgoes the fullness of his or her potential contributions.

When addressing simultaneous priorities for early child development, policymakers also must understand that certain windows of opportunity can never be opened again. In the words of Stephen Hawking, the arrow of time cannot be reversed. This physical principle is true as well for health, disease, and stimulation. Even with neuronal plasticity, far greater effects can be achieved at earlier ages than at later ages, when far greater inputs would be required to achieve the same effects.

As the authors also suggest, ECD programs can enhance, and be enhanced by, other community services. Integration, in this sense, is even broader and includes combining ECD programs with other health, nutrition, and community development efforts.

From still another perspective, fostering an integrated approach implies the need for multiple policies, those that are relevant to specific problems (for example, early child development) and those that shape the institutions responsible for addressing these problems (for example, day-care centers, primary schools). Policies that enhance linkage between home- or center-based ECD interventions and primary schools, for example, are especially needed for effective early child development.

Assuring Universal and Targeted Coverage

Theoretically, ECD programs should be universal (that is, available to all young children), but because of limited resources, they are usually targeted to the most needy children. Every child deserves access to quality education, as well as vaccination, clean water, and good nutrition. Within a country, ECD programs can be designed to meet the needs of all children, reflecting the country's view of children and shared goals. At the same time, programs can be tailored and targeted to reach particularly vulnerable groups and marginalized children within the society.

Messages (for example, information on good childrearing practices) need to be developed for all potential audiences, including middle-income families, but approaches for delivering the messages can be more aggressive for those who live on the economy's margins. All children can be served by ECD programs, but those who are marginalized need to be served first to have the greatest impact. This approach, combining universal *and* targeted coverage, reflects current public health efforts, which target vulnerable and underserved populations within a framework of health for all.

Expanding Local Efforts ("Going to Scale")

Expanding local ECD efforts to national programs (going to scale) is a major issue for many countries. ECD programs tend to be pilot demonstrations and modest in scale, and they rely on external funding. A main issue is how to scale up these programs to address problems of early child development at a national level and, specifically, to promote national coverage for marginalized children.

The possibility of scaling up existing ECD programs depends on the probability of incorporating ECD services into an overall network of national services. Stand-alone ECD services are not permanent, regardless of their innovativeness, excellence, and effectiveness; if they are to survive, they must be part of a broader network of human development services. Creating a new infrastructure for early child development in most countries is not cost-effective. Similar efforts for children, for example immunization, have been successful only when they have been incorporated into existing services.

The possibilities for scaling up quality, effective ECD programs need to be addressed nationally and internationally. Addressing this issue will require close examination and comparison of existing ECD programs within and among countries. Benefits and costs (for example, of formal versus informal programs) must be measured.

Involving Multiple Stakeholders

Children, and their parents, are the main stakeholders, or actors, in early child development; they can tell what they need and what is best for them. Parental responsibility and involvement includes fathers, who can be a major resource for early child development.

Outside of the family, five principal actors are required for implementing any major social change within a country. These five actors are: the government, the private sector and organized labor, nongovernmental organizations (NGOs), the media, and multilateral organizations. To promote early child development, all of these social partners must work together, in synergy, at the national level. International and multinational organizations also can exert influences that may have national impact.

Government

The chapters in this volume well demonstrate that early child development is a service that has both social *and* economic returns. Some national governments are already supporting effective, quality ECD programs, and other governments must be encouraged to do the same. With national policies in place, governments can effectively enlist other stakeholder's support and participation and establish a national focus for organizing a decentralized network of service delivery.

Private Sector and Organized Labor

The private sector is a large, untapped resource for early child development. In recent years this sector has become increasingly convinced of the relationship between the quality of education and the quality of the work force. Communicating a unified message about the importance and value of ECD intervention to the private sector could stimulate this sector's investment and involvement. Very little effort has been made as of yet to engage the private sector in these programs.

Businesses and labor unions will become involved if they are shown that the returns to investment are high. Private companies will respond, for economic or ethical reasons, if they are asked to contribute by influential persons or groups. The private sector is already contributing to education efforts, and several pharmaceutical companies are significantly involved in improving health in developing countries. Expanding these efforts to include integrated child development programs is necessary and feasible.

Early child development presents an enormous opportunity for large corporations and microenterprises to contribute to the development of human capital. Private expenditure for health and education are already as large or larger than public investment in these areas of human capital formation. Both public and private resources for investing in young children, however, still lag behind those for school-aged or older children. More efficient use of total resources can be channeled for services to very young children. Employers can be encouraged to invest in these programs—it is in their self-interest to prevent employees' absenteeism because of childcare responsibilities. Also, family day-care centers are businesses that offer employment. Corporate resources can help ensure the sustainability of ECD programs.

NGOs
Nongovernmental organizations also are an important resource for early child development. Some NGOs (for example, Bernard van Leer Foundation, World Vision, Christian Children's Fund, Plan International, Save the Children) are already collaborating on ECD projects with the World Bank. Fruitful partnerships could be developed between and among various organizations, and including religious groups. Networks of NGOs would be useful for delineating and achieving shared goals. Expanding the involvement of NGOs will increase the number of groups and individuals working toward the ultimate goal of improving children's lives.

Media
The media can play a major role in articulating a unified message and convincing governments to address early child development. Few institutions are as powerful as the media in creating public awareness and in initiating public debate on issues such as early child development. Decisionmakers in both the public and private sectors must be convinced of the importance and value of ECD programs. Ways of engaging the media need to be determined.

International and Multilateral Organizations
Public policy is formed by asserting the public's influence, demonstrating benefits, and highlighting other countries' policies. Concern for children deserves to be at the center of multilateral organizations' broad agendas for human development, poverty alleviation, and economic stability. Multilateral organizations could play a greater role in early child development by incorporating ECD concepts into their lending policies. Also, broader partnerships among these organizations could be forged by identifying shared goals and mobilizing resources for children. How these organizations attend to the needs of children can be a measure of their influence on human and economic development worldwide.

Utilizing Emerging Technologies

New technologies (such as the Internet) can be utilized for enhancing communications among researchers, governments, and organizations and for disseminating ECD information to all areas of the world, reaching communities and children in even the remotest areas. These technological capabilities need to be explored in relation to early child development. Two examples of this enhanced capability are the World Wide Web sites of The Consultative Group on Early Childhood Care and Development (http://www.ecdgroup.com) and ChildWatch International (http://childhouse.uio.io).

Next Steps

Immediate action can be taken in several areas to stimulate increased awareness of the need for early child development. The conference participants suggested that a multilateral organization could meet with groups interested in early child development to organize a strategy group to address the policy issues and implications of early child development. Such a group could initiate broad, but focused, discussions of the differing views of children, definitions of early child development, and goals of ECD interventions. This group would help stimulate national and international attention on early child development.

At the same time, researchers could document comparative data on the effects of ECD interventions. Excellent data are available for demonstrating the benefits of primary, secondary, and tertiary education, and similar data are needed for early child development. Researchers also could initiate systematic analyses of the benefits and costs of ECD programs. These data would provide the information needed to improve existing programs and to design new interventions.

Based on available information, as summarized in this volume, additional ECD interventions need to be initiated and targeted to children and families at greatest risk of compromised development. Health and education professionals in national and international organizations could encourage government officials and policymakers to utilize existing frameworks, some of which are provided in this volume, to organize public discussions on ECD policies. These discussions should include consideration of alternative policies that can have tremendous effect on the quality of children's lives; for example, probably the single most potent intervention for improving school enrollment is enforcement of child labor laws.

Conclusion

The primary issue for early child development is not whether to invest, but how much and at what level. Further consideration of the policy implications of early child development will require reflection on a number of issues, including those summarized above. For individual ECD programs, careful consideration must be given to the balance of priorities; extent of participation; involvement and role of partners; contributions by public and private sectors; need and strategies for empowerment; cultural context; integration of services; quality, coverage, and scale of programs; tradeoffs among services; balance among research, action, and advocacy; and development of culturally sensitive methodologies and outcome indicators and measures.

Research shows that ECD programs offer one of the most powerful tools for breaking the intergenerational cycle of poverty. Because learning begins at birth, and even before, the starting point for involving families in ECD programs must be as early as possible. Special emphasis is needed to focus on those most in need, to reach the unreached, and to both create and respond to demand in a timely manner. When the intervention regards the development of young children, it is never too early, but it can easily be too late.

Knowledge and understanding of ECD programs is no longer the constraint facing early child development. Rather, transforming this knowledge into action is the major limiting factor in implementing ECD programs and requires the combined support of governments, NGOs, the private sector, and the media. The challenge to care for society's youngest members is not just a challenge for a single country or continent; it is a challenge for the entire world community.

Subject Index